NATAL SIGNS
Cultural Representations of
Pregnancy, Birth and Parenting

NATAL SIGNS
Cultural Representations of
Pregnancy, Birth and Parenting

EDITED BY

NADYA BURTON

DEMETER PRESS

Funded by the Government of Canada
Financé par la gouvernement du Canada   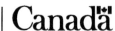 | Canadä

Demeter Press
140 Holland Street West
P. O. Box 13022
Bradford, ON L3Z 2Y5
Tel: (905) 775-9089
Email: info@demeterpress.org
Website: www.demeterpress.org

Demeter Press logo based on the sculpture "Demeter" by Maria-Luise Bodirsky <www.keramik-atelier.bodirsky.de>

Cover artwork: Martina Field, "In the Beginning," 1994, compotina intaglio print, 9 x 6 inches. Artist website: www.martinafield.com.

Printed and Bound in Canada

Library and Archives Canada Cataloguing in Publication

          Natal signs : cultural representations of pregnancy, birth and parenting / editor, Nadya Burton.

Includes bibliographical references.
ISBN 978-1-926452-32-6 (paperback)

          1. Pregnancy--Social aspects. 2. Childbirth--Social aspects. 3. Parenting--Social aspects. 4. Popular culture. I. Burton, Nadya, editor

RG556.N38 2015   306   C2015-906126-1

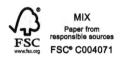

MIX
Paper from
responsible sources
FSC® C004071

As always, for lb and mt

Table of Contents

Acknowledgements
xi

Introduction
Nadya Burton
1

SECTION 1: LOOKING AT PREGNANCY

What to Expect When Your Avatar is Expecting:
Representations of Pregnancy and Parenthood in Video Games
Lauren Cruikshank
19

Masculine Pregnancy:
Butch Lesbians', Trans Men's & Genderqueer
Individuals' Experiences
Michelle Walks
41

That Fat Man is Giving Birth:
Gender Identity and the Pregnant Body
K. J. Surkan
58

Gay Men's Narratives of Pregnancy in the Context of
Commercial Surrogacy
Damien W. Riggs and Deborah Dempsey
73

Crone and Moon, Umbilical Cords/Blood Ties
Brescia Nember Reid
88

Imminent
Jennifer Long
90

Heroes and Villains:
Representations of Midwives in the Late Twentieth Century
Ontario Midwifery Revival
Elizabeth Allemang
94

Spacemaking and Midwifery:
With, Within, Without
Mary Sharpe and Kory McGrath
127

SECTION 2: LOOKING AT BIRTH

Refusing Delinquency, Reclaiming Power:
Indigenous Women and Childbirth
Claire Dion Fletcher and Cheryllee Bourgeois
153

Resistance and Submission:
A Critique of Representations of Birth
Alys Einion
172

Representations of Birth and Motherhood as
Contemporary Forms of the Sacred
Anna Hennessey
194

Does Labour Mean Work?
A Look at the Meaning of Birth in Amish and
Non-Amish Society
Natalie Jolly
218

Representing Birth: An Inquiry into Art Making and
Birth Giving: Implications for Teaching Student Midwives
Jeanne Lyons
232

Birth is a Labour of Art
Marni Kotak 251

Split Open
Ara Parker
265

Flower of My Flesh
Rosie Rosenzweig
267

Birth Shock: Exploring Pregnancy, Birth, and the Transition
to Motherhood Using Participatory Arts
*Susan Hogan, Charley Baker, Shelagh Cornish,
Paula McCloskey and Lisa Watts*
272

Making Meaning of Stillbirth
Kory McGrath and Lynn Farrales
296

SECTION III: LOOKING AT PARENTING

Kids Aren't Cute
Beth Osnes
317

Paternal Loss and Anticipation:
An Artist's Perspective
Rachel Epp Buller
321

Two Mums and Some Babies:
Queering Motherhood
Rebecca English, Raechel Johns and Angela Dwyer
335

Go the Fuck to Sleep Prince George?
Juxtaposing Cultural Representations of Motherhood and
Exploring the Politics of Authenticity
Betty Ann Martin
351

About the Contributors
371

Acknowledgements

The authors join me in thanking the anonymous reviewers of the manuscript for their thoughtful and rigorous critique and feedback. We know our work is stronger for your engagement with our ideas.

I owe a debt of gratitude, as always, to my midwifery colleagues at Ryerson University who invite me so generously into the fold of their midwifery world, embracing the sociologist who works alongside them and is never quite of them. Your insights always make their way into my thinking and reflection about pregnancy and birth, and I thank you for the ongoing critical engagement that is a part of my relationship with each of you. I would also like to especially thank May Friedman (Social Work, Ryerson University) who first encouraged and then mentored me through the process of editing this book.

This book emerges in part from my teaching of a course on cultural representations of the childbearing year with students in the Faculty of Community Services at Ryerson University. I am blessed to have mature, wise, and engaged students who grapple with these issues alongside me, making our learning the inevitably mutual experience that it should be.

Most profoundly and from the deepest part of my soul, to GT, who makes absolutely everything possible.

Introduction

THINKING ABOUT REPRESENTATIONS of pregnancy, child-birth, and parenting is an exciting project in the contem-porary context. Positioned in an era when traditional and historical constraints on representations of these life events have been unsettled, we find ourselves facing a shifting landscape. We are, furthermore, also confronted by evolving economies of cultural production and consumption; not only are we encountering new images, but we are continuing to witness changes in the systems of generation and circulation by which they are produced and consumed.

Although most readily accessible popular representations remain conventional and banal, just as notably we find ourselves increas-ingly confronted by images and representations that pose new questions, unsettle assumptions, and stretch and break boundaries, while opening up new possibilities for what is imaginable. The explosion of visual representations of pregnancy, childbirth, and parenthood over the last few decades thus works in multiple ways. On the one hand, some of these representations continue to centre deeply gendered subjects, reinscribe docile patients and bodies in need of surveillance, bolster medicalized, agency-free experiences, and render these profound life experiences both marginal and mundane. But there are far too many representations out there, and far too many new kinds of representations, for this to be the only story. From reality television to anthologies of birth poetry, from photo essays to sculpture, from online video-sharing to tele-vision sitcoms, over the last half century we have seen pregnancy, childbirth, and parenthood emerge from out of the private and the domestic into the light of increasing public display, cultural reflection, discussion, and analysis. It goes without saying that we may not always like what we see, that at times the vastly expanded terrain poses social, political, and ethical questions. And yet we might be forgiven for feeling as though there has never been a more exciting time to be grappling with these images and ideas; there has never been more fertile ground for analysing, arguing, debating, and tussling over the diverse meanings these new images and narratives offer us. This collection of essays presents us with some of these discussions and reflections, exploring representations of the messy experiences of pregnancy, birth, and parenthood in ways that indeed unsettle and stretch the boundaries of public discourse and that do justice to the diversity of these experiences.

As we look at representations of pregnancy, birth, and parenthood two decades into the twenty-first century, we might be able, as Imogen Tyler suggests, "to imagine that a shift is taking place; a movement from an abject aesthetics towards the creation of a 'life-full' natal aesthetics that cannot be subsumed back within deathly abject paradigms" (3). The perspective of a "life-full natal aesthetics" might help us to recognize and think critically about the generativity of current representations, to think about what kinds of possibilities are given birth to, expanding horizons for thinking, conceptualizing, and becoming other things. The implications of this shift could be significant; changing representations don't merely *reflect* a changing world, they also actively participate in that transformation, generating new forms of visibility and possible action.

The increasing publicity of private and intimate experiences, such as pregnancy, birth, and parenthood, is one notable aspect of a new representational landscape in which the tools of image production and circulation are easily and broadly accessible. From blogs to YouTube to social media sites, we find ourselves with unprecedented access to visual representations of these experiences. Images created are more easily consumed, re-used, and re-purposed than they have been at any previous time. Access to self-representation and to the tools that allow for manipulation and disseminating of images, while not entirely universal, have transformed the landscape of representation of pregnancy, birth, and parenthood. Analyses of representations have long focused on issues of identity: race, class, gender, and other markers of the inequitable distribution of power in our worlds. This sociological framing encourages us to ask important questions about the power both to represent and to be represented. "All colonized/subjugated people," writes bell hooks, "who create an oppositional subculture within the framework of domination recognize that the field of representation ... is a site of ongoing contestation and struggle" (84). hooks writes about the impact of the camera on the capacity of the black community to represent itself and suggests that the power to self-represent is perhaps more important even than the need for desegregation and equal access. The need for this kind of analysis palpably persists as inequity is reduced in some contexts but is increasingly entrenched in others.

FRAMING PERSPECTIVES

In exploring and engaging cultural representations of pregnancy, birth, and parenthood it may be helpful to consider two familiar framing problematics: that of Michel de Certeau and his discussion of the practices of everyday life and the disruptive use of tactics to unsettle the conventional understandings of the distinction between producer and consumer of cultural products; and that of Pierre Bourdieu and his analysis of power as a striating force within social structures (see for example *The Field of Cultural Production*).

Today, the need to nuance and rethink the distinction and relation between the categories of cultural production and cultural consumption arises not only in light of theoretical and practical considerations, such as those that de Certeau analyzes, but also in light of the progressively more accessible tools of cultural production. De Certeau's methods of identifying the users or consumers of the artifacts of cultural production, not as passive recipients but as actors engaged in a form of secondary production or "mode of operation" (de Certeau xi), encourages us to recognize the border separating production and consumption as porous. We need to complicate the dominant image of powerful and active producers of representations and images as well as passive and docile consumers of the same. In challenging the hegemony and the finished nature of the original context of production, we are obliged to ask not simply what does an image *mean*, but how can it be *used*, and what can it be *made* to mean? How might images or representations be deployed in contexts that are generative of additional or possibly contradictory meanings? Thus our interest lies not simply in documenting diverse representations of pregnancy, birth, and parenting, but rather in more fully attending to what it is we *do* with these images and representations as cultural producers and consumers. To read (consume/use) an image is to discover an occasion to either reinscribe dominant meanings or to draw upon productive tactics of diversion. Such a form of creative consumption is "devious, it is dispersed, but it insinuates itself everywhere, silently and almost invisibly, because it does not manifest itself through its own products, but rather through its ways of using the products imposed by a dominant economic order" (de Certeau xii-iii). How do consumers and producers of images of pregnancy, birth, and parenthood engage and utilize available representations to make their own worlds that offer possibilities for social change and transformation through the "innumerable and infinitesimal transformations of and within the dominant cultural economy in order to adapt it to their own interests and their own rules" (de Certeau xiv)?

The ambiguities of the politics of production are further made evident in the altered terrain of the last many decades in which the technologies of image production and manipulation are increasingly available and accessible. The ways in which we make use of these readily accessible tools remains germane and is as central to our discussion as the simple fact of access. While we must not underestimate the value of controlling the means of production and self-representation, we simultaneously cannot assume an easy link between the power to represent and the intention and capacity to engage in liberatory practice. There is no necessity to the political implications or practical outcomes that flow from cultural production; nothing is guaranteed. The degree to which broadened participation challenges or enhances dominant interests and paradigms is continually a matter of negotiation. While we have seen the tools of representation democratized and the commitments of diverse forces of feminism, the politics of identity and the voice of the subaltern utilize these tools to question and unsettle the status quo; the question of what is reinscribed and what is liberated needs to be repeatedly asked in a changing array of circumstances and contexts. The dynamism inherent in this situation reflects the vitality of current forms of cultural representation that generate both the risks and the possibilities we see in current images of pregnancy, birth, and parenthood.

A desire to challenge, unsettle, and offer alternatives to historically dominant representations of pregnancy, birth, and parenthood is a consistent preoccupation of a number of chapters in this book. In light of these concerns, Pierre Bourdieu's complex analysis of the structuring of the cultural field might serve to remind us as well of the ways in which relationships of power "are embedded in the systems of classification used to describe and discuss everyday life—as well as cultural practices—and in the ways of perceiving reality that are taken for granted by members of society" (Johnson 2). As this book demonstrates, we see around us an increasingly prevalent dissatisfaction with the ways in which the unequal distribution of power is entrenched in cultural production. Bourdieu insists that in seeking to engage and understand cultural objects we must operate in multiple sites at the same time: "Literature, art and their respective producers do not exist independently of a complex institutional framework which authorizes, enables, empowers and legitimizes them. This framework must be incorporated into any analysis that pretends to provide a thorough understanding of cultural goods and practices" (Johnson 10).

We find the work of cultural production firmly grounded in and not distinct from the arena of social relations of power. When we look at works and images, we must engage the contexts of production, circulation, and consumption simultaneously. To look at representations of pregnancy, birth, and parenthood is always more than to engage the meaning and value of the work, it is inevitably to engage in and grapple with the ways in which power is distributed in this time and place; and it is precisely this link to and embeddedness within the social and political arenas of our time that make engaging these cultural representations so compelling and indeed important. This is not a benign practice; it is a political one.

ALISON LAPPER PREGNANT

If one were in London at any time between 2005 and 2007, one would likely have stumbled across sculptor Marc Quinn's extra-life-size nude statue *Alison Lapper Pregnant*. Lapper, a British artist born with a condition called phocomelia that resulted in no arms and shortened legs, collaborated with Quinn on the creation of this piece, which generated extensive discussion about public art, disability, and representations of the nude pregnant body, amongst other things. The almost twelve-foot and more than thirteen-ton marble sculpture was exhibited as part of Trafalgar Square's *Fourth Plinth Project*. Conceived as a way of addressing the empty plinth in the square, left statue-less since its construction in the mid-nineteenth century for mundane bureaucratic reasons, the fourth plinth has, since 1999, held a series of rotating and temporary exhibits, mostly sculpture. It is a provocative site for public art in London's most famous and visited square, and although the project was not originally designed to prompt discussions of identity and diversity, almost all of the pieces exhibited have inevitably done so (Sumartojo). Rendered in Carrera marble, the seated figure of *Alison Lapper Pregnant* has been seen to challenge the subject matter of public and monumental art, among the most traditional of artistic and representational forms. The nude body of a seven-month pregnant disabled woman sat for two years amidst tributes to some of Britain's most notable military heroes, and, in this context, the sculpture has been read as everything from sensationalist to subversive.

That the disabled pregnant body has rarely been the subject of public art speaks to issues of exclusion and marginalization and, in this framing, *Alison Lapper Pregnant* can be read to be about visibility and pride, celebration of both disabled and pregnant bodies. Quinn's sculpture might be understood to transgress multiple conventions through the proud display of pregnancy and disability. The sculpture is also often identified as challenging normative understandings of public art and Lapper herself has called Quinn's sculpture an "anti-monument," speaking back, as it were, to the traditional subject matter of the form (Millet). In layering a pregnant and disabled body, Quinn not only endeavours to expand notions of beauty, for the sculpture's seductive aesthetic quality challenges what might traditionally be seen as its doubly "abject" subject matter, it also poses a challenge to the site as a place of such historical and political gravitas. Bringing together the pregnant and disabled body in this context might be understood to subvert notions both of the assumed asexual nature of the disabled body and the disabled nature of the pregnant body: "Popular representations have tended to idealize pregnancy socially, yet they also veil the female pregnant body, reinstating its preferred existence within the proverbial home. Pregnancy is glorified and yet stigmatized, and indeed often considered a disability" (Millet).

The material choice (Carrera marble, referencing classical sculpture) for *Alison Lapper Pregnant* was clearly significant in relation to the context and placement of the sculpture and was a key aspect of its message and impact. But the potent image of a seven-month pregnant Alison Lapper has also moved off the plinth. Repurposed and recontextualized away from its original setting, the image rematerialized to take a central place in the opening pageantry of the 2012 Paralympics in London in a considerably expanded forty-three-foot inflatable version entitled *Breath*. This new version belies the gravitas of the original context and material; here the image, in balloon form, is light and celebratory. Material remains essential and context is everything. It is a powerful lesson in the agile politics of representation. That another version of *Breath* shows up, perched on the edge of the island of San Giorgio Maggiore as part of a Quinn exhibit to coincide with the 2013 Venice Biennale, further highlights the mutable, shifting, and malleable nature of the images we consume today.

PREGNANT THOMAS BEATIE

Cultural representations of pregnancy, birth, and parenting have long been profoundly heteronormative. The diverse reality of who births, and who accompanies those who birth, have not, for the most part, shown up in cultural representations of these events, and so those old questions about representation (who is included and who is excluded in the process of both creating and consuming representations) remain germane.

In 2008, transgendered pregnancy emerged into public consciousness. Photographs of a pregnant Thomas Beatie, circulated widely in the media, were arguably the images that finally undid the impossibility of male pregnancy. The images challenged the stability of what had seemed to most as an unambiguous and unbreachable threshold. Although not the first pregnant man either in cultural representation or in lived experience, Beatie was taken up in the popular imagination in new ways. Like *Alison Lapper Pregnant*, Beatie's representation was and continues to be deployed, re-created, and re-interpreted in a wide range of contexts. It is worth noting that Beatie's trans male pregnant body was also the subject of a Marc Quinn sculpture, raising, as did *Alison Lapper Pregnant*, some of the tensions between the shock value of non-conforming bodies and the project of delivering and engaging the hitherto absent in cultural representation. Celebrated in some settings as doing the liberatory work of gender-transgressing, critiqued in others for its use by (mostly non trans) theorists to highlight the ways in which gender norms are constructed and reinforced (Riggs 159), Beatie's image, again not unlike *Alison Lapper Pregnant*, was recast along a range of political and cultural lines. And although Beatie offers us reimagined social and political possibilities for queer and transgendered pregnancy, birth, and parenting, he also offers us an image whose meanings and effects are malleable, contingent, and diverse. In this way, our reflections on images of Beatie can serve as guides for ways of consuming a wide range of representations of pregnancy, birth, and parenting. In looking at representations of Beatie we can be less prone to pin down meaning and more inclined to see the image as a force full of potential, one that given different circumstances can be made to do many different things. Exploration and criticism of images of queer and transgendered pregnancy, such as those that Thomas Beatie presents, offer among other things "a way to envision and encourage other ways of being, other understandings of existing articulations ... in which our common sense understandings about gender, sex, and sexuality are disarticulated and rearticulated in more contingent arrangements—arrangements that help those 'possibilities for a livable life' for everyone" (Sloop qtd. in Landau 184).

In her introduction to a special issue of *feminist review* addressing birth, Imogen Tyler draws on Hannah Arendt's discussions of the absence of natality in western thinking. This absence, Tyler argues after Arendt, speaks to a missing discourse and a profound fault line in our capacity to both think/theorize and act/make change:

> Hannah Arendt suggests that the absence of this primary fact from histories of thought represents a significant lacuna in political and philosophical traditions. For Arendt natality, the capacity to begin, is the foundational fact of all thought, all politics and all action. Without some fundamental understanding of the place of birth, there can be, she suggests, no social change, no human future. (Tyler 1)

While this book explores representations of pregnancy, birth, and parenting, particularly in cultural (rather than philosophical or political) contexts, the inevitable link between philosophical and political thinking and cultural production is at play. What we can think and speak, conceptualize and articulate, in some ways will always condition what we can represent in culture. And of course, it is not only the arenas of philosophy and political thought that might contribute to a "fundamental understanding of the place of birth," but equally the potent areas of cultural creation. The absence of conceptualizations of the natal, for Arendt, poses problems for the capacity to think and generate change and future. In this book, and scattered liberally through current cultural production, "life-full" natal aesthetics abound. Examining natal signs in the diverse arenas in which they arise and using these explorations to expand our worlds is one aspect of creating change and imagining future.

LOOKING AT PREGNANCY, BIRTH AND PARENTING

This collection pulls together a range of pieces, both creative and theoretical, that together pose questions and challenges to the way experiences of pregnancy, childbirth, and parenting are often represented in diverse cultural contexts. Loosely chronological, the chapters unfold in three sections, starting first with discussions of pregnancy, then birth, and finally parenthood. The stylistic variety of the chapters reflects the interdisciplinary nature of this book, drawing as they do on perspectives that are grounded in anthropology, gender studies, cultural studies, history, sociology, and beyond. The chapters offer us a variety of styles of engagement, thoughtfulness, cultural practice, critique, and resistance. Collectively they demonstrate an exciting range of methods of engaging the issues at stake.

The first section, "Looking at Pregnancy," opens with Lauren Cruikshank's "What to Expect When Your Avatar is Expecting," which explores disembodied (virtual) pregnancy and birth through a study of online gaming worlds. Cruikshank argues that digital spaces that include avatars remain outside the focus of much work on reproductive representation, and her chapter offers us captivating insight into maternity and gaming worlds. She suggests that these sites offer compelling possibilities for examining the ways in which simulated pregnancies and births are both constrained by and may be free to rework dominant social constructions of reproduction. Following Cruikshank we explore representations of pregnancy that widen the traditional frame. Three chapters in this section, those by Michelle Walks, K.J. Surkan, and Damien Riggs and Deborah Dempsey, engage representations of pregnant bodies that don't easily identify or map onto what Walks calls "the cultural fetish of feminine pregnancy." These three chapters highlight the invisibility of masculine and queer pregnancy and encourage a broader understanding of how pregnancy might be experienced and seen. Walks' chapter, "Masculine Pregnancy," emerges from research into and interviews with butch lesbians', trans men's, and genderqueer people's experiences with pregnancy. Seeking to fill a notable gap in the literature, Walks addresses the ways that individuals "who are female but masculine" experience and negotiate pregnancy. Surkan's chapter, "That Fat Man is Giving Birth," highlights the ways in which his own experience as a female-bodied person on the transmasculine spectrum underscores the "social incompatibility of pregnancy and masculinity." Surkan speaks to the impossibility of being a pregnant man and hence being socially read as "fat." Riggs and Demspey's chapter explores male pregnancy from a very different standpoint, that of gay men engaging surrogates to carry and birth a child for them. In "Gay Men's Narratives of Pregnancy," Riggs and Dempsey also seek to fill a gap in the literature, exploring gay men's perceptions of women who act as surrogates and the ways in which gay men navigate a pregnancy undertaken for them. Again expanding ideas of who is entitled to claim pregnancy, Riggs and Dempsey look at male experiences of "disembodied" or vicarious pregnancy.

Two creative works that address pregnancy in visual forms follow. The first, by Brescia Nember-Reid, includes two paper cut-outs. *Crone and Moon* is created by shadows cast as light projected though paper cut-outs and paper puppets. Two characters, moon and old woman, converse, perhaps about the role of both moon and midwife and their relationships to fertility. The second piece by Reid, *Umbilical Cords/Blood Ties*, uses cut-outs in black paper to present a family line of bodies attached by umbilical cords. Room is made for diverse bodies (queer and trans) and the links between ourselves and past generations is highlighted. Jennifer Long delivers us six photographs from her series *Imminent*, a body of work that creates what she calls an "ambiguous psychological narrative" of pregnancy (and in some cases motherhood). Seeking to draw out and express the often-contradictory experiences of moving towards motherhood, Long photographs pregnant and mothering bodies in their domestic environments. Highlighting themes such as confrontation and concealment, reflection and hesitation, Long's photographs give us an intimate visual glimpse of the unromanticzed beauty of the pregnant body.

Two chapters that look at representations of those who care for pregnant and birthing bodies complete this first section, the first by Elizabeth Allemang and the second by Mary Sharpe and Kory McGrath. In her chapter "Heroes and Villains," Allemang traces some of the diverse ways that the modern midwife has been represented, expanding this book's reflections to address not only representations of pregnancy, birth, and parenting, but to include representations of the midwife. Allemang reveals three divergent and at times contradictory representations of Ontario midwives as countercultural mother, feminist activist, and aspiring professional, identifying ways in which each of these representations includes aspects of both the hero and the villain and often revealing as much about who is doing the representing as about the midwives themselves. Posed as a series of reflections and questions, the closing chapter to this section, "Spacemaking and Midwifery" by Sharpe and McGrath, explores the way that spacemaking is enacted in midwifery care. Shifting back and forth from the practical and concrete to the philosophical and intangible, Sharpe and McGrath reveal the ways in which meanings are created in midwifery and birthing spaces (home, clinic, hospital, and birth centre) through actions and representations that can bolster and/or unsettle a midwifery philosophy of care.

The second section of the book, "Looking at Birth," opens with Claire Dion Fletcher and Cheryllee Bourgeois' review of prevalent imagery of pregnancy, birth, and mothering in Aboriginal culture. "Refusing Delinquency, Reclaiming Power," moves from pre-contact self-representation, to colonial imagery, to the current context in which birth and mothering have been taken up as forms of resistance and pride. Understanding the reclaiming of powerful womanhood as one aspect of healing from the effects of colonization, Dion Fletcher and Bourgeois provide examples of artists using their work to strengthen Indigenous community. Alys Einion's paper, "Resistance and Submission," draws compelling parallels between some of the features of representations of women's experiences of intimate violence and representations of childbirth. Relationships between the materiality of the body and the power dynamics inherent in contexts of sexual violence and in the social and institutional practices of medicine are explored. Careful not to equate the experiences of birth and sexual assault themselves, but rather the *representations* of these two experiences, Einion addresses the ways in which resistance and submission are enacted in these two narratives. She speaks to the risks of representations that both mirror and constrain the experiences of birthing women and argues for alternate narrative forms that place the locus of control firmly with the birthing woman. Exploring the ways in which representations of birth may highlight an empowerment that is (controversially) connected to the female body, Anna Hennessey looks to how contemporary birth movement imagery draws on both secular and religious art to centre birth as a source of feminist empowerment. Hennessey explores this birth-focused model of feminism through a study of birth imagery, particularly the use of sacred imagery in secular context and its "re-sacrilization." Hennessey's "Representations of Birth and Motherhood" addresses the ways in which birth, religion, and art interact to understand birth as a rite of passage, while simultaneously acknowledging the problematic links to essentialized notions of the female body. Natalie Jolly's "Does Labour Mean Work?" opens up discussion of the way in which constructions of femininity may impact women's experiences of pain in childbirth and may in turn condition the role of medicalization and surgical intervention as ways to avoid this pain. Looking at a culture of femininity that devalues women's capacity and tends towards separation from physical strength and capability, Jolly suggest that the consequences on women's experiences and understandings of their birthing bodies are notable. Drawing on her ethnographic study of Amish homebirth practices, Jolly provides an alternate construction of femininity in which women's bodies and minds are constituted as strong and capable in such a way that tolerance of the pain of childbirth becomes emblematic of Amish femininity. Jolly asks what alternate conceptions of femininity might engender in the current context of increasingly medicalized and surgical birth.

Shifting focus to the creation of art and representations of birth, Jeanne Lyons explores the education of midwifery students and the links between art making, midwifery, and birth giving. In "Representing Birth," Lyons explores her pedagogical practices as she teaches student midwives to create art as a way of connecting to the work of midwifery and the experience of birth. Marni Kotak takes the connection between childbirth and art making further in her chapter "Birth as a Labour of Art." She discusses her exhibition/performance *The Birth of Baby X*, which presented the lived pregnancy, birth, and mothering of her son as a piece of art "exhibited" at Microscope Gallery in Brooklyn. Kotak writes of the traditional lack of room for motherhood and art making (or other professional practice) to co-exist and pushes for the representation and celebration of pregnancy, birth, and motherhood as intimately linked to the practice of art. Situating her work in a broader context of increased representations of maternal subjectivities amongst a newer generation of artists, Kotak acknowledges that motherhood retains a problematic place in artistic production and that representations of motherhood tend to remain on the margins of art practice. Both Ara Parker and Rosie Rosenzweig use verse to explore and represent experiences of childbirth. Parker's narrative, "Split Open," draws us into the intensity of childbirth, the moment in which the "world itself was changed." Seeking to articulate what she argues is so often rendered silent and invisible, she writes of needing a "feminist framework in which to honour this experience." Rosenzweig writes of two births in her poem "Flower of My Flesh." Watching the "bloom" of first her own pregnancy and birth and then her daughter's pregnancy and birth, Rosenzweig captures the deep pride in birthing her own child and then watching her child "bloom" in turn. Stretching into the future, Rosenzweig touches on the desire to follow the "flowers of her flesh" through her grandson, with the hope of being able to watch his own blooming as he moves into his future.

This section of the book closes with two chapters that explore some of the most painful and challenging moments of childbirth. In "Birth Shock," Susan Hogan, Charley Baker, Shelagh Cornish, and Paula McCloskey present their work on using the arts in participatory workshops designed to enable women to explore their challenging experiences of birth and transitions into motherhood. The chapter highlights the ways in which image making and reflection can serve as meaningful tools to support sometimes transformational experiences in facing and healing from disappointing or traumatizing experiences of childbirth and post-partum depression. In "Making Meaning of Stillbirth," Kory McGrath and Lynn Farrales consider the ways in which words, images, and artifacts are used to represent stillbirth. They reflect on how the use of language, remembrance photography, and mementoes can impact bereaved families' understanding and experience of loss, informing how they make meaning of their experience.

The third section of the book, "Looking at Parenting," begins with Beth Osnes' "Kids Aren't Cute." With poignancy and humour,

Osnes' prose captures the simultaneously mundane and profound experience of parenting young children, irreverently elucidating some of the reasons that kids may be deep, philosophical, racist, selfish, spiritual, and savvy, but not cute. In "Paternal Loss and Anticipation," Rachel Epp Buller presents the work of artist-father Merrill Krabill. Buller explores the idea that negotiating parenthood and artistic creation may have both similarities and differences for mothers and fathers. While efforts to address the relationship between motherhood and art are recent, Buller suggests that explorations of the ways in which fatherhood and art may be intertwined are still few and far between. Noting that explorations of gay and lesbian parenting have increasingly become the focus of study and research, Rebecca English, Raechel Johns, and Angela Dwyer suggest that there has been less exploration of the ways individuals position themselves in relation to different discourses of parenthood. In, "Two Mums and Some Babies," the authors use discourse analysis to explore the ways in which one family challenges heteronormative ways of performing family and positions themselves in terms of queering discourses of motherhood. In the final chapter in the book, "Go the Fuck to Sleep Prince George?" Betty Ann Martin explores some of the tensions between competing cultural representations of motherhood. Looking at a variety of sites of resistance to prevailing and constrained cultural norms of motherhood, Martin suggests that the trend towards alternative representations leaves women to more freely negotiate motherhood.

Natal Signs: Cultural Representations of Pregnancy, Birth and Parenting explores some of the ways in which reproductive experiences are taken up in the rich arena of cultural production. Taken together, the chapters in this collection pose questions, unsettle assumptions, and generate broad imaginative spaces for thinking about representation of pregnancy, birth, and parenting. Indeed, they demonstrate for us the ways in which practices of consuming and using representations carry within them the productive forces of creation. Our hope is that we have offered a diverse and critically engaged set of possibilities for attending to some of life's most meaningful moments in ways that open possibilities in our hearts and minds.

WORKS CITED

Bourdieu, Pierre. *The Field of Cultural Production*. New York: Columbia University Press, 1993. Print.

de Certeau, Michel. *The Practice of Everyday Life*. Berkeley: University of California Press, 1984. Print.

hooks, bell. "Black (and White) Snapshots." *Ms.* 5.2 (1994): 82-87. Print.

Johnson, Randal. "Pierre Bourdieu on Art, Literature and Culture." Editor's Introduction. *The Field of Cultural Production*. By Pierre Bourdieu. New York: Columbia University Press, 1993: 1-25. Print.

Landau, Jamie. "Reproducing and Transgressing Masculinity: A Rhetorical Analysis of Women Interacting With Digital Photographs of Thomas Beatie." *Women's Studies in Communication* 35.2 (2012): 178-203. Print.

Longhurst, Robyn. "YouTube: A New Space for Birth?" *feminist review* 93 (2009): 46-63. Print.

Millett, Ann. "Sculpting Body Ideals: *Alison Lapper Pregnant* and the Public Display of Disability." *Disability Studies Quarterly* 28.3 (2008). Web. 4 May 2015.

Riggs, Damien. "What Makes a Man? Thomas Beatie, Embodiment, and 'Mundane Transphobia.'" *Feminism & Psychology* 24.2 (2014): 151-171. Print.

Sumartojo, Shanti. "The Fourth Plinth: Creating and Contesting National Identity in Trafalgar Square, 2005-2010." *Cultural Geographies* 26.1 (2012): 67-81. Print.

Tyler, Imogen. "Introduction: Birth." *feminist review* 93 (2009): 1-7. Print.

1.
LOOKING AT PREGNANCY

LAUREN CRUIKSHANK

What to Expect When Your Avatar is Expecting

Representations of Pregnancy and Birth in Video Games

WHEN IT COMES TO VIDEO GAMES, much attention is paid to representations of death. Game developers spill considerable digital blood crafting elaborate spectacles of violent demise in death-oriented games, while academics and the popular media spill equally as much ink debating the implications of those virtual fatalities. Avatars, visual representations of human players in these digital spaces, die repeatedly in games, such that experiences of dying become "part of the everyday life in the world" (Klastrup 144). However, in the context of this discussion and a medium in which death has so often been the focus, what about birth?

How are avatars born? Are there games that represent beginnings of life as well as endings? How do games deal with natalities alongside fatalities? What kinds of games explore conception, pregnancy, birth, and postpartum experiences? How is birth enacted and understood within the unique media forms of video games and what can we learn from these representations of avatar reproduction? I consider several interesting game texts here to illustrate how examining reproduction in games can extend existing work on the visual culture of reproduction and contribute to existing media analyses of the procreative body.

Important work has been done on the popular construction of birth and the dominant cultural expectations around expectant bodies in other media contexts, such as film and television. These explorations point to an understanding of the birth process as "ground zero" of gender relations (Russell 255), due in no small part to the ways that motherhood is coupled tightly with femininity, such that "womanhood and motherhood are often outwardly synonymous" (359). In this way, reproduction, as Adrienne Rich tells us, defines "woman" in ways that regulate the lives of all women, whether or not they are mothers, and continues to be a key site for the negotiation of female identities, relations, and activities (Woollett and Boyle 307).

If the media have been and continue to be the major dispenser of the ideals and norms surrounding motherhood, (Douglas and Michaels 11) this mediation of motherhood begins in earnest with portrayals of pregnancy and birth. Even the "topic of getting pregnant is a media obsession" (Angel qtd. in Podnieks 3) and once a pregnancy has begun, the expectant mother is habitually feminized, romanticized, and infantilized in media representations, while also deemed unruly, "in need of constant surveillance," and rendered especially passive by the perceived precariousness of pregnancy and a related relationship of implied deference to medical authority (Morris and McInerney; Russell; Podnieks). As for portrayals of labour and birth:

> Widely distributed films, reality TV programs, and sitcoms stress the time-worn, predictable pattern—the laboring woman's mad rush to the hospital, her fear, screams and hysteria, the unbearable pain, the desirability, indeed necessity, of epidural anesthesia, and the inevitability of a cesarean section. (Pincus 82)

Many of these representations of labour and birth focus primarily on men's distress rather than women's labouring experiences (Elson) until they eventually climax with a carefully framed "money shot" of the baby as it emerges from its mother's body (Russell 262). Regardless of the dramatic trials endured by the labouring mother and anxious father, the birth event as depicted on film and television will almost certainly conclude with "happy endings and warm feelings" all around (Morris and McInerney 138).

These film and television portrayals of birth have been subject to some academic critique, and preliminary work has been done as well on negotiations of birth and motherhood online via blogging, social media, and other online forums (De Choudhury, Counts and Horvitz; Friedman and Calixte; Lopez). However, digital spaces that include avatars, such as video games and virtual worlds, have been largely unstudied as of yet as sites of reproductive representation.

Lisa Nakamura does devote a chapter to avatars and the visual culture of reproduction online in her book *Digitizing Race: Visual Cultures of the Internet*. However, Nakamura intentionally puts aside the avatars of games and virtual worlds to closely analyze the graphical avatars posted by participants on a popular online pregnancy discussion board. The site she examines serves as a forum for women interested in pregnancy to convene and dis- cuss concerns in common, but also a digital space to represent themselves as graphical avatars in signatures below their posts, visually signifying a range of pregnant and non-pregnant states as well as other personal characteristics in the process. Nakamura is interested in the counter to the medicalized gaze upon women's bodies that these women create with their own constructed, dy- namic, and often playful images of their bodies, whether they are attempting to conceive, pregnant, or post-pregnant (158). These avatars exist for Nakamura as a challenge to the female "hyper- real, exaggerated hyperbodies" evident in most mainstream video games, which she suggests have "left the real female body behind in a significant way" (136).

If as Nakamura points out, "the stakes in regards to digital pregnant body avatars are especially high on account of the con- tentious and bitter political and cultural discourse surrounding the status of the maternal body in our culture," (134) what then, of the digital games that do attempt to engage with the visual culture of reproduction? A central question here is how simulated pregnan- cies and birth events might stand to either reinscribe or possibly rework dominant social constructions of expectant motherhood and new parenthood. If "every technology is a reproductive tech- nology" (Sofia 48), then it is the work of this inquiry to examine more closely how video games are reproductive technologies, and what it is they serve to reproduce.

In order to explore these questions, this paper draws on analyses of the reproductive themes in several video game titles and the re- vealing constructions of procreation and negotiations of gender that result. Several games that incorporate conception, pregnancy, and birth are considered, with a specific interest in games that portray human-oriented reproduction. Thus, games such as the *Pokémon* series, the *Viva Piñata* series, or *Spore* games that task players with breeding animals or other fantastical beings are set aside here, although this category of game is intriguing in its own right. Also excluded for this particular case are games that depict parasite/host relationships culminating in the threat of an alien creature bursting out of an ill-fated human's chest, stomach, or head, such as in *Dark Seed*, the *Resident Evil* series, or the *Alien* game franchise. Persistent anxieties around monstrous impregnation, the abject reproductive body, and the horror of the fearful Other as offspring can be read throughout these games and the horror narratives that predate them in film and literature (Creed; Berenstein). However, for the purposes of this study, the alien parasite is set apart from narratives that reflect primarily human reproduction, although there are some interesting crossovers, as we will see.

These criteria yield a list of titles that is relatively small, but is an interesting sample of games across several genres. Representative games include: *Fallout 3, Assassin's Creed II,* and *Beyond: Two Souls,* which could be broadly defined as action/adventure games; role-playing games such as *Fable II, Fable III* and *Dragon Quest V;* and simulation/nurture games such as *My Little Baby,* the *Harvest Moon* series of games, or *The Sims 1, The Sims 2,* and *The Sims 3,* along with the various *Sims* expansion packs. There are also games such as *Silent Hill 3* and *F.3.A.R.* that feature pregnant women birthing hybrid child-creatures as part of their horror narratives, deviating only slightly from the aforementioned parasite alien trope. Other games with birth elements include strategy games that employ heirs, such as the *Crusader Kings* series, and projectile-style birth games, such as *Baby Maker Extreme* and *Big J's Birth Game.* This list is by no means exhaustive, but is intended to give a sense of the range of games that include birth in some way and highlight the ways birth is currently represented in game texts.

CONCEPTION

Where do babies come from in games and virtual worlds? Even in the few games that do depict birth and/or children, it is relatively rare that conception itself is represented. There are a few exceptions, however, and these are interesting to examine. One of the most comprehensive representations of the reproductive experience in popular games thus far occurs in *The Sims* series, the self-described "people simulator" (Bentley) by Maxis / Electronic Arts, which has included a semblance of birth since its first iteration in 2000. *The Sims*, *The Sims 2*, and *The Sims 3*, along with the numerous expansion packs for each version, are so-called "sandbox" games, which allow players to largely define many of their own objectives, modify the world themselves, and play in a number of different ways. The organization of the game series is based primarily on managing individual homes and directing the lives of the avatars or "Sims" that make up each household.

The importance of reproduction and level of detail paid to reproductive processes within *The Sims* series has changed significantly over the various iterations. In the original game, opposite sex Sim couples that engage in passionate kissing and other romantic interactions will eventually prompt the appearance of a dialog box asking, "Should we have a baby?" and a choice to press either "Yes" or "No." The first expansion pack for *The Sims*, called *Livin' Large*, added a "Vibromatic Heart Bed" that allows Sims to choose "Play in Bed" as a possible action that will also prompt the baby dialog choice box for opposite sex couples.

The Sims 2 incorporates aging, pregnancy, and genetics into the game engine in a much more significant way, allowing players to conceive new characters from existing ones, play through Sim pregnancies, help raise the resulting babies to adulthood, and play several generations of Sims avatars successively. With *The Sims 2*, the "Play in Bed" expansion interaction from *The Sims* was incorporated into the main game experience as "WooHoo," available to any two adult Sims with a relationship status strong enough.

In both *The Sims 2* and *The Sims 3*, two romantically linked Sims can get into a bed, change booth, hot tub, or other designated location together and choose from interactions that may include "Cuddle," "Make Out," "WooHoo," or if they are of the opposite sex and the appropriate ages, "Try for Baby." In these games, the "Try for Baby" interaction is available for a pair of male and female "Adult" aged Sims, including male but not female "Elders." If the player selects "WooHoo" or "Try for Baby," an animation of the two Sims moving under the sheets, behind the curtain, or under the water occurs amid audible giggles, growls, moans and yelps. Fireworks or a shower of hearts will eventually go off above the Sims' heads as the activity concludes and if a "Try for Baby" attempt is successful, a short lullaby tune will be then be heard. The "Try for Baby" interaction in *The Sims 2* and *The Sims 3* holds varying chances of conception affected in part by where the interaction took place and possibly other factors, such as a full moon or various fertility treatments, depending on which expansion packs are installed. One interesting variation of note takes place in *The Sims Medieval*, which does not designate a "Try for Baby" interaction. Instead, any "WooHoo" interaction between opposite sex adults Sims carries a random chance of conception.

Recent games in the *Fable* series, including *Fable II* and *Fable III*, also include the possibility of conception after romancing, marrying, and then propositioning a potential partner. After leading a spouse to a bed, players can choose to "sleep," engage in "protected sex" (if a condom has been purchased), or have "unprotected sex." If the player chooses to initiate either sex interaction, the game screen will fade to black while giggles, moans, and suggestive comments can be heard. Interestingly, a player can initiate sex with in-game characters of either gender, in or out of wedlock, or by engaging the services of a prostitute. However, pregnancy will only result if sex is unprotected, partners are of the opposite sex, and partners are married. If these three conditions are met, the interaction carries a high chance of resulting in a pregnancy, indicated by a post-coital comment by one's spouse such as, "I hope you want to be a dad, because there's a little one on the way," (*Fable II*); "Well, you've done it... I'm pregnant!" (*Fable III*); "Look at the size of you! We're going to be parents!" (*Fable II*); or "You're pregnant! This is.... It's just so incredible! I've never been so happy!" (*Fable III*).

A completely different and much darker representation of conception occurs in the *F.E.A.R.* series of first person shooter horror games. In the concluding sequence of *F.E.A.R. 2: Project Origin*, cutscenes interspersed with gameplay reveal Alma, a supernatural female entity and the game's main antagonist, attempting to rape the male protagonist Becket. Alma conceives as a result of this attack, setting the scene for the next game in the series. The game concludes with Alma, naked and heavily pregnant, placing Becket's hand on her swollen stomach, while an eerie child's voice whispers "Mommy...."

Of course, sex plays a lesser or greater role in these portrayals of conception depending on the intended player demographics. *The Sims*, a game series with a teen rating, represents sex acts with euphemisms and hearts, whereas M-rated games such as *Fable II*, *Fable III*, or *F.E.A.R. 2* include more overt audio and/or visual sexual references as part of their procreation narratives.

Both *The Sims* series and the *Fable* games also incorporate the pleasures of alea, or "chancing," into the conception gameplay (Caillois 17). The randomized possibility of conceiving through choosing "Unprotected Sex" or "Try for Baby" serves as a gambling mini-game built into the larger gameplay. In *The Sims 2* and *The Sims 3*, we can assume that players choose "Try for Baby" in the hopes of conceiving, since the "WooHoo" action is otherwise identical and available at no cost. In *Fable II* and *Fable III*, however, condoms must be purchased in advance at a small cost in order for the "Protected Sex" interaction to be available to the player. Along with pregnancy, sexually transmitted diseases can also be contracted via "Unprotected Sex" in these games, lending conception a somewhat negative connotation as one of two consequences of not purchasing a condom in advance and spending that item during the sex interaction. This difference in each series' orientation to conception is also reflected in the terminology for each action, since although both game series have interactions that carry a chance for conception or no chance for conception, "Try for Baby" frames the action in terms of a desire to conceive, while "Unprotected Sex" implies more of a gamble and a risk of unintended negative consequences.

PREGNANCY

As for pregnancy itself, one of the most common ways that pregnant states are represented in games is not at all. In other words, there are a host of games that either begin a procreation game element with the birth event itself (*Fallout 3, Assassin's Creed II, Baby Maker Extreme, Big J's Birth Game*) or skip over an implied period of pregnancy altogether, such as the kiss to bassinet transition seen in *The Sims* first iteration and the instant appearance of a baby after sex in *Fable II* and *Fable III*. Only slightly more game focus is devoted to depictions of pregnancy in games such as *Dragon Quest V* and many of the titles in the *Harvest Moon* series, which include a female character suddenly fainting shortly after getting married and, after examination by a doctor, discovering she is pregnant. In these particular examples, no physical trace of pregnancy is evident in the character's appearance or acknowledgement of the character's pregnancy made again until her labour begins later in the game.

The most comprehensive inclusion of pregnancy again occurs in *The Sims 2* and *The Sims 3,* where a Sim's pregnancy lasts throughout three days of game time, an approximation of the three trimesters of pregnancy. A pregnant Sim won't have many physical indications of her pregnancy for the first trimester (about twenty-four hours in game time or twenty-four minutes in real time), although she may run to the toilet to be sick, after which a thought bubble with a pacifier and a question mark in it will appear above her head. After a day of game time has passed, the avatar will watch in surprise as her belly suddenly bulges. She will begin walking with a slight waddle, experience more hunger, fatigue, and bladder urgency, and her clothing will now become default maternity clothes. If she has a job, she will also receive a message around this time indicating that she is now on leave to prepare for a baby and should "get some rest." After a second day of game-time, a pregnant Sim's belly will bulge further and she will move much more slowly and with a pronounced waddle. Her hunger, fatigue, and bladder will again become more challenging for the player to manage and she may experience cravings for specific food items, mood swings, or a sore back. Other Sims can also engage with a pregnant Sim through special interactions such as "Rub Belly" and "Talk to Belly" in *The Sims 2* or "Feel Tummy," "Listen to Tummy," and "Talk to Tummy" in *The Sims 3*. Pregnant Sims in *The Sims 3* can also "Announce Pregnancy" to others, "Ask to Feel Tummy," or can approach another Sim who is advanced in the medical career path and "Ask to Determine Gender of Baby" before he or she is born.

Other features of pregnancy in the later Sims games include being able to influence the number of babies born and their gender by having a pregnant Sim eat certain foods, watch children's television, listen to children's music on the stereo, read pregnancy books, or use one of several other fertility-enhancing rewards and actions present in the game. In addition, pregnant Sims are subject to restrictions on their in-game actions that other Sims do not experience, including not being able to leave the house in *The Sims 2*. They are also unable to change their appearance, do yoga, work out to music, and make use of the hot tub, diving board, or waterslide. Pregnant Sims in *The Sims 3* may not be not able to drive, take a taxi, or swing on a swing set at certain points in their pregnancy. However, they can still down multiple shots of espresso, drink champagne or other alcoholic drinks, and get into physical brawls with other Sims, activities that would subject actual pregnant women to considerable public scrutiny and criticism.

LABOUR AND DELIVERY

Despite the scarcity of games that represent conception and pregnancy in any substantial manner, there are a larger number of games that portray labour and birth, often in ways that suggest childbirth is difficult, dangerous, and painful. Games such as *Beyond: Two Souls, Dragon Quest V, F.3.A.R., Assassin's Creed II, The Sims 2, The Sims 3* and some versions of the *Harvest Moon* series all represent a mother in labour that involves pain or intense effort. In all of these examples, the labouring mother is represented suddenly and dramatically in the throes of the active labour stage and this process triggers alarm, distress, or intense concern in the other characters around her. For example, Tuesday in *Beyond: Two Souls* is visibly sweating while she grimaces, screams, swears, clutches at her stomach, and describes herself as "wracked in pain"; Maria in *Assassin's Creed II* grits her teeth, screams, and pants; mothers-to-be in *Dragon Quest V* and some titles of the *Harvest Moon* series huff, pant, or exclaim "Ow!" while labouring; and pregnant Sims in *The Sims 2* and *The Sims*

3 cross their eyes, double over, and hold their stomachs amid gasps, grunts, and groans that come and go in an approximation of frequent painful contractions. *Fallout 3* begins from the baby's point of view just after birth, so no labour is heard or seen, but blood in the visual field and the weak, winded voice of the baby's mother reference the strain of childbirth. Moments after being born we hear the mother suffer cardiac arrest and are later told that she did not survive the ordeal.

However, the most dramatic representation of painful labour for game purposes can be found in *F.3.A.R.*, which represents Alma's supernatural labour with not just painful screams, but accompanying powerful contraction waves that act as explosions, rippling through the game-world, tinting it red, setting objects on fire, building increasingly dense fog, and spawning waves of enemies. Despite this dramatic labour, the birth of Alma's baby at the end of the game is comparatively understated. The male protagonist walks over and bends down near the prone mother to lift up an already swaddled baby from somewhere below the camera's view. The grotesque figure of Alma serves as the shock value in this scene instead, angrily staring up at us while lying naked, bloody, and vulnerable on the floor. She is audibly panting and whimpering even after giving birth, presumably under the strain of her still massive stomach, a glowing and distended red orb stretched taut to the point of tissue transparency and horrifically strung-up by artery-like glistening cables. Once the baby is delivered, one possible ending for the game sees Alma close her eyes, stop breathing, and burn up from within, disappearing in a sphere of red light and providing another variation on death caused by childbirth. Depending on the game played, childbirth is frequently framed as dangerous or potentially deadly, either for the mother (*F.3.A.R.*, *Fallout 3*, *Beyond: Two Souls*, *Harvest Moon*), the baby (*Assassin's Creed II*, *Beyond: Two Souls*), or indeed all of humanity (*Silent Hill 3*, *F.3.A.R.*).

In the context of this framing of childbirth and risk are the choices made by game designers to represent birth in a hospital environment, home environment, or other location with helpful attendants present or not. Many games examined here represent birth occurring in a medical environment, including a hospital or medical clinic (*Fallout 3*, *Baby Maker Extreme*, *Big J's Birth Game*, *Harvest Moon*), while other games, especially those that take place in a historical or fantasy context, portray birth taking place at home with female attendants (*Dragon Quest V*, *Assassin's Creed II*).

An interesting exchange about the decision to go to a hospital and the riskiness of birth occurs in *Beyond: Two Souls*, when homeless mother Tuesday goes into labour under a bridge, prompting another homeless character, Walter, to exclaim, "We need an ambulance! We need a whole god-damned hospital!" Tuesday responds, "No! No hospital! They'll take my baby! No... No one's gonna take my baby!" Walter retorts with "Jesus Christ, girl! We ain't got nothing here! Ain't got as much as a blanket... hot water! We got nothin'!" This sequence prompts the protagonist Jodie to venture out with group leader Stan, asking him, "What are we gonna do? Do you know a doctor?" to which Stan replies, "No. Besides, we don't have any money to pay for it anyway." The pair proceeds to break into a nearby supermarket to steal supplies, including towels, scissors, and diapers. After Tuesday is helped to a nearby abandoned building, she asks everyone to leave except Jodie, who protests that she has "never done anything like this before." When Tuesday insists, Jodie says, "Ok, don't worry, We're going to figure this out... I mean, how hard can it be?" Jodie helps Tuesday remove her jeans and places towels underneath her, reassuring and coaching her through the pushing stage until baby Zoey is delivered. Jodie then cuts the cord and wraps the newborn in a towel before handing her to her mother.

This sequence is interesting not only for the discussion of hospital birth as simultaneously safer and riskier for the marginalized characters in the game, but also for a more comprehensive portrayal of childbirth than most of the other games provide. Although the scene begins with Tuesday already in what appears to be advanced stages, at least ten minutes of game time is devoted to her labour process, depending on how the game is played—a relatively long time in game time. Comforting the labouring mother is built into gameplay and the game is the only one from the sample studied to include an umbilical cord, which must be cut by player actions.

Like *Beyond: Two Souls*, the birth scene in *Assassin's Creed II* includes effort, pain, female attendants, and a baby born realistically tinged with blood and other fluids. Although one of the two Italian midwives attending the birth motions in a way that may represent cutting the cord out of view, the baby does not show any trace of a cord despite a discernable navel when it is held, limp in the midwife's arms. The midwives exchange a concerned look in response to the baby's lifelessness just as the father, Giovanni, bursts in the door. Upon seeing the limp baby, Giovanni confidently instructs the midwife to "Give him here," which she does. "Giovanni," the baby's mother Maria says in a despondent voice, to which he replies, "Shhhh, my love. It will be alright." He holds the baby up and in Italian tells the child, "You are an Auditore. You are a fighter. So ... fight!" One of the midwives clutches at her heart and casts her eyes down in despair. The player is then given instructions from the baby's point of view to move one's legs, arms, and head, spurring the newborn to kick, swing his arms, and eventually to cough and cry, no longer lifeless. The scene resumes with Giovanni proudly exclaiming, "Listen to him! A fine set of lungs!" Maria asks, "And what shall we call him, my love?" Giovanni replies, "Ezio! Ezio Auditore da Firenze!" lifting the crying child high in triumph.

In contrast to these dramatic portrayals of childbirth, there are games that represent childbirth in ways intended to be humorous, with varying levels of tastefulness. On the ridiculous end of the spectrum are *Baby Maker Extreme* and *Big J's Birth Game,* which both reinterpret childbirth as a projectile game. In *Baby Maker Extreme,* an independent game available via the Xbox Live Marketplace, players see the lower half of a white pregnant woman on a hospital table, her feet in stirrups and a white doctor in gown and mask standing in front of her. The player is then tasked with pressing controller buttons in time with the sounds of quickening heavy breathing while a syringe fills with liquid. Once it is full, the player is instructed to "mash" the B button as the syringe empties and a temperature gauge rises. With a pained cry from a female voice and a popping noise, a baby tucked into the fetal position is launched through the air from between the woman's legs to the sounds of rock music and applause, knocking over people and objects as it flies throughout different rooms in the hospital in an attempt to remain airborne as long as possible.

Big J's Birth Game is an online Flash game that operates on much the same premise, with the player initially pressing "Z" to keep Big J "supplied with gas and air.... The more you give me the larger my breasts become (!) and the further my lovely babies will go" (*Big J's Birth Game*). Players pump air into the gas mask of the white topless mother lying motionless on a hospital bed to inflate her breasts and then launch babies from between her legs, attempting to aim each launch so that the babies land in the strollers of three fathers passing by, preferably by matching the colour of each baby to the race of the father.

These games employ highly exaggerated notions of childbirth as a simple projectile game mechanic for cheap laughs, tapping into sexist, racist, and sexualized tropes about birth and expectant women in the process. They also reflect a literal joke on the notion common in popular culture that childbirth involves "popping out" a baby, or that an expectant mother is "about to pop" or "about to blow."

Although treated quite differently, the onset of labour in *The Sims 2* and *The Sims 3* is also largely represented as comic, with exaggerated huffing and puffing and bulging crossed eyes as Sims experience contractions. If there are any other Sims around at this time they will run to the pregnant Sim's side and "panic," excitedly pointing, looking scared, dancing from foot to foot, and gasping. Finally, the pregnant Sim will straighten into a neutral standing pose and a birth animation will play. In *The Sims 2* this sequence shows the green prism above the pregnant Sim's head twitch, bulge, and split into two in a cascade of fireworks. A diapered baby will drop from this animation into its mother's arms and she will catch it, hold it up, coo affectionately at it, and nuzzle her nose to its nose. In *The Sims 3*, the pregnant Sim will spin around and reach down around her waist to lift into the air a swaddled baby that appears in a swirl of sparkles. In both versions of the game a text screen will accompany this animation asking the player to name the new baby and revealing its gender. Occasionally, a twin or triplet will be born, with the same animation repeated. In both cases the birth sequence occurs while the pregnant Sim is fully clothed and standing upright, and without intervention or help from attendants—in fact, Sims often give birth at home completely alone. After the animation ends, the baby or babies appear in the family profile and regular Sim life resumes.

One interesting difference from previous versions is the inclusion in *The Sims 3* of an option to go to the hospital once a pregnant character's labour begins. This prompt will often spontaneously appear as an automatic action for the pregnant Sim to "Go to Hospital," which she will do unless the "Go to Hospital" actions are actively cancelled by the player each time they pop up. This design choice codes in an expectation that babies will be born in the hospital, but it also highlights home birth as a more meaningful option in the Sims world than it previously was, set up in contrast to a default hospital birth as a conscious choice players can decide to make.

If the pregnant Sim is directed to go to the Hospital by the player or the action appears autonomously, her labour pains will stop and she will calmly get into a car or taxi, travel to the hospital, and walk normally through the hospital doors. After this point, quiet ambient hospital noises such as beeping monitors and intercom paging announcements can be heard, but no audible continuation of labour. The text box announcing the baby's arrival will eventually appear and the mother will then walk out of the hospital doors with the new baby in her arms, get into a vehicle, and travel home to resume her Sim life.

ANALYSIS: THEMES AND PATTERNS

These games provide a wide range of portrayals of conception, pregnancy, and birth with some noteworthy patterns emerging across the various texts. It comes as no surprise that the video games examined here largely replicate the misrepresentations, distortions, deletions, and exaggerations around birth that occur in other media portrayals. Some of these reinforced again here include: the contemporary expectation of control over conception; the omission of many of the physical aspects of pregnancy and delivery; the speed of childbirth; the portrayal of labour as sudden, dramatic, and painful; the focus on male experiences of the process; and the passivity of the mother in the context of a medical setting and/or male characters, usually labouring lying on her back in a bed. Expectant parents in these games are usually white and heterosexual, and in at least three cases, must be married to become pregnant. Absent from these portrayals are representations of early gentle labour, waters breaking, different labour positions, an umbilical cord (in all cases but one), any mention of the delivery of a placenta, perineal trauma, breastfeeding, or a recovery period. No non-heterosexual parents are depicted and fathers are either not present to assist labouring mothers or are not useful at all in the labour process.

When looking at video games in comparison to other media, however, it is also essential to consider the uniqueness of this particular medium. Video games vary widely, but one key characteristic is that games are interactive in non-trivial ways. Games require players and their input to co-create the gameplay and variety of possible experiences (Apperley). It is telling, then, that most of the moments of birth depicted in games are not interactive. Birth takes place most often in game cutscenes, which are animation sequences during which players simply watch or hear a scene unfold without being able to exercise any influence. In many games, players can name a baby or choose a few characteristics for the new arrival once the birth is complete, but cannot exercise any control during the labour or birth itself. The one notable exception to this rule is the role that Jodie plays in *Beyond: Two Souls*, assisting Tuesday as a birth attendant. As Jodie, the player selects actions such as placing towels underneath Tuesday, comforting her, coaching her, catching the baby, and cutting the umbilical cord. These moments are interspersed with cutscenes, so that in many ways the interaction is intended to trigger each subsequent scene and move along the narrative in pre-determined ways. A similar technique is used in *Assassin's Creed II*, where the player is tasked with moving one's arms, legs, and head from baby Ezio's point of view in order to revive oneself and live.

In both cases if players do not complete the required steps when prompted, the game in question will not progress. In other words, although the player has some interaction with the game during these birth scenes, these moments do not involve any opportunities to make meaningful choices. Computer scientists Alexandra Holloway and Sri Kurnaiwan share this observation in their review of video games involving childbirth, noting: "When birth scenes do exist in games, the available actions, or affordances, to the player are minimal at best."

In addition, when birth scenes in games involve interaction, this interaction is primarily available from the point of view of someone other than the labouring mother. In other words, birth is non-playable from the role of the one giving birth. Players can engage with the game from the father's point of view in *Dragon Quest V*, the baby's point of view in *Fallout 3* and *Assassin's Creed II*, a brother's point of view in *F.3.A.R.*, or a female birth attendant's point of view in *Beyond: Two Souls*. In the projectile birth games, the player appears to be placed in a hybrid role that alternates between the perspectives of medical attendants administering drugs, the birthing mother building up power or aiming to launch a baby, and the babies themselves as they fly through the air. In both games however, only portions of the mother's body can be seen, she is motionless and her face is not visible, rendering her more of a static background image than a protagonist. In contrast, babies, doctors, and fathers have visible faces and are animated, making the mother a passive launcher prop in the game play.

This removal of interactivity during birth events positions labour and delivery as a dramatic spectacle in games, but does not acknowledge or incorporate the potential agency, power, or perspectives of a character giving birth. Instead, these characters are objectified as conduits for delivery meant to be looked at by players, instead of active decision-making subjects for players to embody as they engage with the challenges and choices involved in the work of childbirth.

In the *Harvest Moon* series, *The Sims* series, and the *Fable* series players can play as either parent. Nevertheless, in each of these games female avatars giving birth are once again not responsive to player interactions while they are in labour or during delivery, although fathers are playable during a birth scene in most cases. The one exception is in *The Sims 3*, which allows labouring mothers to accept or delete one action, the "Go To Hospital" option.

Another very interesting aspect of birth in *The Sims 2* game is that it is also possible for men. If aliens abduct a male character during the game, he will return pregnant in a few days time. He will then experience all of the same symptoms and processes of pregnancy that female Sims do, except that when the child is born, it may have green skin, "alien" facial features, and possibly red or yellow eyes. The birth sequence is also different—an alien baby appears by levitating in a spiral around the male Sim as he shields his eyes until it lands in his arms. He will then hold the alien baby away from himself in disgust until he takes a second look, relaxes, and then smiles and cuddles the newborn to him.

As previously mentioned, the alien abduction and subsequent pregnancy is a trope rife with cultural resonance around seizure and penetration that conjures up familiar sci-fi fears about the permeability of the body. It is interesting to note that it is adult male Sims with the "knowledge" aspiration and science careers who have the highest chance of getting abducted and impregnated, not, for example, those with the "family" aspiration. As well, although females can get abducted, they won't return pregnant, whereas men always will. In one fell swoop, male alien birth in this game collects the comic, horrific, and sentimental tints toward birth we have seen separately in the other game representations together into one short animation.

The concept of male birth is also in line with the cultural imaginary that has long toyed with the possibilities for ectogenesis, or genesis outside the womb. Stories about efforts to displace birth from women's wombs and create life "not of woman-born" are nothing new, certainly. From Frankenstein and Pygmalion through artificial intelligence and cloning technology, attempts to play mother abound in the myriad mythological and technological endeavours intended to rework how humans are made. We could argue that creating avatars is also a direct descendant of this tradition. If avatars reflect this desire to self-replicate and reproduce technologically, games often encourage us to do just that via character creation applications, the in-game body shops and face factories for designing and assembling avatars that act as a kind of workaround of the womb, that original body shop.

Elizabeth Grosz tells us that this history of circumventing or denying the power of the womb is "a tendency in phallocentric thought to deny and cover over the debt of life and existence that all subjects, and indeed, all theoretical frameworks, owe to the maternal body" (121). One useful antidote to this tendency is to acknowledge natality in each instance that we can. In her critique of a philosophical tradition that has long been concerned with mortality, Hannah Arendt reminds us that the other side of this coin is natality, and the possibility of bringing forth a new world each time we commence action. A birth reminds us that all social worlds are not given, but humanly scripted, and that they also promise to renew with each new participant. As Patricia Bowen-Moore elaborates, "Birth is indeed a worldly phenomenon—the appearance of a new creation who in turn creates" (32). Those newly born are estranged from the world's previously established ways and as they become more familiar, can initiate action and change that world.

In this light, some of the most intriguing and non-traditional portrayals of pregnancy and birth in video games and virtual worlds have occurred through player-participant initiative, intervention, or modifications of existing games. For example, players of *The Sims* series have shared downloadable objects for the game to make same-sex pregnancies possible, including offspring that share genetic characteristics of both parents. There are also player-created modifications for the fantasy role-playing game *The Elder Scrolls III: Morrowind* that allow players to add menstrual cycles, pregnancy, birth, and babies to the game, creating playable female characters that can accomplish quests while visibly pregnant or toting babies strapped to their backs. *Second Life*, a virtual world that encourages players to create custom content, has many player-created reproduction experiences, including pregnancies without the baby, babies without a pregnancy, clinic visits, ultrasounds, animated labour and child-carrying poses, pregnancies of varying lengths, interactive talking bellies, Lamaze classes, various exotic delivery experiences, partner interactions, animated food and maternity health supplements, due date timers, and a spectrum of highly customizable newborns, including a wide range of non-human babies (Cruikshank and Kennedy).

These user-created game modifications act as in-game reproductive technologies that both highlight and challenge not only the absence of reproductive possibilities in most games, but also the conventional and limited notions of conception, pregnancy, and childbirth often reproduced in games when they do appear. If Western dominant discourses around motherhood position mothers "too often as objects rather than subjects, as absences over presences and as spoken *for* instead of speaking themselves" (Podnieks 5), player participation and modification of games is one way to talk back in order to challenge stereotypical or problematic portrayals. Nakamura suggests that the "radical possibilities that new media offers to digitally create 'other' bodies, other iterations of 'woman' and 'man' that elude the dichotomies between interior and exterior, white and non-white, and female and male are especially evident in digital visualizations of bodies, that is to say, avatars" (160). After all, given that the spaces of video games and virtual worlds are entirely designed environments, any number of worlds and avatars to populate them is possible.

The birth stories scripted within these digital worlds, as well as those absent, model a powerful, specific, and persuasive digital visual culture of reproduction. These "reproductions of reproduction" often work to legitimize common stereotypical ideas about pregnancy and childbirth, but they are also capable, as we begin to see here, of resisting and reworking these commonly held assumptions and misrepresentations in new and progressive ways as well. We would be wise to remember that our human natality assures us that new worlds are always possible. After all, as Arendt reminds us, we were born to change the game.

WORKS CITED

Apperley, Thomas H. "Genre and Game Studies: Toward a Critical Approach to Video Game Genres." *Simulation & Gaming* 37.1 (2006): 6-23. Print.

Arendt, Hannah. *The Human Condition.* Chicago: University of Chicago Press, 1958.

Assassin's Creed II. Montreal, Quebec: Ubisoft, 2009. Video game.

Baby Maker Extreme. Toronto: Stegersaurus Games, 2010. Video game.

Bentley, Tom. *The Sims* (Game Manual). Redwood City, CA: EA-

Games, 2001. Print.

Berenstein, Rhona. "Mommie Dearest: Aliens, Rosemary's Baby and Mothering." *The Journal of Popular Culture* 24.2 (1990): 55-73. Print.

Beyond: Two Souls. Paris, France: Quantic Dream/Sony, 2013. Video game.

Big J's Birth Game. Ganges.com, 2014. Video game.

Bowen-Moore, Patricia. *Hannah Arendt's Philosophy of Natality.* New York: St. Martin's Press, 1989. Print.

Caillois, Roger. *Man, Play, and Games.* Champaign, IL: University of Illinois Press, 2001. Print.

Creed, Barbara. "Horror and the Monstrous-Feminine: An Imaginary Abjection." *Screen* 27.1 (1986): 44-70. Print.

Cruikshank, Lauren and Tracy Kennedy. "Where (Virtual) Babies Come From: Conception, Consumption and Reproduction in Games and Virtual Worlds." *Internet Research 12: Performance and Participation.* Association of Internet Researchers. Seattle, WA. October 2011. Conference presentation.

Dragon Quest V: Hand of the Heavenly Bride. Tokyo: Square Enix/Nintendo, 2009. Video game.

De Choudhury, Munmun, Scott Counts, and Eric Horvitz. "Major Life Changes and Behavioral Markers in Social Media: Case of Childbirth." *Proceedings of the 2013 Conference on Computer Supported Cooperative Work.* ACM, 2013. Print.

Douglas, Susan and Meredith Michaels. *The Mommy Myth: The Idealization of Motherhood and How It Has Undermined All Women.* New York: Simon and Schuster, 2005. Print.

The Elder Scrolls III: Morrowind. Rockville, Maryland: Bethesda, 2002. Video game.

Elson, Victoria L. Dir. *Laboring Under an Illusion: Mass Media Childbirth vs."The Real Thing."* Birth Media.com, 2008. Film.

Fable II. Redmond, Washington: Lionhead Studios, 2008. Video game.

Fable III. Redmond, Washington: Lionhead Studios, 2010. Video game.

Fallout 3. Rockville, Maryland: Bethesda Game Studios, 2008. Video game.

F.3.A.R (F.E.A.R. 3). Chicago, Illinois: Day 1 Studios, Warner Bros,

2011. Video game.

F.E.A.R. 2: Project Origin. Kirkland, Washington; Monolith/Warner Bros, 2009. Video game.

Friedman, May, and Shana L. Calixte, eds. *Mothering and Blogging: The Radical Act of the Mommyblog*. Bradford: Demeter Press, 2009. Print.

Grosz, Elizabeth. *Space, Time, and Perversion: Essays on the Politics of Bodies*. New York: Routledge, 1995. Print.

Harvest Moon (series). Tokyo: Victor Interactive/Marvelous, 1996-2014. Video game.

Holloway, Alexandra, and Sri Kurniawan. "System Design Evolution of The Prepared Partner: How a Labor and Childbirth Game Came to Term." *Meaningful Play*. 17 October 2010. Web. 10 May 2014.

Klastrup, Lisbeth. "What Makes World of Warcraft a World? A Note on Death and Dying." *Digital Culture, Play, and Identity: A World of Warcraft Reader*. Ed. Hilde Corneliussen and Jill Walker Rettberg. Cambridge: MIT Press, 2008: 143-166. Print.

Lopez, Lori Kido. "The Radical Act of 'Mommy Blogging': Redefining Motherhood Through the Blogosphere." *New Media & Society* 11.5 (2009): 729-747. Print.

Morris, Theresa, and Katherine McInerney. "Media Representations of Pregnancy and Childbirth: An Analysis of Reality Television Programs in the United States." *Birth* 37.2 (2010): 134-140. Print.

Nakamura, Lisa. "Avatars and the Visual Culture of Reproduction on the Web." *Digitizing Race: Visual Cultures of the Internet*. Minneapolis: University of Minnesota Press, 2008. 131-170. Print.

Pincus, Jane. "Review: Laboring Under an Illusion: Mass Media Childbirth vs. The Real Thing." *Birth: Issues in Perinatal Care* 37:1 March 2010, 82-83. Print.

Podnieks, Elizabeth. Introduction. "Popular Culture's Maternal Embrace." *Mediating Moms: Mothers in Popular Culture*. Montreal: McGill-Queen's Press, 2012. 3-32. Print.

Russell, Dominique. "The Reality of TV Labour: *Birth Stories*." *Mediating Moms: Mothers in Popular Culture*. Ed. Elizabeth Podnieks. Montreal: McGill-Queen's Press, 2012. 253-267. Print.

Second Life. San Francisco: Linden Lab, 2003. Virtual world.

Silent Hill 3. Tokyo: Konami, 2003. Video game.

The Sims. Redwood City, CA: Maxis/EA Games, 2000. Video game.

The Sims 2. Redwood City, CA: Maxis/EA Games, 2004. Video game.

The Sims 3. Redwood City, CA: The Sims Studio/EA Games, 2009. Video game.

The Sims: Livin' Large Expansion Pack. Redwood City, CA: Maxis/ EA Games, 2000. Video game.

The Sims Medieval. Salt Lake City, Utah: The Sims Studio/EA Games, 2011. Video game.

Sofia, Zoe. "Exterminating Fetuses: Abortion, Disarmament, and the Sexo-Semiotics of Extraterrestrialism." *Diacritics* 14.2 (1984): 47-59. Print.

Woollett, Anne, and Mary Boyle. "Reproduction, Women's Lives and Subjectivities." *Feminism & Psychology* 10.3 (2000): 307-311. Print.

Masculine Pregnancy

Butch Lesbians', Trans Men's & Genderqueer Individuals' Experiences[1]

I confess that I have this womanly desire, an animal urgency, to make a baby. Would they [the other butches] see me as less of a butch [if I got pregnant]? (Jiménez 161)

People just couldn't wrap their heads around [a butchy/masculine-presenting person being pregnant]. [It's like], "these two things do not go together"—you know like that Sesame Street thing [singing], *One of these things is not like the other. One of these things just doesn't belong.*" (Cathy)[2]

BETWEEN FEBRUARY 2011 AND APRIL 2012, I conducted research in British Columbia focused on butch lesbians', trans men's, and genderqueer[3] individuals' experiences with pregnancy and infertility. I came to this research topic as a queer femme who had heard first-hand from butch, trans, and genderqueer-identifying friends of their diagnoses of infertility, and also (from both different and the same friends) of their desires to experience pregnancy. I was aware that in Canada, when a baby is born and seen as having a vulva, the child is labelled as "female," and there is a cultural expectation for that baby to grow up and become a feminine heterosexual mother. I knew that not all of those babies become feminine, heterosexual, or mothers, and yet culturally we continue to link pregnancy with femininity. As Robyn Longhurst noted with respect to her work with heterosexual first-time expectant mothers in Hamilton, Aotearoa/New Zealand:

> Pregnant bodies are produced in ways that assume particular gendered norms and a particular coherence.... Pregnant bodies and the regulatory regimes that prohibit and enable them to perform in specific ways are temporally and spatially located, and are socially coded through a range of competing gendered discourses. (456)

Further, the idea that one is not truly a "woman" until or unless she is a mother persists in Canada, and "women's bodies are represented in medical discourses as bodies that are waiting for babies" (Longhurst 460). While the focus of much academic work on mothering and womanhood has been on people who are recognized as women and mothers, there is a dearth of research in the area of how individuals who are female but masculine negotiate these decisions and experiences. All the while, there is growing scholarship focused on queer parenting and reproduction.

My research is situated within this emerging scholarship, and was influenced by three particular works focusing on mothering and queer reproduction. First, Ellen Lewin studied lesbian mothers in the United States from the 1970s through to the early 1990s. Her research covered many issues, but mainly focused on how lesbian mothers negotiated being both a lesbian and a mother at a time when the two identities were seen as oxymoronic. Second, Jacquelyne Luce studied how lesbian/bi/queer women conceived (of) families in British Columbia. Her research considered policy and practice of assisted insemination, adoption, parenting, and infertility from the 1980s through to the early 2000s. Third, Rachel Epstein specifically considered butch lesbians who got pregnant and became mothers. Epstein pointed out that according to mainstream social expectations, "Butches are not supposed to be mothers, and mothers are not supposed to be butch. When butches mother they denaturalize both terms and transform both subjectivities" (55). While Epstein's "Butches with Babies: Reconfiguring Gender and Motherhood" was published in 2002, Canadian mainstream culture has had limited representations of masculine desires and experiences of pregnancy,[4] aside from Thomas Beatie's fairly public pregnancies (in 2008, 2009, and in 2010).

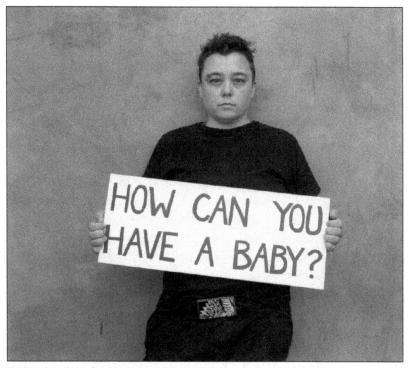

Illustration 1: "How Can You Have a Baby?" From the photography project "A Series of Questions," that "explores the power dynamics inherent in the questions asked of transgender, transsexual, genderqueer, gender non-conforming, and gender-variant people" (Weingarten n.d.). Artist: L. Weingarten © Permission granted by artist.

In fact, regarding queer/masculine individuals' experiences of pregnancy, a common question that comes to people's minds is, "How can you have a baby?" (see Illustration 1, "How Can You Have A Baby?"). To address the dearth of attention given to trans/masculine individuals' experiences and desires for pregnancy, this chapter focuses on two particular questions: One, how do butch lesbians, trans men, and genderqueer individuals balance or make sense of their masculinity with their desire for and experiences of pregnancy in a culture that only represents and recognizes pregnancy as a feminine? And two, how does our culture react to these individuals' desires and their experiences of pregnancy? Moreover, the approach of this chapter is a *queer* one, one that "makes the things we otherwise take for granted suddenly unpredictable, uncooperative, and unexpected" in part through its "[disruption of] the normative practices of kinship and culture" (Gibson 1). This chapter, thus, makes a unique contribution by focusing on butch lesbians', trans men's, and genderqueer individuals' desires for pregnancy, their negotiation and experiences with clothes during their pregnancy, and, lastly, the impossibility of being recognized for who they are during pregnancy.

RESEARCH METHODS

I undertook this study guided by queer, feminist, and Pagan epistemologies, and used anthropologically-based research methods. I conducted 22 face-to-face interviews, and distributed two types of questionnaires among self-identified butch lesbians, trans men, and genderqueer individuals, and health care professionals in British Columbia. I also engaged in participant observation at various Pride, LGBTQ*, and family-oriented events in the southern half of British Columbia. Of the 22 interviews, ten were with various types of health care professionals (HCPs; that is, interviews were with midwives, perinatal nurses, and physicians who specialize in trans health, among others), and 12 were with butch lesbians, trans men, and genderqueer individuals (BTQs) who had either experienced or been diagnosed with a condition linked to infertility (n=4) or who had experienced a successful pregnancy (n=8). Of the two questionnaires I designed, 46 eligible individuals completed and returned the one designed for BTQs, and 28 completed and returned to one for HCPs (most of these were completed by nurses, physicians, and midwives), for a total of 74 eligible returned questionnaires. Of the 96 total participants, there were two or more from each of British Columbia's five health regions. BTQ participants ranged in age from 19 to 60, with an average (mean) age of 32. In terms of ethnicity, 78 individuals identified as White or Caucasian, seven as mixed ethnicity, five as Asian, two as Jewish, and one as Indigenous. Some of the "mixed" individuals identified themselves as being part Asian, Indigenous, Arab, South Pacific, and/or Caucasian, or simply "mixed." Additionally, 3 did not specify their ethnicity.

The data presented in this chapter stems from multiple sources. Most significant to this discussion are the narratives derived from the seven interviews I conducted during my Ph.D. research with butch lesbian and genderqueer individuals who had previously experienced a successful pregnancy. Some narratives from the four individuals I interviewed about their experiences or diagnoses of infertility also contribute to this chapter. This is in addition to questionnaire responses from and interviews with midwives and physicians, as well as BTQ individuals.

Below, I draw attention to some of the effects of the everyday social experiences that butch lesbians, trans men, and genderqueer individuals face in a culture where they and their reproductive desires, choices, and experiences are ignored and misunderstood, even by their friends, family, and communities. This was apparent in the narratives of desire and dissonance regarding pregnancy, as well as in the discussions of what the interview participants wore when they were pregnant, in addition to how they were seen (and not seen) when they were pregnant.

PREGNANCY: DESIRE AND DISSONANCE

Pregnancy is an incredibly public experience for women. "The everyday behaviours of pregnant women tend to be policed by strangers.... People frequently regard themselves as societal supervisors of pregnant women's behaviour" (Longhurst 468). Pregnancy as a public experience is expected to be feminine. For all but one[5] of the butch lesbians and genderqueer individuals with whom I spoke who had experienced pregnancy, their narratives clearly articulated both their desire to experience pregnancy and their feelings of tension or awkwardness with being perceived as feminine. For Bryn, Cathy, Vanessa, Joy, Imogen, Quinn, and Lou—and even for AJ who had yet to be pregnant, but desired that experience—gender, and more specifically femininity, was not connected to their desire.

While they acknowledged that pregnancy is typically understood to be a feminine thing, these individuals' desires to experience pregnancy were not connected to gender. Thus, instead of it being a feminine desire, the people I spoke with linked their desire to their love of children, human biology (as in DNA or the biological clock/"yearning"), or simply that an innate desire could not really be explained.

Moreover, Vanessa, Bryn, and Joy, as well as the other butch lesbian and genderqueer parents who came to experience a pregnancy, were comfortable with the idea of experiencing pregnancy, as it did not present itself as a uniquely or necessarily feminine experience to them. They still, however, had to negotiate their own sense of how to fit their gender (identity and expression) together with an experience typically thought of as feminine. For Joy, this realization happened when reading Rachel Epstein's article "Butches with Babies," which she read a couple of years before experiencing pregnancy herself:

> When I read [that article], it started making me think about my own [future] experience. I was quite a bit younger then, and I wanted a child. I wanted to carry a child. ... And it got me thinking about [my gender] presentation. And the fact that I was very comfortable with who I'd become, and very comfortable with my body, but knowing this would raise issues for me in the future. So, whenever I think about—[the topic of your research]—I mean, I think about my own experience as well—but it often goes back to that moment of realization, that there was going to be dissonance there for me at some point.

Clearly, the fact that butch lesbians and genderqueer individuals are not "feminine" presented a challenge to their thoughts about and experiences of pregnancy. It, of course, also presented a challenge to those they encountered.

The individuals I spoke with were sometimes surprised by the reactions of others to their desires and experiences of pregnancy, as well as frustrated by their need to justify and prove themselves. Bryn talked at length about needing to justify her desires for pregnancy with her butch/genderqueer identity. Bryn told me, "I've always been clear to my family and friends that I wanted kids," and yet before conceiving, she felt she had to weigh her desire to experience a pregnancy against her need to be recognized and accepted as a "butch" by fellow queers. Once she was pregnant, Bryn found her friends and family critical of her experience and committed to the discordance between being butch and pregnant.

Bryn provided examples relating to how friends, family, and strangers could not fathom pregnancy as anything other than feminine; she commented on how people made inaccurate assumptions about her pregnancy and her gender identity. For example, Bryn revealed to me that her parents were convinced that her being pregnant meant that she was *finally* embracing femininity. She explained that her family had always been accepting of her being gay, but her masculinity "dumbfounds them"; they continued to say, "Your hair would be so much nicer if you grew it out." Thus, "When they found out I was pregnant, it was a big hurray! ...It was like, 'You are finally acting like you should be acting.'" Similarly she noted how her friends were sometimes unable to see beyond the status quo and imagine pregnancy as something someone "butch" could do. Once pregnant, a masculine gender identity became even more of a challenge when faced with figuring out what to wear.

MA(N)TERNITY CLOTHES

Before engaging in this research I was quite aware of the overtly feminine nature of maternity clothes—mainly quite frilly, floral, and often in socially-deemed feminine colours and cuts—yet I gained a new perspective on maternity clothes from the research participants. When I asked Tracy about her reaction to finding out she was pregnant—after she inseminated on a lark with a little semen that was left in the syringe after her girlfriend tried inseminating at home—she noted: "I was shocked. What was I going to wear? ... [There is] nothing that I'm going to freakin' wear!" At the time of the research as well as at the time of the participants' pregnancies, there was a notable lack of anything but feminine-deemed clothing available in stores in British Columbia. Since this time, a few clothing lines have introduced more androgynous and masculine styles, cuts, and colours available for those who are pregnant. Only one of the seven interviewees who had experienced pregnancy noted that she felt comfortable in the available, notably feminine, maternity wear. The six others endured being uncomfortable in maternity wear, wore larger sizes of the typical men's wear they were used to but that did not fit their growing bodies quite right, or wore a mix of both.

Vanessa admitted that pregnancy "was probably the first experience that I had that did make me feel more feminine," and she did not consider that as positive. Vanessa compared her experience of pregnancy to when she was a pre-teen: "It was like I was eleven again, and being forced into clothes that didn't work, and I was so frustrated. I would scour the internet for shirts that would work." Further, Vanessa's experience of pregnancy was reminiscent of the contrast between the girls she went to high school with and herself. Other interviewees shared examples of how they made clothes work for them—as best they could—during their pregnancies.

Before becoming pregnant, and early in her pregnancy, Bryn was unsure about what she was going to wear when she was visibly pregnant and if she would still be recognized by others in the queer community. While for most of her pregnancy Bryn wore the same clothes as before she became pregnant, just in larger sizes, at a certain point she needed maternity pants. At this point she found that not only were the men's (regular) pants not comfortable, but they were not staying up either. Thus, she had to give in to the more feminine maternity wear. While Bryn felt she had to "give-in" at the end, Tracy, Quinn, and Cathy did not find that wearing maternity clothes was a choice for them at all, and found ways to wear larger sizes of men's clothing. Part of this lack a choice, at least for Cathy, was the fact that she could not get the help she needed when she did enter a maternity wear store.

Choices of what to wear, thus, were not just about comfort, but also about being able to access clothes that fit. While Vanessa turned to the internet for other choices in maternity wear, Cathy, Bryn, and Joy attempted to find appropriate clothes at local maternity stores. There, however, they were ignored by the sales associates. Being ignored or not recognized as (potentially) pregnant, it turned out, was not limited to experiences with sales associates, but is a matter of cultural norms and gendered expectations.

INVISIBILITY OF MASCULINE/QUEER PREGNANCY

One of the most surprising findings from this research was the degree to which the individuals I spoke with were not seen, when pregnant, for who they were: a pregnant masculine individual. Sometimes this was a result of what they wore when they were pregnant, and sometimes even they could not explain why this might have been the case. Their invisibility might be explained by the fact that, as questionnaire respondent Isabella (40s, Asian, butch) noted with regards to Thomas Beatie being "a pregnant man," "Pregnancy seems discordant to being masculine. [Pregnancy] seems contradictory to the idea of a trans man. In this light, the title 'the pregnant man' seems inaccurate." Regardless of this perspective, Bryn, Cathy, Joy, Imogen, Quinn, Vanessa, and AJ experienced pregnancy as butch lesbians or genderqueer individuals. Their invisibility as such was most explicitly illustrated in their narratives of trying to buy clothes in a maternity wear store.

Joy, Cathy, and Bryn each recounted stories of the misunderstandings and invisibility they experienced while trying to purchase maternity wear. Joy had immigrated to British Columbia from outside Canada and spoke with a different accent. She was unsure if her negative experience stemmed from the fact that she was masculine-appearing or because the sales associate really did not understand what Joy was saying.

> *I had a really uncomfortable encounter at a maternity wear store where I went in and said [that] I was looking for shirts. And [the sales associate] said, "I don't understand what you mean." And I said, "Shirt, like a button shirt," and she said, "I don't think we have shirts." And so I kind of repeated, thinking surely is it my accent? I mean, how is it you don't understand the word "shirt"? And eventually she said, "Oh you mean a blouse!" And I don't know if it was a deliberate "you don't look the part" or if she literally didn't understand what I was saying, but, um, I mean, it was bizarre. And so I felt like whenever I went into a maternity wear store that I was, I just didn't look the part. I didn't—none of the clothes made me feel comfortable. In my general life shopping I've found a couple of stores that will always have the clothes that I need, and I don't deviate. I hate shopping. And I go to these places, and I*

get my clothes, and I get out as quickly as possible. And
suddenly I was thrust back into [the] generalized shopping
world ... into the ones that are about being feminine.

Since two other interview participants also noted feeling hints
of unease and difficulty with getting the help they needed at
maternity stores, I believe that what Joy felt was not just in her
mind. Both Cathy and Bryn felt like they were ignored or not
recognized as potentially pregnant individuals by store staff
when they sought to buy clothes that would (better) fit their
bodies when they were pregnant. What became evident in the
narratives of their pregnancies was that there is an invisibility
of "the pregnant lesbian."

While femme lesbians are often invisible as lesbians in their
daily life, and thus it is not surprising that when pregnant they
are recognized as "straight," I was surprised to find out during
the interviews that none of the interview participants felt that they
were recognized as lesbians (and they all identified as such) during
their pregnancy. This was despite the fact that almost every one
of them experienced pregnancy while living in East Vancouver, a
neighbourhood recognized as a lesbian mecca. Tracy, Quinn, and
Cathy, who wore larger sizes of men's clothes, each noted that
publicly they were very rarely, if ever, recognized as pregnant, but
instead perceived as men with a beer belly. Tracy noted: "I still got
called man or sir—[people thought I had a] beer belly." Similarly,
Cathy and Tracy noted how even at eight months pregnant, their
co-workers could not fathom that they were pregnant. Their embodied masculinity denied any possibility of pregnancy.

In contrast, those who wore typical maternity wear were con-
tinuously recognized as "straight." Pregnancy was the first time in
many years that Imogen was perceived as a straight woman; Bryn
and Gayle also noted similar experiences. Gayle, a white butch
questionnaire respondent in her forties, noted:

When [I was pregnant and out] with my wife I was constantly
frustrated with people trying to figure out our relationship
cause being a lesbian couple didn't make sense to them.
We were sisters or friends or something else.

While strangers had a hard time seeing Gayle, Bryn, and Imogen as anything but straight, Bryn's friends could not understand her being pregnant, unless it could be justified it in terms of her femme-identified partner being unable to get pregnant.

Thus, Bryn recounted a few occasions when her friends had made comments that made her realize that they did not understand that *she* was pregnant. Sometimes upon telling her friends that she was pregnant, they would respond by saying, "What the hell? We thought you were butch! Why can't [your femme wife] Kait have a kid?" Two particular situations exemplify this point. First, Bryn noted:

> *We were at a friend's dinner party—I even said, "Oh I am pregnant," and [my friend] said, "Oh that's great," and later she offered me a drink. When I said no, she said, "So big of you not drinking when your partner is pregnant."*

Another example demonstrated the awkward position that Bryn was put in as a result of her friends' disbelief and questioning.

> *Even when I was showing [visibly pregnant], one of my best friends didn't get that it was me [who was pregnant, so I said to them], "Like do you see that it is me?"*
>
> *"Like, what? It is you? I thought it was Kait! I just thought you were getting stuffier."*
>
> *Like over and over again with my friends, they just wouldn't get it: "What, you're pregnant? Oh there must be something wrong with Kait."*
>
> *And I felt awkward about it too. ... Cause then, when they realized there is nothing wrong with Kait—that I fought for this—I felt like I had to get into the details of the relationship that I wasn't even comfortable talking about.... But no, thank you very much, Kait is okay. They just assumed there [were] fertility issues there.*

Even though Bryn's friends did not want to hurt her feelings or invade the privacy of her relationship with her wife, they did. They were caught up in the cultural fetish of feminine pregnancy.

FEMININE PREGNANCY AS CULTURAL FETISH

What has come out of this research for me is that, similar to New Zealand-based human geographer Robyn Longhurst who has studied heterosexual women's experiences of pregnancy, "I want to displace the alignment of pregnant with a particular gendered construction of femininity" (457). I recognize that in part, this displacing involves recognizing what Quinn called the "cultural fetish of pregnancy being associated with femininity." Despite Quinn telling me this during our interview, it took me a while to understand the layers to what she'd said. At first her statement seemed easy enough to agree with and accept as an everyday statement, but upon hearing Quinn's words repeated as I went back to the digital recording and transcript, I realized that her concept of "cultural fetish" is more appropriate than my initial classification of feminine pregnancy as simply being expected. The experiences narrated to me in the interviews I conducted were not just about cultural *expectations*. Instead, they exemplify the West's cultural obsession with feminine pregnancy as a cultural fetish.

When I first heard the words "cultural fetish," I dismissed the "fetish" aspect as hyperbole or a humorous use of words from someone in the queer community. It was only in being reflexive about why I did that, and thinking about what came to my mind as "fetish," that I really *heard* what Quinn was saying. The word "fetish" is loaded with meanings. In the queer community, the word "fetish" often conjures up ideas and practices related to something that is sexually stimulating. To the general public, a "fetish" may be seen as an obsession. For anthropologists, "fetishes" are items or idols with supernatural or religious significance or powers. For Marx, "commodity fetishism" renders subjects and actions into objects with economic value. Put together, it is revealed that a cultural fetish is something that is valued not necessarily for its original use or for its base use or parts' value, but something with added sexual, spiritual, aesthetic, or commodity (for commodity's sake) value.

Feminine pregnancy is a cultural fetish in mainstream Euro-American cultures. *Women* who are pregnant become *pregnant bodies* that are objectified and sexualized. Pregnant women and bodies are no longer private entities; instead, they are under the surveillance of both strangers and people they know. The view and treatment of pregnant women and their bodies is part of the larger cultural rendering of women into objects, whether it be through the medical and scientific discourse as "bodies that are waiting for babies" (Longhurst 460) or through popular culture's display of women as sexually stimulating heroines in latex or leather skin-tight outfits as "fighting fuck toys" (Newsom). Pregnant women/bodies are cherished icons, and understood to be fragile and in need of protection (provided by men). The cultural value of pregnant women/bodies is both economic and beyond economic. Economically, pregnant women and bodies are a valuable commodity, both to use in advertising and as a market to direct advertising towards. Beyond economic value, pregnant women and bodies hold cultural value for their reproductive power. That power, however, is recognized as exclusively a feminine one. The cultural fetish is one not simply about pregnancy, but about *feminine* pregnancy.

Choosing and experiencing pregnancy as anything other than feminine is challenging, due to the cultural fetish surrounding feminine pregnancy. The fact that family, friends, and strangers could not acknowledge the reality that they were presented with illustrates this. In Canada, we have come a long way to recognizing lesbian and gay parents, but it is important to note that sexuality and gender are different. Breaking gender boundaries and expectations related to pregnancy and parenting is not likely something that can be done in a short amount of time. Moreover, butch lesbians, trans men, and genderqueer individuals are not the only ones who are uncomfortable in overtly "feminine" maternity wear. Undoubtedly, many heterosexual women are also repulsed by the obligatory feminine wear available to them when pregnant. Thus, I argue that the first part in creating change, and being more aware of the diverse experiences of pregnancy, is in consciously recognizing that "We have this cultural fetish of pregnancy being associated with femininity."[6]

Recognizing the cultural aspects that affect people's desires and experiences of pregnancy is important, just as it is important to recognize their individual desires and urges. While many people see butches, trans men, and genderqueer individuals as being in opposition to experiences of pregnancy, Gayle Rubin explains otherwise—at least with respect to butch lesbians—noting that, "Butches vary in how they relate to their female bodies. Some butches are comfortable being pregnant and having kids, while for others the thought of undergoing the female component of mammalian reproduction is utterly repugnant" (474). Moreover, for those who grow up perceiving themselves as masculine while in a female body, reproduction and desires for parenting can be quite confusing. For example, for Ulric, a white FTM questionnaire respondent in his thirties, his female sex and desire to be a father confused him as an adolescent. He noted, "[As a teen] I thought about becoming a father, but I didn't know transition resources existed, so I assumed I was crazy." If Ulric told anyone else of his desires, they too would likely have thought he was crazy, quite literally. Hank (30s, white, trans man) had a similar response when I asked him in our interview, "And as a teen or young adult, was there a time when you thought you might become a mother or parent?" He responded, "Parent, yes. Mother, no. Like I said, [I've] had no inkling to birth.... [Never] a birthing parent. But I didn't grow up thinking I was going to be a dad [either]." Even after Thomas Beatie's pregnancies, masculinity and pregnancy are not recognized—at least by mainstream culture—as potentially coexistent, and thus they are not represented in popular culture, with the exception of Beatie. Individuals, however, certainly are recognizing the potential for these two (formerly mutually exclusive) traits to coexist. In the meantime, so many other people get caught up on the elements of gender and cannot see desire for pregnancy and parenthood as a personal or human desire instead of a necessarily gendered one.

[1]This chapter is a shorter, edited version of the chapter "Desiring and Achieving Parenthood: expectations and experiences" from my doctoral dissertation *Gender Identity and In/Fertility*. A much smaller version appeared as "Feminine Pregnancy as Cultural Fetish" in *Anthropology News*.

[2]Pseudonyms are used for the participants of my research.

[3]While these gender identities are increasing discussed in popular culture, I define them here so the reader knows how I am using them. As I have noted elsewhere (Walks, "Stratified Reproduction" 87), Butch lesbians are one of the two main stereotypes of lesbians, with 'femmes' being the other (more feminine) stereotype. Historically, butches were recognized as 'the lesbian' seen as "not a woman but rather an 'invert,' or the embodiment of some third and anomalous gender category" (Lewin "On the Outside Looking In" 106-7). I define them generally as women who are sexually attracted to other women, and who often identify or express themselves in a more androgynous or masculine manner (though, certainly there are many exceptions, as noted by Bergman and in Coyote and Sharman). Despite being categorized as 'female' at birth, trans-men identify and present as male. They often (or plan to) take testosterone, have one or more surgeries to alter their chest, and/or have a hysterectomy. They may or may not desire to or alter the appearance of their genitals. "Genderqueer is a term and identity less familiar to many people. Genderqueer individuals explicitly challenge gender norms, and thus sometimes call themselves 'gen-derfucking,' or, using more politically correct language, 'gender variant' or 'gender non-conforming.' Genderqueer individuals may simply present as androgynous, or they may also purposefully mix stereotypical masculine and feminine signifiers. As an example, they might confidently have a beard while at the same time wearing a pink dress or skirt, or alternately, breastfeed their child while sporting a moustache" (Walks, "Stratified Reproduction" 87). That said, in terms of gender identity, for the purposes of this research project, I let people self-define or self-identify.

[4]The only transmasculine Canadian to be highlighted in mainstream media related to issues of reproduction is Trevor MacDonald, who has become known for his successful challenging of La Leche League's "mother's only" policy ("Breastfeeding Group"; Tapper, "Breastfeeding" and "Transgender").

[5]Tracy was the only person to experience a pregnancy without wanting to experience it. This was due to the fact that she and her former partner acted on a lark on Tracy's birthday. After assisting her (then) partner with an at-home insemination, her (then) partner then emptied the remaining semen in the syringe into Tracy. They

figured that given the amount of semen in the syringe, there was no chance of it taking, but instead they were both surprised (and disappointed to some extent) to find out a couple of weeks later that Tracy, and not her (then) partner, was pregnant. Tracy never had a desire to be pregnant, aside from its "use value" of bringing a child into her family because her partner was not able to.

⁶My argument, which some might consider a theory of feminine pregnancy as a cultural fetish, is a work in progress. For the purposes of this paper I suggest readers consider feminine pregnancy to be a cultural fetish and focus on what can be done to change this fetish. At this time, my preference is not to theorize cultural fetish, but to remain grounded in people's experiences rather than in theories. The theorization of feminine pregnancy as cultural fetish, I defer to a future article. I am grateful to the reviewers for their input on this issue.

WORKS CITED

Bergman, S. Bear. *Butch is a Noun*. Second Edition. Vancouver: Arsenal Pulp Press, 2010. Print.

"Breastfeeding Group Rejects Transgender Dad's Leadership Bid." *CBC News Canada*. CBC. August 20, 2012. Web. August 20, 2012.

Coyote, Ivan E. and Zena Sharman, eds. *Persistence: All Ways Butch and Femme*. Vancouver: Arsenal Pulp Press, 2011. Print.

Epstein, Rachel. "Butches with Babies." *Journal of Lesbian Studies* 6.2 (2002): 41-57. Print.

Gibson, Margaret. "Queering Motherhood in Narrative, Theory, and the Everyday." *Queering Motherhood: Narrative and Theoretical Perspectives*. Ed. M. F. Gibson. Bradford, ON: Demeter Press, 2014. 1-23. Print.

Jiménez, Karleen Pendleton. *How to Get a Girl Pregnant*. Toronto: Tightrope Books, 2011. Print.

Lewin, Ellen. *Lesbian Mothers: Accounts of Gender in American Culture*. Ithaca, NY: Cornell University Press, 1993. Print.

Longhurst, Robyn. "'Corporeographies' of Pregnancy: 'Bikini Babes.'" *Environment and Planning D: Society and Space* 18 (2000): 453-472. Print.

Luce, Jacquelyne. *Beyond Expectation: Lesbian/Bi/Queer Women and Assisted Conception.* Toronto: University of Toronto Press, 2010. Print.

Newsom, Jennifer. Dir. *Miss Representation.* 90m. Girls' Club Entertainment, 2011. Film.

Rubin, Gayle. "Of Catamites and Kings: Reflections on Butch, Gender, and Boundaries." *The Transgender Studies Reader.* Eds. S. Stryker and S. Whittle. New York: Routledge, 2006. 471-481. Print.

Tapper, Josh. "Breastfeeding Dad Wins Support from Parenting Community. *The Star.* August 20, 2012. Web. August 20, 2012.

Tapper, Josh. "Transgender Man Can Be Breastfeeding Coach." *The Star.* April 25, 2014. Web. April 25, 2014.

Walks, Michelle. "Feminine Pregnancy as Cultural Fetish." *Anthropology News* 54.1-2 (2013): 12. Print.

Tapper, Josh. *Gender Identity and In/Fertility.* Diss. U. of British Columbia, 2013. Web. [add date of access]

Tapper, Josh. "Stratified Reproduction: Butch Lesbians', Transmen's, and Genderqueer Individuals' Experiences in British Columbia." *Fertile Ground: Exploring Reproduction in Canada.* Eds. S. Paterson, F. Scala, and M. Sokolon. Montréal: McGill-Queen's Press, 2014. 99-119. Print.

K. J. SURKAN

That Fat Man is Giving Birth

Gender Identity, Reproduction and the Pregnant Body

"**D**ID YOU ALWAYS WANT TO BE PREGNANT?" The social worker peered across the room at the two of us, but the question is directed to me, since I am the patient. My partner and I are sitting in an office in a prestigious urban teaching hospital, on a floor dedicated to reproductive medicine. On any given day in this location, scores of women emerge from the elevator, sit in waiting rooms, have vital signs checked, undergo blood tests, ultrasounds, and internal exams, and consult with doctors, nurses, social workers, and patient coordinators—all in the attempt to have a baby.

These women, the prospective mothers, are often "older" by reproductive standards, meaning they are over thirty and fertility is on the wane. Most are accompanied by husbands or male partners in these initial consultations; less frequently do lesbian couples or single women appear in the fertility clinic. But things are changing; it is, after all, 2006 and we are in Massachusetts. Gay marriage has just been legalized, and these newly minted, newly legitimized couples are increasingly seeking out medical help in starting a family. For some, assisted reproductive technology is a necessary part of the process of conceiving and bringing a pregnancy to term. But the mechanics of sexed reproduction are very different from the highly gendered social meanings attached to pregnancy, fertility, birth, and lactation. As a female-bodied person on the transmasculine spectrum navigating fertility treatment, pregnancy, and birth, my gender presentation and its reception throughout the process highlight the social incompatibility of pregnancy with masculinity. The figure of the pregnant trans man challenges gendered assumptions in such a profound way that it is often impossible for transgender and genderqueer pregnancies to be understood as such. Instead, it is often easier for those embodiments to be read as "fat men."[1] The degree to which transgender and gender non-conforming people experience gender dysphoria in pregnancy varies dramatically and can be deeply impacted by conflicting cultural interpretations of their gestating bodies.

It goes without saying that pregnancy is a phenomenon strongly associated with being female; at the same time, it involves dramatic change to the physical body in ways that challenge conventional cultural associations with femininity. For this reason, there is an enormous amount of effort in shoring up the cultural signification of the pregnant body as female and feminine, from representations of pregnancy in popular media, to maternity wear, to the discourse produced by and about pregnant women. Although necessarily temporary, being pregnant is more than a "condition"—it becomes an identity, and one that is bound and even policed by gender expectations.

The social worker's question gave me pause. I hadn't thought much about *pregnancy* itself; my focus had been on the larger questions of whether to have a child and how to add that new person to our relationship, taking us from being a couple to a family. I realized that my answer had to be "no, never"—pregnancy per se had never been on my bucket list of somatic experiences. Neither, it seemed, was it something my cisgendered female partner wanted, though she was not opposed to the idea of having a family. I, for one, really wanted to be a parent, and was profoundly curious about who a child of mine would turn out to be. Given the biological realities of my conventional female embodiment and reproductive system, pregnancy seemed to me to be a necessary nine-month expedition I would take, a temporary transformation of the body that would be a mere blip on the larger road trip of life.

In many ways I was right; the necessarily temporal aspect of pregnancy means it is an identity position one moves through, rather than a permanent embodied identity. At the same time, there is no denying the profound physical changes that occur in pregnancy (and even prior to that, the effects of elevated estrogen and progesterone levels as a result of fertility treatment). My subsequent decision to breastfeed meant that I was more often read as a masculine woman after giving birth. But in some ways, the biggest transformation I encountered post-pregnancy was not somatic at all; it was the shift into parenthood. My new social identity as "Papa" to two children reflects my gender identity, and has forever changed my life for the better.

Prior to my pregnancies, I was frequently perceived as androgynous, and was used to encountering gender confusion as people alternately read me as a middle-aged butch woman or teen boy (and sometimes in LGBT communities, I could be understood in line with my self-identification as a genderqueer trans man), depending on their assumptions and the social context. I did not know how pregnancy would affect my gender presentation, but I was hardly prepared for the degree to which gender would figure in my pregnancy experience. The pregnant man was an oxymoron; either I could be read as pregnant, or male, but never both simultaneously. As my belly grew bigger around my gestating fetus, paradoxically, my pregnancy became in some contexts more invisible; I could only be seen as a fat man.

WOMAN OR MAN?
READING THE GENDERED FAT/PREGNANT BODY

Because I had not undergone any steps toward medically transitioning from female to male, my androgynous experience as a pregnant man resonated heavily with S. Bear Bergman's description of himself in his essay "Part-Time Fatso": "Whether I'm fat depends on whether the person or people looking at me believe me to be a man or a woman" (139). Bergman's lived experience of being at the receiving end of radically different reactions to his[2] size demonstrates how gendered our perception of fat really is. As he points out, "a man can be much, much fatter than a woman and still be viewed as comfortably within the standard deviation" ("Part-Time" 139). Jerry Mosher echoes this observation in "Setting Free the Bears: Refiguring Fat Men on Television," writing that unlike fat women, "the fat man's depiction as 'ordinary' suggests that fat men are held to a standard less severe and more forgiving" (167).

An individual assigned female at birth but identifying as both "a butch" and "transgendered," Bergman recounts being treated extremely differently by others based on their perception of his gender: encountering respect as a "big dude" but being reviled as a fat woman. Ordering food in restaurants becomes a gender test, as servers reading him as female selectively forget parts of his order and bring him diet Coke when he orders regular ("Part-Time" 141), effectively policing his weight. "I am sometimes ... reduced to asking for a Coke just to see for sure what gender someone thinks I am," he writes ("Part-Time" 142).

Julia Serano describes a parallel experience in the first year of her transition from male to female:

> What I found most striking was how other people interpreted my same actions and mannerisms differently based on whether they perceived me to be female or male.... [I]t was not merely my behaviors that were interpreted differently, it was my body as well: the way people approached me, spoke to me, the assumptions they made about me, the lack of deference and respect I often received, the way others often sexualized my body. All of these changes occurred without my having to say or do a thing. (192-193)

These testimonials by transgendered people are incredibly helpful in making sense of my experience as an ambiguously gendered pregnant person, and why—as impossible as it seemed—my pregnancy was simply *not seen* by so many as I moved through the world.

The gendered disparity between acceptable size parameters is rooted in a socially policed feminine ideal that Cecilia Hartley refers to as the "tyranny of slenderness" (60) in which women are required to be thin and take up little space. "This model of femininity suggests that real women are thin, nearly invisible," Hartley writes (61). Pregnancy creates an exception to this unwritten rule, a form of embodiment in which women necessarily take up more space, eat more food, and require larger clothing to accommodate the presence of a growing fetus. In order for this seeming contradiction to be resolved, a great deal of effort is put into the association of pregnancy with femininity. Michelle Walks describes this as "the cultural fetish surrounding pregnancy" in her groundbreaking study of pregnant people with masculine or genderqueer gender identification, writing that "our culture is only able to recognize pregnancy as feminine ... and the desire to experience pregnancy as a feminine one" (Walks "Feminine Pregnancy as Cultural Fetish" 12).

For me, gender perception, fatness, and pregnancy were inextricably tied together; whether I was pregnant or merely fat depended a lot on whether I was perceived to be male or female, *and vice versa*: being perceived as pregnant meant for most people that I was necessarily a woman, whereas being fat made me even more androgynous and more likely to be read as a man. The extraordinary inability (or unwillingness) of people to see "the elephant in the room" (me!) reflects the degree to which societally we have internalized the gender binary and indeed rely on it for a sense of stability in the world. For most people, the pregnant man represents an impossibility that cannot be reconciled within a normalized sex/gender binary of feminine female and masculine male. The pregnant butch, like the fat woman, is abject, a gender representation that fails to conform to the standards of idealized femininity. Finally, the pregnant fat woman is both abject and experiences the loss of visibility in her pregnancy, doubly masked as it is by her size and the cultural fetish of feminine pregnancy.

FAT, PREGNANT, AND TRANSGENDER ABJECTION

The abjection of fat women is taken up in Le'a Kent's essay "Fighting Abjection: Representing Fat Women" in which she locates cultural processes of abjection in the late 1994 resurgence of "the presentation of fat bodies as pathological" in media generally and weight loss advertisements specifically (132-133). In particular, her analysis of the prevalence of the "before" picture in these ads resonates with the dichotomous cultural representation of trans identity in before/after pictures.[3] "The before-and-after sequence gets to the heart of mainstream fat representation and the resulting paradoxes and impossibilities of fat identity," she writes. The contrast between the abject "before" picture and the normalized "after" picture, which is held up as the representation of the "true self," demonstrates how "the fat body is once again caught up in a narrative of erasure" (134-5).

The abject fat woman's body is, Kent argues, "that which must be expelled to make all other bodily representations and functions, *even life itself*, possible" (135; emphasis mine). In the pregnant body, this expulsion of the abject literally coincides with the production of new life, through birth. The pregnant body is itself therefore a kind of nine-month enactment of the before-after depiction of weight loss; abjection is deferred (or at least tolerated) with the naturalization of pregnancy in anticipation of the birth that ultimately promises to restore the body to its feminine ideal.

There is an interesting overlap between the somatic experience of fatness and pregnancy, as well the societal and cultural rules and taboos around reading a body of size. Mostly this translates into intense cultural anxiety about whether a person is pregnant or "merely fat," and how one can tell the difference. Blog posts as well as celebrity and tabloid news routinely engage in the "pregnant or fat" game in which women's bodies are publicly scrutinized and discussed in an effort to classify them in one category or the other. The dilemma of correctly reading the fat female body became the focus of a BBC news magazine article in 2010, "Is that woman pregnant or fat?" Described as "a minefield of mixed signals, indecision, guilt, and offence," the piece considers the problem of when and whether to give up a seat on public transportation to a woman of substance.

Faced with "nagging doubt—is she pregnant, fat, or just wearing a baggy top?"—the BBC article offers seven tips to ascertain whether someone is actually pregnant or merely fat, including shortness of breath, belly- or back-rubbing, swollen feet and ankles, and a "waddling walk" among other signs. Remarkably, there is no discussion whatsoever of the gender dynamics involved in the ostensibly chivalrous gesture of offering up a seat, and never is the assumption that only pregnant women deserve to be the beneficiary of a seat questioned in any way. Also unaddressed are issues of class, race, and femininity, all of which also play a significant and intersectional role in determining whose bodies qualify for rescue and whose are abject and repulsive in their corpulence.[4] Despite the fact that many fat people also suffer from shortness of breath, swollen appendages, and difficulty walking, they are not to be accommodated in this way, unless actually pregnant. Indeed, the "minefield" occurs precisely because the act of giving up one's seat itself indicates an acknowledgement of non-normative embodiment that is usually studiously ignored. Only in the context of pregnancy is one socially permitted to notice fatness or comment on it without being considered offensive.

Even when publicly acknowledged to be pregnant, the scrutiny of female bodies doesn't end—and this is particularly true for celebrities, as Emma Gray notes in her blog post "Kim Kardashian Pregnancy Weight Fat-Shaming: Why You Really Should Care":

> Both the volume of stories about Kardashian's body and what headlines say about it remind us how acceptable it has become to talk publicly about an individual woman's appearance in terrible ways. They also demonstrate how having a female body that is anything other than thin— whether it be average, overweight or simply pregnant—is being cast as both a crime and a punishment. (Gray)

The public fascination with and policing of the fat/pregnant body demonstrates a deep cultural anxiety about its deviation from the normatively feminine. Pregnancy has the potential to rescue women from fat abjection, provided the pregnant woman doesn't gain too much, tipping her back into the realm of "fat," and that she loses any residual post-partum weight within a short time after giving birth.

Kent examines what she calls counterabjection in fat-positive publications such as the quarterly magazine *FaT GiRL: The Zine for Fat Dykes and the Women Who Want Them*, which includes political action tips to empower fat women. Interestingly, one such tip directly engages the very issue raised by the BBC article, framed here as harassment "about being fat or looking pregnant" (Kent 141). The suggested response in the zine is to theatrically "act out a monstrous birth," pulling a bloody Barbie doll or tampon as if from the body in what Kent describes as "a parodic abject birth" (142). Such a performance denaturalizes the pregnant body by embracing the conflation of pregnancy with the embodiment of the fat woman. In the monstrous fake birth, the fat woman confronts the fat-shaming harasser, demonstrating that the "problem" is deeper than the "fat or pregnant" binary suggests: even pregnancy would not resolve the problem of abjection once femininity (and correspondingly heterosexual desirability) has been called into question through the ambiguously fat body.

INVISIBILITY OF PREGNANCY

Even without a trans or non-binary gender identification, being fat can render pregnancy invisible. In "Fat and Knocked-Up," Megan McCullough writes about her experience as a fat pregnant woman:

> I found that even in the waiting room at my obstetrical practice, my body rarely figured as pregnant.... Most women assumed I was there for an annual exam. On several occasions when I clarified that I was pregnant, there would be an uncomfortable pause and often the conversation would end or switch tracks, as a social mistake had occurred. (225)

Like McCullough, the invisibility of my pregnancy also extended even to the clinic, though in my case I put it down to the incongruence of my gender presentation with my newly-acquired baby bump. As I have described it previously, this made for some quite humorous encounters with medical staff:

> We go to a prenatal appointment in my second trimester. The nurse hands the urine cup to my tall, slender partner, saying "Your husband can wait over there." She looks aghast when my partner informs her that it is not she but the shorter and fatter "husband" who is pregnant. (Surkan "FTM")

For what it was worth, the nurse recovered quickly; she turned to me and thrust the cup in my direction. "Well, then, I'll need the urine specimen from you, in that case."

As it turns out, my experienced invisibility of masculine pregnancy was not unique; it was also reflected in Michelle Walks' findings in her doctoral research study *Gender Identity and In/Fertility*, in which she interviewed and surveyed members of what she terms "the BTQ community": butch lesbians, transmen, and genderqueer individuals in British Columbia who had experienced pregnancy and/or infertility. As discussed earlier, Walks argues that "BTQ individuals who experience pregnancy and breastfeeding explicitly challenge *the cultural fetish associating femininity with reproduction* (including pregnancy, breastfeeding, mothering, and fertility)" (*Gender Identity* ii; emphasis mine).

The invisibility effect of this relentless cultural fetishization of pregnancy as feminine for the seven subjects interviewed who had experienced pregnancy in Walks' study was two-fold and diametrically opposed: either there was a failure to recognize masculine-presenting women as pregnant at all or, conversely, there was an automatic reading of pregnant women as heterosexual and normatively feminine, regardless of their actual sexual or gender identity. If masculine individuals were somehow recognized or known to be pregnant, the association of pregnancy with femaleness trumped other gender cues, resulting in the perception that they were "straight." Walks writes, "What surprised me to find out during the interviews was that none of the interview participants felt that they were recognized as lesbians during their pregnancy" (*Gender Identity* 124).

In particular, butch or masculine respondents described an inability of others to recognize their pregnancies at all, which Walks characterizes as "microaggressions, including misunderstandings and invisibility among friends, family, and strangers" (122). She connects this pivotally to the problem of maternity wear, which is by and large designed to promote connotations of femininity and as such was rejected by most of her subjects: "Only one of the seven interviewees who had experienced pregnancy noted that she felt comfortable in the available maternity wear. The six others either endured being uncomfortable in maternity wear, or wore larger sizes of the typical men's wear they were used to, or a mix of both" (117).

As a result, those wearing men's clothes "noted that publicly they were very rarely, if ever, recognized as pregnant, but instead perceived as men with a beer belly ... even at eight months pregnant, their co-workers could not fathom that they were pregnant. Their embodied masculinity denied any possibility of pregnancy" (124). My own experience at the end of my first pregnancy echoed this finding:

> I go from being a somewhat androgynous guy to a distinctly fat man. About a week away from birth with a 9-pound baby, my partner and I go to a plant show sponsored by the local horticulture society. It is late summer in Philly and a million degrees out and I blend in perfectly with all the other middle-aged fat men wearing oversized shorts and giant button-down short-sleeve shirts over their beer bellies. The woman cashier asks me, "Do you need a bag, sir?" when I buy a small plant for our front yard. "Please," I say. She doesn't look at me twice. (Surkan "FTM")

Interestingly, fashion and maternity clothing is also indicated as problematic for fat women as well; McCullough points to "the new celebrity culture around revealing and consuming images of celebrity's pregnancies and maternity clothing" as a key element in the invisibility of fat pregnancy (224). "As fat bodies are not considered attractive, fat women are not encouraged to show off their pregnancies and maternity clothing for fat women is hard to find," she writes (225).

Whether a problem of size or a problem of gender presentation, the narrow options for maternity clothing reflect cultural ideas about the proper way to be a pregnant woman. In 2014, Vanessa Newman and Michelle Janayea decided to change that, making media headlines with Butchbaby & Co., a company offering a new line of "alternity wear" for "androgynous and masculine-identified parents-to-be" (Kaitlyn). Newman and Janayea describe alternity wear as "the alternative to the hyperfeminine, heteronormative, eurocentric maternity wear that only exists today ... the only androgynous, all-inclusive apparel for pregnant masculine, trans, and queer individuals of all race, sizes, and class" (Butchbaby).

With the tagline "Don't change, just because your body does," the Butchbaby & Co. vision offers a glimpse of a different future for representation of the pregnant body, one that resists prescriptive femininity:

> Pregnancy does not have to be hyper-feminine. Pregnancy belongs to all those who can carry a child; regardless of sexual orientation or gender presentation. You can be butch, you can be stud, you can be non-gender conforming, you can be trans, you can be lesbian, you can be bisexual, you can be queer, you can be straight, and you still have a right to bear children. You still have a right to be mom, mommy, mama, maddy, moddy, dommy, daddy, dad, whatever you feel comfortable being called; you have a right to choose pregnancy and feel comfortable.... We aim to make pregnancy all inclusive of gender, sexual orientation, presentation, race, and class. (Butchbaby)

The Butchbaby & Co. business model aims to fill the void expressed by Walks' masculine subjects of their experience struggling to find something to wear in pregnancy.

GENDER, SIZE, AND THE VARIABLE EXPERIENCE OF PREGNANCY

How do we characterize the experience of the gender non-conforming individual in pregnancy? There is no universal answer, given the rich diversity of gender expression and personal relationship to highly gendered somatic experiences. As Gayle Rubin so clearly articulates, "there are many different ways to be masculine" (474), and similarly, she notes that different people have different reactions to and relationships with their masculine female bodies in pregnancy: "Butches vary in how they relate to their female bodies. Some butches are comfortable being pregnant and having kids, while for others the thought of undergoing the female component of mammalian reproduction is utterly repugnant" (474).

This observation is borne out in Walks' interviews with her research subjects, though it is not limited to butches—trans men also express very different comfort levels with pregnancy, some experiencing intense gender dysphoria and others none at all. For example, the recent article "Real Men Give Birth" follows two gay couples comprised of a cis man paired with a trans man. In each case, the trans man was birth parent to the couple's child—yet despite these parallels in family structure and common identification as gay men, their experiences with pregnancy were extremely different (Graff).

Sion Jesse, who was just twenty-one when he decided to have a child, "hated being pregnant so strongly that he emphatically wants *never* to do it again." Stephen Stratton, on the other hand, was thirty-two and had already been on hormones for ten years. "His gender dysphoria had peaked right after puberty and through his early years in college.... Being a man, he says, made it possible for him to tolerate pregnancy" (Graff). Both men discontinued testosterone in order to achieve pregnancy; for Sion, who was younger and had less androgen exposure, this meant that he was routinely identified as a lesbian throughout his pregnancy and the subsequent time he spent nursing his son. Stephen, who had previously had top surgery, was never mistaken for female, but was not always recognized as the birth parent who had actually carried his daughter.

In "Real Men Give Birth," more emphasis is placed on the hormonal effects of pregnancy than weight gain, which may be a function of the concerns of the gay (and perhaps trans) male blog audience in imagining male pregnancy and its potential to disrupt masculinity. Butches, in contrast, are more inclined to focus on maternity clothing and weight gain as significant issues contributing to the invisibility of their pregnancies. Nevertheless, both trans men and butches express a great deal of variation in their acceptance of pregnancy and perhaps even the degree to which they even perceive it as necessarily coded female/feminine in the first place.

Most difficult for all across the butch-FTM spectrum is the invisibility of masculine pregnancy, which can make it challenging to locate services and support and can especially make the navigation of highly gendered spaces particularly difficult for butch, trans, and genderqueer pregnant bodies. Not least of these is access to public (and nearly always gendered) bathrooms, which as any person experiencing pregnancy knows is even more critically necessary than usual, especially as the due date nears. I stopped worrying about entering the women's bathroom while heavily pregnant, figuring that my pregnant shape would be reassuring to women in that space. For the most part it did, until I was confronted one day by an alarmed elderly lady as I came through the door, belly and all. "Sir—you are in the women's restroom." I didn't hesitate in my response. "Ma'am—I'm pregnant."

[1]See Gilman for an in-depth consideration of fat masculinities and their representations in various cultural and literary contexts.
[2]I use masculine pronouns in referring to Bergman, in accordance with his preference as stated on his website ("Frequently Asked").
[3]I have discussed the significance of before/after photos and images of the bifurcated face in representing transgendered bodies in more detail in "Passing and the Tropes of Masculinity," chapter two of my dissertation, *Passing Rhetorics*.
[4]A. K. Summers captures this perfectly in her graphic novel *Pregnant Butch* in a depiction of the pregnant butch on the subway, surrounded by men and utterly invisible to them: "Imagine how often you're offered a seat when most people take you for just another fat guy on the subway."

WORKS CITED

Bergman, S. Bear. "Frequently Asked Questions." *S. Bear Bergman.* N.d. Web. 10 February 2015. Web

Bergman, S. Bear. "Part-Time Fatso." *The Fat Studies Reader.* Eds. Esther Rothblum and Sondra Solovay. New York: NYU Press, 2009. 139-142. Print.

Butchbaby & Co. "Vision." *Butchbaby & Co.* 3 December 2014. Web. 10 February 2015.

Gilman, Sander L. *Fat Boys: A Slim Book.* Lincoln: University of Nebraska Press, 2004. Print.

Graff, E.J. "Real Men Give Birth." *Gays With Kids.* 4 February 2015. Web. 10 February 2015.

Gray, Emma. "Kim Kardashian Pregnancy Weight Fat-Shaming: Why You Really Should Care." *HuffPost Women.* 26 March 2013. Web. 10 February 2015.

Hartley, Cecilia. "Letting Ourselves Go: Making Room for the Fat Body in Feminist Scholarship." *Bodies Out of Bounds: Fatness and Transgression*. Eds. Jana Evans Braziel & Kathleen LeBesco. Berkeley, CA: University of California Press, 2001. 60-73. Print.

"Is That Woman Pregnant or Fat?" *BBC News Magazine*. 9 June 2010. Web. 10 February 2015.

Kaitlyn, "Butchbabay & Co. Brings Maternity Wear Out of the Women's Section." *Autostraddle*. 20 December 2014. Web. 10 February 2015.

Kent, Le'a. "Fighting Abjection: Representing Fat Women." *Bodies Out of Bounds: Fatness and Transgression*. Eds. Jana Evans Braziel and Kathleen LeBesco. Berkeley,CA: University of California Press, 2001. 130-150. Print.

McCullough, Megan. "Fat and Knocked-Up: An Embodied Analysis of Stigma, Visibility, and Invisibility in the Biomedical Management of an Obese Pregnancy." *Reconstructing Obesity: The Meaning of Measures and the Measure of Meanings*. Eds. Megan B. McCullough and Jessica A. Hardin. New York: Berghahn Books, 2013. 215-234. Print.

Mosher, Jerry. "Setting Free the Bears: Refiguring Fat Men on Television." *Bodies Out of Bounds: Fatness and Transgression*. Eds. Jana Evans Braziel & Kathleen LeBesco. Berkeley, CA: University of California Press, 2001. 166-193. Print.

Rubin, Gayle. "Of Catamites and Kings: Reflections on Butch, Gender, and Boundaries." *Transgender Studies Reader, Vol. 1*. Eds. Susan Stryker and Stephen Whittle. New York: Routledge, 2006. 471-481. Print.

Serano, Julia. *Whipping Girl: A Transsexual Woman on Sexism and the Scapegoating of Femininity*. Berkeley, CA: Seal Press, 2007. Print.

Summers, A. K. *Pregnant Butch: Nine Long Months Spent in Drag*. Berkeley, CA: Soft Skull Press, 2014. Print.

Surkan, K. "FTM in the Fertility Clinic: Troubling the Gendered Boundaries of Reproduction." Oxford: Inter-disciplinary Press, Forthcoming in 2015.

Surkan, K. *Passing Rhetorics and the Performance of Gender Identity: (Auto)biographical, Visual, and Virtual Representations of Transgender Subjectivity and Embodiment*. Diss. University of Minnesota, 2003. Print.

Walks, Michelle. "Feminine Pregnancy as Cultural Fetish." *Anthropology News* 54.1-2 (2013): 12. Print.

Walks, Michelle. *Gender Identity and In/Fertility*. Diss. Simon Fraser University, 2013. Print.

DAMIEN W. RIGGS AND DEBORAH DEMPSEY

Gay Men's Narratives of Pregnancy in the Context of Commercial Surrogacy

HISTORICALLY, GAY MEN HAVE PRIMARILY become fathers in the context of heterosexual relationships, or for some men through foster care, adoption, or co-parenting arrangements as sperm donors (Riggs and Due). Since the beginning of the twenty-first century, however, gay men living in western countries have increasingly made use of commercial surrogacy services (Everingham, Stafford-Bell, and Hammarberg). The increased use of these services has become possible as a result of legislative change in countries such as the U.S. (in which many states now allow for the contracting of surrogacy services), in addition to the provision of services in countries where the regulation of commercial surrogacy has not occurred until relatively recently (such as India and Thailand). The rapid growth in the use of commercial surrogacy services by gay men has been shaped by factors such as 1) a desire for genetic relatedness between children and at least one of their fathers (in a couple), 2) the perception that commercial surrogacy allows men to have greater control over the process of having a child, and 3) the perception that commercial surrogacy arrangements offer greater legal security to gay men (Murphy; Tuazon-McCheyne).

At the same time as this boom in the use of commercial surrogacy services by gay men, there has been a rapid increase in academic research and publishing on the topic of commercial surrogacy focused primarily on women who act as surrogates. Arguably, this research is divided into two camps: 1) research primarily undertaken in countries such as the U.S. where women who act as commercial surrogates are depicted as making agentic choices and experiencing primarily positive relationships with the people for whom they carry children (e.g. Markens), and 2) research focusing on countries such as India where it has been argued that there is a considerable risk of the exploitation of women who act as commercial surrogates, women who may experience surrogacy as conflicting with their cultural beliefs and who are typically estranged from those for whom they carry children (e.g. Pande; Rudruppa). Recent legislative changes in countries such as Thailand and India would suggest that potentially the latter framing of commercial surrogacy has played something of a role in informing legislative decisions about whether or not to allow for commercial surrogacy and who is eligible to use surrogacy services.

Despite the now considerable body of research on commercial surrogacy—as noted above primarily focused on the experiences of women who act as surrogates—relatively little research has been undertaken specifically focusing on gay men who are intended parents. What research does exist in this area has primarily focused on 1) the functioning of gay families formed through commercial surrogacy (Bergman et al.), 2) gay men's decisions about having children through commercial surrogacy arrangements (Greenfeld and Seli), and 3) how gay men negotiate decisions about genetic relatedness (in the context of gay couples) (Dempsey, "Surrogacy").

A small number of papers have explored gay men's experiences of pregnancy and birth in the context of commercial surrogacy arrangements, and these indicate that men's participation in the pregnancy and birth is to some degree formative for their parental identities. Drawing on interviews undertaken with twenty gay fathers (of whom five had children through surrogacy arrangements), Berkowitz and Marsiglio suggest that her participants "discussed living vicariously through the actual pregnancy" (377). They did this by staying in close contact with the woman carrying their child throughout the pregnancy, including attending medical appointments and scheduling regular telephone conversations or emails so as to learn about the progress of the pregnancy. Lev too discusses from her own interview research how some gay men wish to stay in close contact throughout the pregnancy with the woman carrying their child, although Lev emphasizes that for some men this is about a concern to ensure that the woman is taking adequate care of the child she is carrying. More recently, Ziv and Freund-Eschar have studied the emotional experiences of gay men becoming parents through overseas surrogacy. They found that the men experienced some frustration and anxiety because of their physical distance from the pregnancy and the lack of opportunity to "bond" with the developing fetus. All of the men in this study felt their lack of physical proximity to the woman carrying their child and developing fetus hindered the development of their parental identities pre-birth. Finally, Riggs, Due and Power found that Australian gay men felt emotionally unsupported by offshore surrogacy clinics with regard to issues associated with the pregnancy and birth. The men reported that clinics did not consult them in decisions about how and when the surrogate would give birth, and also believed clinical staff could be insensitive to the emotional impact of a pregnancy loss on intended parents.

To add to this growing body of research on the topic of gay men negotiating pregnancies in the context of commercial surrogacy arrangements, the present chapter provides an analysis of a small sample of books written by gay men documenting their experiences of commercial surrogacy. The books were identified through a search of the website Amazon.com utilizing the search term "gay surrogacy." A total of eight books were identified, however four of these were "how-to" guides not written by gay men or not including gay men's own narratives. The data included in the analysis below were derived from the remaining four books written by gay men who had undertaken a commercial surrogacy arrangement:

- *Dads: A Gay Couple's Surrogacy Journey in India* (Hirschi)
- *A Gay Couple's Journey through Surrogacy: Intended Fathers* (Menichiello)
- *The Journey of Same-Sex Surrogacy: Discovering Ultimate Joy* (Warner)
- *Our 'Journey': One Couple's Guide to US Surrogacy* (Westoby)

These four books were read with a focus on the chapters within each book that specifically addressed the topic of pregnancy. Of the books, three document gestational commercial surrogacy arrangements undertaken in the U.S. by U.S. citizens (Menichiello; Warner; Westoby) and one documents a gestational commercial surrogacy arrangement undertaken in India by Swedish citizens (Hirschi). All of the authors were in a gay relationship when their child was conceived and born.

To a degree reflecting concerns raised by the literature outlined above in regards to how women who act as surrogates are represented, three of the books very clearly spoke of women who act as surrogates in ways that reduced them to functional objects. Indeed, this was even the case when one of the women was a close friend of the gay fathers (Warner). The fourth book provided something of a more critical reading of the ethics of commercial surrogacy, though as we shall see below ultimately resorted to a narrative that legitimated commercial surrogacy through an emphasis on the financial benefits it is presumed to provide to women (Hirschi).

ANALYSIS

For this chapter, the four books were analysed in terms of discursive repertoires. Discursive repertoires may be understood as ways of thinking or talking about a topic that provide a particular framework through which to understand the topic and a particular language through which to speak about it (Wetherell and Potter). Two particular discursive repertoires were identified through repeated readings of the book chapters. The first discursive repertoire was the claiming of the pregnancy by the men, such as through the use of the pronouns "we" and "our." The second discursive repertoire was one in which women who act as surrogates were positioned as an almost troublesome imposition upon the lives of gay intended parents. Each of these two discursive repertoires are now discussed in turn.

Claiming the Pregnancy

In 2014, actress Mila Kunis (who was pregnant at the time) appeared on *Jimmy Kimmel Live* and performed a rehearsed skit in response to Kimmel's statement that he and his wife were pregnant. In the skit, Kunis emphasized that whilst men in heterosexual relationships are typically involved in creating a child (i.e., through heterosex), and whilst they may support their partner during the pregnancy, they are never at any time pregnant and therefore do not personally experience pregnancy in an embodied way. Predictably, the skit evoked strong responses from media commentators—particularly heterosexual men—with pieces appearing on the *Good Men Project* (Denkenberger) and in the *Huffington Post* (Schwem). Both of these responses were premised on the claim that in a heterosexual relationship there may indeed be many embodied activities undertaken jointly by both people in respect to the pregnancy and that claiming that only the woman is pregnant is disrespectful to men.

This example provided by Kunis' skit and the responses to it—of men making a claim to a pregnancy as their own—was apparent in the extracts now presented in this first discursive repertoire. Researchers have noted the use of shared pronouns since the 1990s (e.g., Longhurst), and have suggested that it has the potential to contribute to the erasure of women's embodied experiences in regards to pregnancy. Specifically in regards to gay men, Lewin notes many instances where her participants, when talking about a pregnancy undertaken in the context of commercial surrogacy, claimed the pregnancy as their own, such as by saying, "I'm pregnant" (Phillip in Lewin 175). In the four books examined for this chapter, the notion of a pregnancy being shared by gay men who commission a commercial surrogacy arrangement was a common trope, one that was never problematized or questioned by the authors. Examples within the book include: "Could it be that we were pregnant on our first attempt?" (Westoby), "Today marks the 35th day of our pregnancy … we have completed our seventh week of pregnancy" (Hirschi), and "The holidays were just around the corner. We also just entered our second trimester" (Warner 43).

When examined in the abstract, it is possible to view these types of comments as the authors staking a claim to *their* child, a claim that arguably is important in regards to their future relationship with the child. At the same time, however, these comments typically appeared with sole reference to the male couples. In other words, whilst in the broader social phenomenon the claim that "we're pregnant" is made by heterosexual men and women, in the examples provided above the claims were made by male couples *solely about the couple*, thus in effect excluding the woman who was actually pregnant.

The use of particular pronouns to stake a claim to the pregnancy was not the only way in which the authors did this. They also made possessive claims about the women who were carrying their child, such as: "You really have to put a huge amount of trust in your surrogate" (Westoby). This example demonstrates how particular descriptions of pregnant women in the context of commercial surrogacy reduce such women to being the property of intended parents: "your surrogate." Another example of the reduction of women to their role in carrying a child appears as: "Thing is, when our child is growing inside a womb 10,000 kilometres away, it's hard to wrap around the concept" (Hirschi). In this example a pregnant woman in a commercial surrogacy arrangement becomes just "a womb." Concern about this type of reductive logic has been repeatedly raised specifically in reference to Indian women who act as surrogates and how the logic of "wombs for rent" serves to reduce women to their reproductive capabilities (Rudruppa).

Women as Troubling Impositions

Whilst it could be argued that the examples provided in the previous repertoire are indicative of the authors drawing upon culturally available discourses about men and pregnancy, the extracts included in the second discursive repertoire more clearly depict women in negative ways. Three of the authors spend considerable portions of their chapter/s on pregnancy discussing how challenging they found their relationship with the women who carried a child for them. It is of course understandable that, as with any relationship, stress may at times place individuals in antagonistic relationships with one another. This may be particularly the case where the woman who acts as a surrogate is not a friend of the intended parents prior to the surrogacy arrangement.

Yet the extracts included below, it is argued here, go beyond the simple expression of antagonism in a stressful situation and extend to the depiction of women who act as surrogates as troubling impositions upon the lives of gay men.

In the text that preceded the first extract below, the author had reported that the woman who was acting as the surrogate—who was a friend of the author—had expressed a desire for a vaginal birth. The author then went on to say, however, that:

> In all honesty, we really would have preferred for her to have agreed up front to have a C-section. Not because we are 'too posh to push', but because it would enable us to plan all of the logistics around when the children were going to be born. (Westoby)

Putting aside the rather odd comment about not being "too posh to push" (given this claim is normally made about women's decisions in relation to their own bodies, not about men's decisions or bodies), the author's seemingly mundane emphasis upon wanting to "plan all of the logistics" is perhaps rather less mundane if we consider the position of the men, who do not have full "access" to their child until s/he is born. Indeed, it is one thing for two men to wish to "plan all of the logistics" related to the birth of a child, but it is another thing altogether to be the woman who is giving birth, for whom logistics may be just one of many concerns. Reducing the pregnancy and birth (and thus the woman undertaking both) to simply a series of logistics potentially contributes to the marginalizing of her experiences as a pregnant woman, specifically as a pregnant woman who in this case had previously given birth vaginally to her own children.

These types of marginalizing comments are amplified in the following three extracts, all from the same author. This author spent a considerable amount of time in his chapter on pregnancy writing negatively about the woman who carried his child, a woman who, like the woman in the previous extract, was also married and had children of her own. In the first extract from this author the woman who acted as the surrogate—Michelle—is depicted as mercenary and as making poor decisions:

Michelle has been doing a lot of complaining about money lately. First it was the compensation checks, now it's that her maternity allowance check is late. I keep wondering if it would be different if she had kept her job.... She's also been talking a lot about how they've been spending the compensation money and I am feeling strange about that. (Menichiello)

It is important to note that this was a commercial surrogacy arrangement involving a contract and schedule of payments. To depict Michelle as "complaining about money" is, in effect, to ignore the inherently fiscal nature of the arrangement: It is only Michelle who is depicted as mercenary, rather than all parties depicted as potentially mercenary. The author then implicitly dismisses Michelle's "complaints about money" by inferring that, had she kept her job, she wouldn't have money troubles. He then further emphasizes this claim by talking about how she has been spending money received as part of the contract. Indeed, a paragraph is later devoted to outlining what Michelle had spent money on, with items such as holidays implicitly depicted as a waste of money.

The presumed binary of women who act as surrogates being either altruistic or mercenary has been identified in previous research (Roach Anleu), and indeed research on gay men and surrogacy has indicated that a majority of gay men seek women who fall within the former category (Ressler et al). As the next extract from the same author again demonstrates—this time when reporting on a conversation with his partner—the emphasis upon altruism as a desirable characteristic potentially serves to allow some gay men to claim that women who act as surrogates should submit to the needs of gay men, rather than vice versa: "'It has been hard, I know. It's almost as though we're married to Michelle and James [Michelle's husband], isn't it,' I asked. 'Whatever they do, whatever decision that they make directly affects us, and it's a feeling I can't get used to'" (Menichiello).

This analogy to marriage mirrors analogies made by gay men in research by Scholz and Riggs on the topic of sperm donation to lesbian recipients. This research found that such men heterosexualise their relationship to lesbian recipients in order to claim

a right to decision-making about children conceived of their do-
nations. Whilst the analogy in the case of surrogacy doesn't per
se heterosexualise the relationship between the gay men and the
woman carrying a child for them (and her husband), it does remove
the relationship from the realms of commercial surrogacy, instead
locating it in the realm of the familial. Yet this appears to only
work one way: the men are depicted as problematically impacted
by the woman and her husband, yet the woman and her husband
are not in turn seen as impacted by the gay men. The source of
tension, then, is again the woman, not the surrogacy arrangement
itself and the men's desire for it. Below, in the third extract from
this author, the depiction of women who act as surrogates as a
troubling imposition is most clearly stated:

> Our first thought was that there was no way that we could
> let Michelle pack up and move to Arizona being eight
> months pregnant with our child. It was way too risky. I
> put a call in to the same attorney who had been helping
> us with our prebirth order. "I wouldn't let her move,"
> our attorney said. "She's doing something wonderful for
> you, yes, that's a given, but there comes a time when you
> just have to put your foot down and say no, you're not
> moving." (Menichiello)

Prior to this extract the author had spent several pages discussing
his anger at the fact that Michelle was moving to another state. In
this extract both he and his male attorney are reported as sharing
the view that, despite the contract not including terms preventing Michelle moving, the author should insist upon it. This was
despite awareness that the move was important for Michelle and
her family. This belief that intended parents should have the right
to determine the movements of women who act as surrogates explicitly reduces such women to the role of service providers who,
upon entering a contract to undertake a commercial surrogacy
arrangement, relinquish rights to their own autonomy. Whilst this
was the most extreme example of such a belief, it was also evident
in other books where a placenta previa meant that the woman was
restricted to bed rest.

In the final extract below, the author who had negotiated with a friend to act as a surrogate comments on how the friendship was an imposition upon his experience of the pregnancy:

> Being friends with the surrogate has its advantages in so many ways, but it also definitely comes with its challenges. I wanted the pregnancy to be a beautiful experience. I wanted to cherish each step and each moment. However, it was very difficult to enjoy it when Mary was always feeling sick and exhausted. This affected her in many ways, not to mention her being hormonal because of being pregnant, and trying to be there for her was exhausting. I felt guilty and responsible and, at times, thought, *It would be so much easier if the surrogate just lived somewhere else and I wasn't having to go through all of this with her.* Being my surrogate's friend was often difficult for me. (Warner 41, original emphasis)

In this extract, whilst the author acknowledges the positives of a commercial surrogacy arrangement undertaken in the context of a friendship, his primary emphasis is on the negatives of such an arrangement. Specifically, whilst he reports empathy for the effects of the pregnancy upon Mary, his concern appears to lie primarily with the difficulties the friendship presented to him. Arguably, what is implied is that undertaking a surrogacy with someone he did not know would have allowed him to care less about the woman and to instead focus on his own feelings. Again, such a desire depicts women who act as surrogates as an imposition on men who commission surrogacy arrangements.

Whilst it is important to acknowledge the often complex journeys that gay men undertake to become parents, this discursive repertoire has highlighted that it is also necessary to be aware of the ways in which gay men's desires and beliefs may lead to the reduction of women who act as surrogates to paid employees who must submit to the will of their employer. Whilst this may not be the intention of the gay men analysed here, it is certainly a potential consequence of some of the ways in which they talk about the women who had acted as surrogates for them.

CONCLUSION

In their research with gay men who had undertaken a commercial surrogacy arrangement, Berkowitz and Marsiglio suggest that "a fascinating feature of gay men's procreative identity is how it becomes intertwined with the real or imagined identity of the child's birth mother" (377). Our argument in the present chapter has been that, at least for the four authors analysed here, there is less of an intertwining of a real or imagined identity with the women carrying their children and perhaps more of an overwriting of their identity. In other words, the two discursive repertoires identified suggest that in many ways the four authors not only distance themselves from the women carrying their children but also potentially attempt to replace them, or at least minimise their role to a paid biological function.

Importantly, this is not to suggest that such constructions of women who act as surrogates were necessarily intended by the authors to dismiss the role of women. Nonetheless, the authors are men living in the context of patriarchal societies and hence are not outside of normative discourses of women and repro-ductivity. At the same time, we must acknowledge that the men live in homophobic social contexts where gay men are seen as inadequate parents who "fail" to provide their children with a mother, a stereotype that the men may have been attempting to refute by focusing attention away from the women who carried their children. Research on lesbian women who have utilised donor sperm has suggested that such women similarly feel an expectation to account for the "lack" of men in their children's lives (Clarke). Yet despite this, it is much less common that lesbian women entirely discount the contribution that men make to the conception of a child through the donation of their sperm, even in cases where there are disputes between women and donors (Dempsey, "Donor"). Indeed, it is far more common that men who act as sperm donors to lesbian recipients demand a return upon their "investment" (Scholz and Riggs).

Whilst the findings presented here may not necessarily represent the beliefs of all gay men who enter into commercial surrogacy arrangements, they certainly align to a significant degree with accounts of women and reproductivity in general and commercial surrogacy specifically. As the persistence of these accounts would suggest, they are not likely to disappear simply by critiquing them. Instead, it is suggested here that wider conversations must be undertaken about gay men's reproductive desires. Indeed, one of the authors (Hirschi) spent a chapter outlining how he disagrees with commercial surrogacy and believes that gay men who wish to become parents should foster or adopt. In his context (Sweden) this is not possible, but his argument was that it should be and that this may reduce the demand for surrogacy services. Whether or not this would be the case is a matter of debate—given the desire for genetic relatedness identified in previous research (e.g., Murphy; Dempsey, "Surrogacy")—but it is certainly a line of thinking that warrants further attention.

To conclude, gay men, as is the case with most men, do not have an embodied relationship with pregnancy: it is something most men experience vicariously. This does not mean that gay men do not have an important role to play in supporting women throughout a pregnancy in the context of commercial surrogacy. Rather, it means that gay men should be encouraged to actively consider how their narratives of surrogacy and pregnancy may, even if unintentionally, dismiss or marginalize the embodied experience of pregnancy.

We would like to begin by acknowledging the sovereignty of the Kaurna and Wurundjeri people, the First Nations people upon whose land we live and work. Thanks must go to Clare Bartholomaeus for editorial work on the chapter. The research reported in this chapter was supported by an Australian Research Council Discovery Grant, DP110101893.

WORKS CITED

Bergman, Kim, Richie J. Rubio, Robert-Jay Green, and Elena Padron. "Gay Men who Become Fathers via Surrogacy: The Transition to Parenthood." *Journal of GLBT Family Studies* 6 (2010): 111-141. Print.

Berkowitz, Dana, and William Marsiglio. "Gay Men: Negotiating Procreative, Father, and Family Identities." *Journal of Marriage and Family* 69 (2007): 366-381. Print.

Clarke, Victoria. "'Gay Men, Gay Men and More Gay Men': Traditional, Liberal and Critical Perspectives on Male Role Models in Lesbian Families." *Lesbian and Gay Psychology Review* 7 (2006): 19-35. Print

Dempsey, Deborah. "Donor, Father or Parent?: Conceiving Paternity in the Australian Family Court." *International Journal of Law, Policy and the Family* 18 (2004): 76-102. Print.

Dempsey, Deborah. "Surrogacy, Gay Male Couples and the Significance of Biogenetic Paternity." *New Genetics and Society* 32 (2013): 37-53. Print.

Denkenberger, Paul. "Open letter to Mila Kunis: A response to taking the 'we' out of pregnancy." *The Good Men Project.* 18 June 2014. Web. 19 February 2015.

Everingham, Sam G., Martin A. Stafford-Bell, and Karin Hammarberg. "Australians' Use of Surrogacy." *MJA* 201(2014): 1-4. Print.

Greenfeld, Dorothy A., and Emre Seli. "Gay Men Choosing Parenthood through Assisted Reproduction: Medical and Psychosocial Considerations." *Fertility and Sterility* 95 (2011): 225-229. Print.

Hirschi, Hans M. *Dads: A Gay Couple's Surrogacy Journey in India.* Yaree AB, 2014. Kindle Edition.

Lev, Arlene Ishtar. "Gay Dads: Choosing Surrogacy." *Lesbian and Gay Psychology Review* 7 (2006): 73-77. Print.

Lewin, Ellen. *Gay Fatherhood: Narratives of Family and Citizenship in America.* Chicago: University of Chicago Press. 2009. Print.

Longhurst, Robyn. "Trim, Taut, Terrific and Pregnant." *Pleasure Zones.* Eds. David Bell, Jon Binnie, Ruth Holliday, Robyn Longhurst, and Robin Peace. New York: Syracuse University Press, 2001. 1-28. Print.

Markens, Susan. *Surrogate Motherhood and the Politics of Reproduction.* Berkeley: University of California Press, 2012. Print.

Menichiello, Michael. *A Gay Couple's Journey through Surrogacy: Intended Fathers.* New York: Haworth Press, 2012. Print.

Murphy, Dean A. "The Desire for Parenthood: Gay Men Choosing to Become Parents through Surrogacy." *Journal of Family Issues* 34 (2013): 1104-1124. Print.

Pande, Amrita. "Commercial Surrogacy in India: Manufacturing a Perfect Mother-Worker." *Signs: Journal of Women in Culture and Society* 35 (2010): 969-992. Print.

Ressler, Ilana B., Danielle Bessett, Julie M. Sroga, Sarah Rompola, Rachael M. Ferrari, Michael A. Thomas, and Steven R. Lindheim. "Perspectives among Gay Male Couples Choosing Fatherhood Using Assisted Reproduction." *Fertility and Sterility* 96 (2011): 12-15. Print.

Riggs, Damien W., and Clemence Due. "A Review of Research on Gay Fathers' Reproductive Journeys and Parenting Experiences." *Journal of Family Planning and Reproductive Health* 40 (2014): 289-293. Print.

Riggs, Damien W., Clemence Due, and Jennifer Power. "Gay Men's Experiences of Surrogacy Clinics in India." *Journal of Family Planning and Reproductive Healthcare* 41.1 (2014): 48-53. Print.

Roach Anleu, Sharon. "Surrogacy: For Love but not for Money?" *Gender and Society* 6 (1992): 30-48. Print.

Rudrappa, Sharmila. "India's Reproductive Assembly Line." *Contexts* 11 (2012): 22-27. Print.

Scholz, Brett, and Damien W. Riggs. "Sperm Donors' Accounts of Lesbian Recipients: Heterosexualisation as a Tool for Warranting Claims to Children's 'Best Interests.'" *Psychology and Sexuality* 5 (2014): 247-257. Print.

Schwem, Greg. "Sorry Mila Kunis, but We Are Both Pregnant." *Huffington Post.* 18 June 2014. Web. 19 February 2015.

Tuazon-McCheyne, Jason. "Two Dads: Gay Male Parenting and its Politicization - A Cooperative Inquiry Action Research Study." *Australian and New Zealand Journal of Family Therapy* 31 (2010): 311-323. Print.

Warner, Jason. *The Journey of Same-Sex Surrogacy: Discovering Ultimate Joy.* Tennessee: Zygote Publishing. 2013. Print.

Westoby, Richard. *Our Journey: One Couple's Guide to U.S. Surrogacy.* CreateSpace, 2013. Kindle Edition.

Wetherell, Margaret, and Jonathon Potter. *Mapping the Language of Racism: Discourse, the Legitimation of Exploitation.* New York: Columbia University Press. 1992. Print.

Ziv, Ido, and Yael Freund-Eschar. "The Pregnancy Experience of Gay Couples Expecting a Child through Overseas Surrogacy."

The Family Journal: Counseling and Therapy for Couples and Families. 23 (28 December 2014): 158-166. Print.

Crone and Moon, Umbilical Cords/Blood Ties

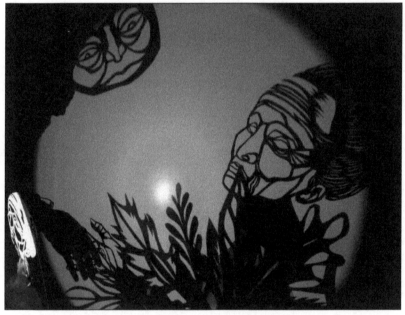

Brescia Nember Reid, "Crone and Moon," 2013, Shadows, cast by paper cut-outs.

This image is made by projecting light through a paper cut-out shadow puppet. We see here an elderly person gazing at the face of the moon. The figure could be a wise and experienced midwife, nearing the completion of her life. She appears as to be conversing with the moon, long thought to have a powerful and mysterious influence on cycles of menstruation and fertility, much as the moon pulls the tides of the oceans. Perhaps she is being pulled through to the next phase in the cycles of life and death.

The subsequent illustration, cut-out in black paper, offers a depiction of the intergenerational continuum of birth. This work imagines a family line, with umbilical cords still attached, a snapshot of multiple generations seen at once, in non-linear time. Centering a representation of queer birthers, including trans folks and LGBT-TIQ2S people, is integral to this web of generations. Homage is

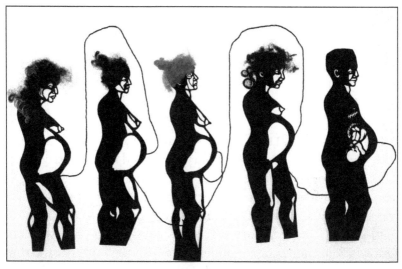

Brescia Nember Reid, "Umbilical Cords/Blood Ties," 2014,
Paper cut-out & string, 2.5ft x 1.2ft.

paid to the curious reality of human reproductive physiology—a fetus with ovaries is born containing their entire life's supply of "eggs" (Moore, Persaud, and Torchia 269). This means that the eggs that were fertilized to become each of us were present in the tiny fetal gonads of our mother/the person who birthed us, while they were within the wombs of our maternal grandmothers (Coad and Dunstall 106).

WORKS CITED

Coad, Jane, and Melvyn Dunstall. *Anatomy and Physiology for Midwives*. 3rd ed. London: Elsevier/Churchill Livingstone, 2012. Print.

Moore, Keith L., T. V. N. Persaud, and Mark G. Torchia. *The Developing Human: Clinically Oriented Embryology*. 9th ed. Philadelphia: Saunders/Elsevier, 2013. Print.

Imminent

OR OVER FIFTEEN YEARS, my artistic practice has explored issues of doubt, vulnerability, perceived ideals, and communication within the context of interpersonal relationships. Working with constructed narratives and a feminist lens, I describe the emotions and quiet moments of everyday life. Touch, gesture, and gaze all play significant roles as conduits of conscious and unconscious modes of communication. My artwork parallels my life experiences and has recently concentrated on pregnancy and mothering through the series *Swallowing Ice, Fold,* and *Imminent. Imminent* began as a series of self-portraits that visually articulated my reflections of being pregnant and the primary caregiver to a two-year-old. Empowered by my personal past, conversations with close friends, and maternal theory, I wanted to voice my experience of a metaphorical loss of a former self and the surreal transformation of my body, intertwined with a fierce sense of love.

Imminent has expanded to an on-going body of work involving numerous pregnant women photographed in their homes. Using the domestic environment, body language, and in some cases mother-child relationships, I aim to create portraits with an ambiguous psychological narrative. The resulting scenes of hesitation, reflection, confrontation, and concealment suggest some of the contradictory emotions and thoughts driven by the journey of becoming a mother. Through the use of simplified colour pallettes, fabricated scenes, and minimal sets, the photographs carry a weight to them—ordinary circumstances hold a trace of the uncanny. My positioning of the lens invites viewers into intimate moments,

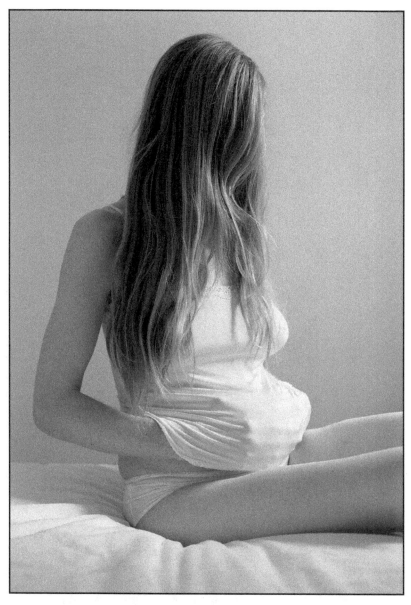

sharing the perspective of the subject or lover. A woman's gaze upon herself, the public's gaze at her, and the power dynamics involved in looking intrigue me. I aim to discuss this and other such complex and layered aspects of pregnancy and perception, including themes of sexuality, judgement, voyeurism, ambivalence, identity loss, beauty, and empowerment.

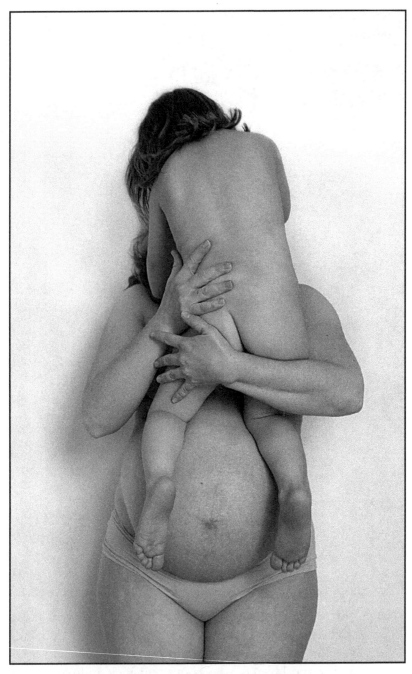

Previous page, Jennifer Long, Untitled, from the series *Imminent,* 2012, colour photograph, 115 x 76 cm. Above, Jennifer Long, Untitled, from the series *Imminent*, 2012, colour photograph, 40 x 60 cm.

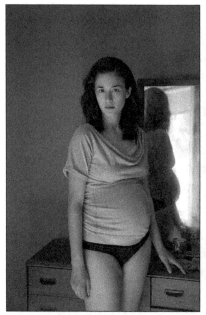 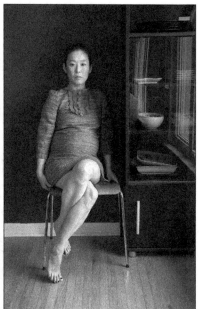

From left to right, Jennifer Long, Untitled, from the series *Imminent,* 2013, colour photographs, both 115 x 76 cm.

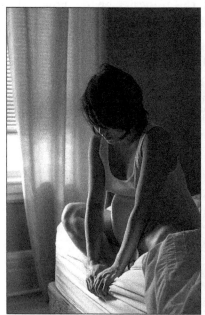 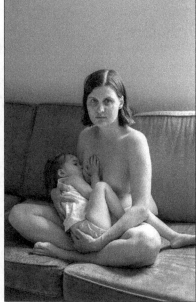

From left to right, Jennifer Long, Untitled, from the series *Imminent,* 2013 and 2012, colour photographs, both 115 x 76 cm.

ELIZABETH ALLEMANG

Heroes and Villains

Representations of Midwives in Ontario's Late Twentieth Century Midwifery Revival

CONTRARY TO THE POPULAR BELIEF that midwifery is one of the oldest female professions, midwifery is considered a "new" profession in Canada (Shroff 11). Throughout much of the twentieth century, Canada was the only western industrial nation and one of only nine of the 250 World Health Organization member countries without legal provisions for midwifery (Barrington 14-5). While the majority of babies around the world are born into the hands of midwives, the modern Canadian maternity care system was built on the model of a doctor-nurse team without the presence of the midwife as an expert in normal birth (Biggs, "Rethinking History" 36). Societal knowledge about midwifery was eroded by the growing monopoly of professionalized medicine and nursing in childbirth over the course of the twentieth century.

In 1994, Ontario became the first province in Canada to legalize midwifery as a self-regulating profession and integrate midwives into the publicly funded maternity care system as primary health care providers for healthy childbearing women and their newborn babies (Tyson et al.). A small group of formally and informally trained midwives had been practicing in Ontario without legal status for almost twenty years prior to the enactment of midwifery legislation as part of a North American resurgence of midwifery as a counter-practice to mainstream maternity care. They were working on the margins of official health care, providing midwifery care to women seeking childbirth alternatives, attending home births, and providing labour support in hospitals (Barrington). These Ontario "pre-legislation" midwives, the first midwives in Canada to undergo legal reform, are often portrayed in dramatic and contradictory ways. In this chapter, I will analyse three dominant representations of midwives that infuse the large body of popular and scholarly literature on North American midwifery revivals, with particular attention to Ontario pre-legislation practice: the counterculture mother, the feminist activist, and the aspiring professional of the white middle class. For each of these representations, midwives are portrayed in heroic and villainous ways. How midwives are represented can tell as much about the interpreter as about the midwives themselves, providing insight into the tensions regarding midwifery public policy during this period.

Like anthropologist Margaret MacDonald, I argue for a "more nuanced analysis" of midwifery representations (MacDonald, *At Work* 7-8) and recognition of the partiality of perspectives (24). I come to this analysis not only as a history scholar, but also as an Ontario midwife and activist whose life and work is reflected in portrayals of pre-regulation midwifery. This combination of perspectives gives me a particular lens through which to analyse representations of midwives. In critically examining the common representations of midwives, I am not implying that other scholars have "got it wrong." Rather, as time has passed since midwifery's transition from a grassroots movement to a regulated profession, it is possible to bring new perspectives to the understandings of midwives who practiced in the late twentieth century midwifery revival. I conclude by sharing a summary of findings from my own oral history research with Ontario pre-legislation midwives that adds to the literature that unsettles and complicates these dominant representations ("Alegal Midwives").

Ontario's *Midwifery Act* represented the first comprehensive regulatory framework for midwifery in the modern Canadian health care system (Eberts et al. 29-33; Government of Ontario). Aboriginal midwives were formally exempt from the legislation, enabling them to provide traditional midwifery services to Aboriginal communities and use the title Aboriginal Midwife (Couchie and Nabigon 48). Over the first twenty years of regulated midwifery, the number of Ontario registered midwives has grown over ten times, from approximately 65 midwives in 1994 to 700 in 2014 working in 100 clinics in urban, rural, and remote communities;

the number of midwife-attended births in Ontario has shown a parallel rise during this period from 18,00 to 240,000 (Weston 3). Midwifery is now regulated in most, yet not all, provinces and territories in Canada. Midwifery education has been established at seven Canadian universities at the baccalaureate level: the University of British Columbia; Mount Royal University in Alberta; the University of Manitoba; Laurentian, McMaster, and Ryerson Universities in Ontario; and L'Université du Québec à Trois-Rivières. Midwifery education also occurs in several programs based in Aboriginal communities: in Nunavut via Arctic College, in Nunavik through the Inuulitsvik Health Centre, and at the Tsi Non:we Ionnakeratstha Ona:grahsta' Birth Centre in Six Nations of the Grand River. In addition, bridging programs at Ryerson University in Toronto and a multi-jurisdictional program coordinated by the Canadian Midwifery Regulators Consortium have provided internationally educated midwives opportunities to qualify for practice in Canada (Association of Ontario Midwives; Canadian Association of Midwives; Canadian Midwifery Regulators Consortium).

Historical research into Canadian midwifery paralleled midwifery's modern practice renewal, supported by developments in the burgeoning field of women's social history. Beginning in the late 1970s, interdisciplinary researchers began to uncover evidence of longstanding Canadian practices of midwifery, both official and unofficial, that flourished in indigenous and immigrant communities prior to the rise of professionalized medicine and nursing (Benoit, "Midwives and Healers"; Benoit and Carroll; Biggs, "Case of the Missing Midwives"; Biggs, "Rethinking History"; Buckley; Epp, "Midwife-Healers"; Epp, *Mennonite Women*; Jasen; Laforce; Langford; Mason, "A History of Midwifery"; O'Neil and Kaufert). Researchers also documented diverse patterns of midwifery's uneven decline over the course of the twentieth century (Connor; Mitchinson 69-103; Oppenheimer; Rushing, "Market Explanations"). Midwifery in Canada in the late nineteenth and early twentieth centuries suffered an inability to grow and to establish itself, in contrast to the growing organizations which made medicine and nursing central to Canadian health care. Medicine claimed pregnancy and childbirth within its scope of practice and began to gain public favour, without being challenged by the organization and professionalization of midwives that occurred in many other countries. Geographic, linguistic, and cultural barriers are often cited as reasons why Canadian midwives did not organize and professionalize during this period. Despite limited persistence of midwifery in geographically remote regions and within distinct religious and cultural communities, midwifery had all but disappeared in Canada by mid-century (Biggs, "Rethinking History" 36).

Midwifery reappeared in Canada in the late twentieth century as a counter-practice to mainstream maternity care. Childbearing women dissatisfied with the predominance of childbirth technologies in postwar North American maternity care sought out "natural childbirth" alternatives that configured pregnancy as a normal healthy life event rather than pathological and potentially dangerous requiring medical interventions (Karmel; Thomas). Some women reclaimed the traditional practices of home birth and midwifery outside official health care as means to take control of their childbirth experiences and redefine technological and institutional practices that had come to dominate North American maternity care (Rothman, *In Labor* 78-110). Women with a range of political and philosophic perspectives were attracted to midwifery and home birth as alternatives to normative maternity care, including traditionalists with conservative family values, women from distinct religious communities, and feminists seeking reproductive control and empowerment (Klassen 63-96; Rothman, *In Labor* 100). Not only did dissatisfaction with mainstream maternity care stimulate interest in these childbirth alternatives, it also inspired some women to learn and practice midwifery outside the law (Barrington 43-5; Burtch 98-9; Kay et al.).

Consumer led home birth and midwifery movements were evident in western Canada, Ontario, and Quebec by the second half of the 1970s, inspired and informed by similar practices that emerged in the United States earlier in the decade (Barrington 34-8; Daviss, "Reforming Birth" 70-86). It is estimated that less than 200 midwives took up practice on the margins of official health care in Canada in the two decades prior to midwifery's legal reform (Barrington 13, 38; Burtch 19). Their training and legal status were varied. Some had formal education in international midwifery programs and nursing; others were self-trained or had apprentice training with family physicians or practicing midwives. Midwifery was defined as part of the practice of medicine in some provinces and not in others (Barrington 137-41; Burtch 158-89). Midwives in Ontario interpreted their status as "alegal," that is without legal status, in contrast to midwives in other parts of the country who were seen to be illegally practicing medicine without a license (Burtch 11).

As the first province to legally recognize midwifery, the Ontario midwifery revival garnered intense public interest and scrutiny by the media, government, medical and nursing professions, the international midwifery community, and academic researchers. The focus of academic attention centred on midwifery's outsider status and its transition from an unofficial practice to a legally recognized profession, largely from a social science perspective (Bourgeault, "The Evolution of the Social Science of Midwifery" 4-8). The voices of midwives are included in this scholarly work in two ways, both as the subjects of scholarly research (in works by Bourgeault; MacDonald; Nestel) and as researchers themselves engaged in developing a scholarship of their own profession (in works by Daviss; James; Sharpe; Van Wagner). Theoretical under-standings of midwifery and its practitioners are deeply entwined with historical and contemporary writings on midwifery in other North American settings (Bourgeault and Fynes, "Integrating Lay and Nurse-Midwifery"). Literature on midwifery's late twentieth century revival in North America highlights the formative influence of counterculture and feminist ideologies, portraying practitioners of the new midwifery pre-eminently as counterculture figures and later as feminists across a spectrum of feminist ideologies (Beckett and Hoffman 131).

THE COUNTERCULTURE MIDWIFE

Midwifery's renewal in late twentieth century North America is commonly attributed to the influence of progressive social move-ments of the sixties and seventies that challenged mainstream authority and institutions. Pre-legislation Ontario midwifery is typically portrayed as part of a North American grassroots, counterculture movement for childbirth reform. The social milieu of the counterculture provided a conducive environment for the emergence of childbirth practices that lay outside official health care. Home birth and female midwifery were seen to be compatible with counterculture ideals of self-sufficiency and traditional ways of living. The counterculture's valorization of the "natural" challenged medical constructs of the pregnant female body as mechanical and pathological by redefining childbirth as a healthy life event (Davies 13; De Vries 256-57; Lemke-Santangelo 82-85).

In the prolific body of "alternative birth literature"[1] that accompanied midwifery's modern renewal in the United States and later in Canada, midwifery is defined as a counterculture practice in opposition to medicine. Midwives' support of mothers in community-based, natural birth alternatives is typically posed as a radical challenge to institutionalized maternity care and medicine's impersonal and mechanistic management of childbirth. Advocates saw in these practices the opportunity to reclaim aspects of the childbirth experience seen to be lost in mainstream maternity care, such as humanism, respect for nature, and spirituality. American midwife Ina May Gaskin constructs female midwifery as a "revolutionary" counterculture practice honouring the sanctity of birth in her foundational text of the North American midwifery revival *Spiritual Midwifery*:

> The knowledge that each and every childbirth is a spiritual experience has been forgotten by too many people in the world today, especially in countries with high levels of technology. This book is revolutionary because it is our basic belief that the sacrament of birth belongs to the people and that it should not be usurped by a profit-oriented medical system.... We feel that returning the major responsibility for normal childbirth to well-trained midwives rather than have it rest with a predominately male and profit oriented medical establishment is a major advance in self-determination for women. (11)

In her 1975 critique of American childbirth, *Immaculate Deception*, American journalist Suzanne Arms contrasts midwifery's grounding in normal or natural birth with medicine's scientific interventionist stance:

> The science of obstetrics is a very recent development, a profession made necessary by the advance of civilization and its introduction of new problems into birth.... [T]he midwife begat the obstetrician, as it was the midwife who practiced for thousands of years in a world where birth was regarded as a natural and normal function of the human body.... She has merely had to attend nature and watch and protect the normal process from interference. It is out of respect for the natural process that the midwife has traditionally worked with only her hands and the simplest of tools....I call the midwife the protector of normal and the conscience of the doctor. (151-52)

Arms' claims to midwifery's superiority and her nostalgic interpretation of childbirth history rest on the binaries of female/male and nature/science that permeate narratives of midwifery's modern North American renewal. While female midwifery is seen to facilitate women's ability to give birth "naturally," male medical science is seen to subvert the natural process of childbirth.

Midwifery manuals written by American "lay" midwives that appeared in the 1970s and 1980s (for example, Baldwin; Davis; Gaskin; Lang) were formative reading for Ontario pre-legislation midwives (Allemang, "Alegal Midwives" 211-15; MacDonald, *At Work* 54-60). These texts played a key role in reinforcing this tension between nature and science and a gendered dichotomy of midwifery and medicine, as highlighted by medical statistician and childbirth consumer advocate David Stewart in his introductory remarks to American midwife Elizabeth Davis' *Guide for Midwifery: Heart and Hands*:

> Midwifery is an art, not a science; and childbirth is an experience, not an experiment.... Today's obstetrics is an attempt to apply science to a process that is beyond science—the process of childbirth. It tries to reduce to masculinely objective routines the management of a process that

is femininely subjective and which defies management. ...
Midwifery is an art; its basis, feeling and intuition. Midwifery is personal attunement by a caring professional. (vi)

This juxtaposition of caring midwifery against impersonal scientific medicine was formalized by social scientists and practitioners
of the new midwifery over the final decades of the twentieth century
into dichotomous models of care that influenced public policy
debates about midwifery (Bourgeault, *Push!* 149-187; Rothman,
In Labor 23-25; Sullivan and Weitz 68-79; Van Wagner, "With
Women" 2-4). American sociologist Robbie Davis-Floyd has
written extensively on dichotomous models for midwifery and
medicine, configuring midwifery as "wholistic" and medicine as
"technocratic" (*Birth* 154-186) and posing female intuition as a key
component to skillful midwifery practice (Davis-Floyd and Davis).

Essentialist and heteronormative representations of counterculture
midwives as wives and mothers figure prominently in accounts of
North American midwifery revivals (Lenskyj 9-13). In the dominant
representation of midwifery's renewal as a grassroots movement,
midwives are typically portrayed as mothers reclaiming the traditional practices of home birth and midwifery. Their motivations
to support other women in childbirth are tied to their personal
experiences of childbirth and becoming mothers. Midwives who
experienced medically managed birth are seen to be driven by personal feelings of dissatisfaction to assist other women to give birth
without technological interference, whereas those who experienced
natural births are seen to be inspired to share this transformative
experience (Barrington 42-43). In her popular guide for aspiring
midwives that remains in print today, Elizabeth Davis offers an
essentialist interpretation of the transformative potential of natural
birth for childbearing women and aspiring midwives:

The potent lesson of natural childbirth is the revelation of
essential feminine force. The experience of birthing calls
on a woman to shed her social skin and discover a definite
feminine power in flowing, accepting and surrendering to
natural forces. Ultimately, giving birth to her child will
transform her, renew her, strengthen her faith and deepen

her identity. Her ensuring change in perspective (so appropriate for becoming a loving mother) is revolutionary because it is antithetical to that of our outwardly focused, control oriented society.... [M]ost practical midwives are mothers who have experienced just such an "awakening" themselves. (2)

"Maternal nurturance" (MacDonald, *At Work* 60) is considered to have played a key role in women's suitability to become midwives and their pathways into practice. Midwifery is widely referred to in historic and contemporary writings as a "calling." It is conceptualized similarly to other forms of women's caring work, notably nursing and teaching, as a natural extension of women's domestic caring and healing roles (Abel and Nelson 11-22). Those suited to midwifery's calling are typically represented as mothers who embody exceptional caring qualities and who are dedicated to the feminine ideals of service and altruism, as described by Davis:

So evolves the practice of midwifery as an art of service—recognizing, responding and cooperating with natural forces.... The most common profile of the midwife is probably the mother with children (often home-born).... The service and self-sacrifice that are such a big part of midwifery cannot be overestimated.... In order for a person to stay with such demanding and responsible work, it should feel more like a calling. (6-7)

There is only muted acknowledgement that non-mothers could make suitable midwives. Similar hesitation is expressed about whether those who are formally trained as nurses or midwives could embody the exceptional caring qualities necessary to this "calling" (Arms 155-160).

In the first major publication documenting midwifery's modern emergence in Canada, Canadian journalist Eleanor Barrington similarly configures midwifery as a calling predicated on female caring and community. Mirroring the prolific American alternative birth literature, Barrington identifies motherhood and nurturance as key qualities for midwifery practice: "All that the midwives have in common is motherhood. The only prerequisites are life experience, quick intelligence, a giving personality, and a passion for birth" (41). She also ties midwives' personal childbirth experiences to their motivations to become midwives: "The provocations to learn midwifery are particular to individuals, but there are a few recurring themes among midwives' professional histories. The most obvious is the enduring impact of a very good, or very bad, [personal] birth experience" (42). Barrington expands the notion of a midwifery calling to incorporate neighbourliness, portraying midwives as chosen by other mothers in an informal network of women supporting one another in childbirth alternatives:

> The first "new midwives" emerged from among ... questioning parents. Mothers, who explored and experimented first for themselves, shared their newfound skills and experience with their neighbours. They gave birth at home, and whoever knew more offered help. Most were reticent to accept the title of midwife until it was thrust upon them by others. (13)

Jutta Mason's representation of the early Ontario midwifery community in her 1990 publication *The Trouble with Licensing Midwives* closely resembles Barrington's portrait of midwifery's informal female network of mothers helping other mothers. She describes the modern revival of midwifery as a "neighbourly venture, a gradually expanding net of womanly connections between friends" (7) where "the link between midwife and labouring woman lay in the shared experiences of being female and being mothers" (5). Mason draws parallels between the historical decline of the neighbour midwife as a non-scientific figure working in a distinct female "popular birth culture" under threat from a rising male medical profession with the midwife's modern emergence as a counterculture symbol for humanizing childbirth ("Midwifery in Canada" 122).

The heroic narrative of counterculture midwifery as a movement to humanize North American childbirth, while dominant, is not universal. Other interpretations of modern midwifery can be found in the media and the health professions literature that similarly portray an oppositional stance between midwifery and medicine, yet assert the superiority of medical science. Unofficial midwifery is portrayed as a dangerous, fringe movement of uneducated and irresponsible individuals (Taylor and Nesdoly 21-2). Concern about midwifery's outsider status is captured in the position statement of the College of Physicians and Surgeons of Ontario published in 1983 that warns against medical practitioners cooperating with unregulated practitioners to provide home birth care (5). Negative perceptions of midwifery in Canada were magnified by a series of Coroner's inquests and criminal prosecutions into the deaths of infants following midwife-attended births in the 1980s (Burtch 167-176). The publicity surrounding a high profile 1985 inquest into the death of baby Daniel Mc-Laughlin-Harris, born at home with midwives in Toronto, was prolific and embodies polarized representations of midwifery and medicine (Bourgeault *Push!* 107-15). Headlines in the Toronto press portray the tensions between the midwives and their supporters and the Crown and its medical experts, using terms such as "witch hunt" and a "battleground" of gender and of nature versus science (Ferguson G5; Hossie 14; Sweet G5; Tedesco 1; Van Wagner, "Women Organizing" 116). Comments made to the *Toronto Star* by Ontario Medical Association representative Dr. James Milligan reinforce the critique of Ontario pre-legislation midwives as unprepared and irresponsible: "For the sake of safety, [midwives] need to be trained and adhere to very high standards. At the moment, a lot of people call themselves midwives and they have virtually no training" (Sweet G6). In public policy debates about Ontario midwifery's legal recognition that followed the McLaughlin-Harris inquest, provincial nursing and medical organizations stated their position that midwifery was unnecessary in the formal health care system but that if it were to recognized, it should be structured as a hospital-based specialty of nursing under the supervision of medicine (Fynes 112-13, 118-120). This position stood in stark contrast to the autonomous, self-regulating profession that was promoted by Ontario midwifery professional and consumer organizations and subsequently recommended by the Ontario government's Task Force on the Implementation of Midwifery in Ontario (Bourgeault and Fynes, "Delivering Midwifery in Ontario" 242-44; Kaufman 100-03.).

THE FEMINIST MIDWIFE

Representations of midwives as feminists or women's health activists entered popular and scholarly writings of the North American midwifery revival with the evolution and diversification of second-wave feminism and the woman's health movement (Rushing, "Ideology" 57-60). Feminist representations, like those of the counterculture, define the "new" North American midwife by her female gender and her status as an outsider to mainstream maternity care and professionalized medicine. Despite early theories linking motherhood to women's oppression (for example, de Beauvoir 774-75; Firestone 238; Friedan 363-34), second-wave feminism politicized childbirth and mothering as sites for female empowerment and social justice (Rich 285-86; Umansky 132-158). With growing recognition of the personal and political significance of mothering in the lives of women, feminists embraced midwifery as a feminist issue. American sociologist Barbara Katz Rothman characterized midwifery as "feminist praxis," largely in reference to its woman-centred model of care that is aligned with feminist principles of female autonomy and bodily integrity (*Recreating Motherhood* 169).

The reclamation of midwifery as a nurturing female activity supporting the natural process of birth resonated across a spectrum of feminist ideologies (Adams and Bourgeault 84-87). Feminist perspectives on mothering and childbirth expanded and transformed the counterculture representations of home birth and midwifery that valorized essential femininity and nature. Feminism gave new meanings to the figure of the North American midwife that are both consistent with and divergent from the counterculture figure. Midwifery was embraced by feminists who accentuated gender differences and valorized women's nurturance, both as midwives and mothers. A maternal feminist midwife figure embodying traditional femininity was conflated with the traditional counterculture midwife. Elizabeth Davis' essentialist portrait of midwives as feminist "rebel" figures remains true to midwifery's countercultural roots while integrating a new maternal feminist perspective. Like Gaskin, Davis sees the everyday act of midwifery as inherently political, yet at an individual, rather than a structural, level:

She is a rebel and a female one at that! So like it, or not, the midwife these days has a decidedly political position. She is almost invariably typed feminist. This, because the potent lesson of natural childbirth is the revelation of essential feminist force…. Hence the midwife, essentially peace-loving guardian of the natural birth process, is thrown into political dichotomy for facilitating this awareness. This is an awkward position for many of the midwives I know. At most a midwife might consider herself an "evolutionary agent" (Timothy Leary's phrase) or feminist in the sense of furthering the individual, non-violent awakening of each women' spirituality. (2)

In contrast, a feminist midwife that conceptualized childbearing as integral to women's reproductive rights was seen to challenge the maternalist midwife figure (Rothman, *In Labor* 32). Those who embraced midwifery as form of social or political activism for women's reproductive control not only recognized the transformative potential of how women gave birth, but also their choice to be pregnant, including safe access to abortion and contraception (Van Wagner and Lee).

These dual representations of feminist midwives reflect tensions regarding essentialism and reproductive rights that are well documented in narratives about modern North American midwifery movements (Ruzek 197; Van Wagner, "Women Organizing" 117). In her analysis of North American midwifery, American sociologist Beth Rushing notes that modern practices of midwifery commonly embody a feminist ethic of care, even for midwives who do not overtly identify as feminist. Rushing uses the term "subtle feminism" to refer to the work of midwives who situate midwifery's women-centred philosophy at the level of the individual rather that at a structural level for political change ("Ideology" 57-60). Barrington observes that traditionalist midwives and their supporters increasingly embraced the feminist principles of reproductive control and empowerment, while rejecting women's reproductive right to abortion that had become a divisive issue in the Canadian midwifery movement (151-153). Midwives of diverse feminist orientations shared a common commitment to women's empowerment in childbirth, care that asserted the normalcy of birth, and women's autonomy to direct their own care (Sullivan and Weitz 60; Van Wagner, "With Women").

Historical theories of midwifery's past played a role in constructing and reinforcing the midwife as a feminist hero reclaiming normal birth. Feminist narratives of midwifery's demise and renewal provided inspiration to the fledgling late twentieth century midwifery movement by highlighting gender and professional rivalries with male medicine. Modern midwives working on the margins of official health care saw resonance in the proto-feminist historical figure of the powerful female healer struggling to resist the male medical takeover of childbirth, most prominently portrayed by Barbara Ehrenreich and Deidre English in their 1973 history of women healers, *Witches, Midwives and Nurses*. Ehrenreich and English paint midwifery's modern emergence as a reclamation of traditional female knowledge and resistance to hegemonic male medicine. Although *Witches, Midwives and Nurses* has been critiqued as polemical and unsubstantiated (Green 489-493), the dichotomy of skilled female midwifery and interventionist male medicine persists in historical and modern narratives of unofficial midwifery and continues to inform theories of North American midwifery's decline and renaissance.

The common narrative of the feminist midwife as an outsider to official care was used to both forward and to discredit North American midwifery, much like the counterculture midwife. The feminist midwife figure, however, was seen as a more vocal advocate of women's reproductive rights and critic of "medicalized" childbirth (Adams and Bourgeault 87). The linking of midwifery to reproductive rights, particularly abortion rights, adds a layer of complexity to the hero-villain binary of midwives by infusing a narrative of divisiveness within the midwifery community itself.

THE ASPIRING PROFESSIONAL

Literature written about the Ontario pre-legislation period is dominated by contested debates about the legal recognition of midwifery, both from within and outside the community of midwives and their supporters. The prolific body of popular and scholarly literature

ELIZABETH ALLEMANG

that accompanied the growth and development of the Ontario
midwifery movement accelerated at the end of the twentieth century
with the passage and enactment of the Ontario Midwifery Act.
These publications contribute another representation of midwives
that dominates the record of Ontario pre-legislation midwifery,
that of the aspiring professional. While there is some discussion
of midwifery's legal reform in other regions of Canada and the
United States (Burtch; Butter and Kay; Davis-Floyd and Johnson;
De Vries; De Vries and Barroso; Foley and Faircloth; Hough; Lay
and Dixon; Solares; Sullivan and Weitz 97-111), the discussion of
midwifery's professionalization is dominated by events in Ontario
given its unique status as the first province to legalize midwifery
in Canada. Attention from critics and supporters, particularly
in the field of social science, focuses on midwifery's transition
from a grassroots movement to a regulated profession. This was
a time of uncertainty and ambivalence for Ontario midwifery, as
a movement that arose as a counter-practice to normative maternity care was being shaped into a regulated profession. Early
accounts of the Ontario midwifery revival that were celebratory
of midwifery's growing popularity and acceptance as a legitimate
part of the health care system were increasingly overshadowed by
critiques that predicted midwifery's loss of autonomy and expertise
in normal birth with its integration into formal systems of health
care, education, and the law. Representations of midwives who
worked for legal reform shifted from heroic tales of their abilities
as skilled and effective lobbyists for childbirth reform (Adamson,
Briskin, and McPhail 176-190; Bourgeault, *Push!* 265-66) to
vilifying their motivations as self-interested and their impact as
undermining midwifery's counterculture roots in normal birth
and woman-centred care (Benoit, "Professionalizing Canadian
Midwifery"; Bourgeault, "Delivering Midwifery"; Burfoot; Daviss,
From Social Movement; Neilans; Paterson, "Ontario Midwives";
Paterson, "Feminizing Obstetrics"; Spoel and James). Class and
race analysis added to the critique of Ontario's professionalization,
highlighting the homogeneity of the Ontario midwifery revival as
a white, middle-class movement (Nelson 295-96; see Nestel; Van
Wagner, "Women Organizing" 115).

Barrington's *Midwifery is Catching* appeared in the early decades of the Canadian midwifery movement at a pivotal juncture of state, professional, and public interest in midwifery. The respectability of midwifery was under question given the predominance of professionalized medicine and nursing in the maternity care system and midwifery's roots outside official health care. Barrington's expressed intent was to promote midwifery as a legitimate maternity care profession. *Midwifery is Catching* has been influential in informing a lasting representation of who took up unregulated midwifery practice in Canada (Nestel, *Obstructed Labour* 23). Its portrayal of midwives' lives and their work is deeply embedded in subsequent research and writing on Canadian midwifery; the book has largely been seen as the authentic narrative of pre-legislation midwifery.

Midwifery is Catching's story of pre-legislation midwifery in Canada is celebratory and optimistic about the impact of professionalizing midwifery for humanizing maternity care. Barrington's account blends the narratives of midwives as counterculture mothers and feminist activists with a compelling portrait of midwives as highly capable and intelligent women to counter what she identifies as a series of common "Myths and Misconceptions" that characterize midwives as ill-prepared and irresponsible (16). She appeals to midwives' maturity, their privileged social position, and their educational status to bolster her argument for the social and legal acceptance of midwifery: "By 1980, the majority of midwives and their clients belonged to the middle class. Today's 'wise-woman' is likely to be about 35, raised in a suburb, and university educated" (16). Barrington concludes that, although there was "no prescribed career path" to midwifery, her "informal survey of a dozen practising midwives reveals a curious array of past lives: one actress, three nurses, two journalists, a teacher, an occupational therapist, a weaver, an X-ray technician, a massage therapist, and a bookkeeper" (41). She describes midwives as typically coming to midwifery as "a second career... that comes after post-secondary education, some other occupation, and usually parenthood" (16).

Barrington's uncritical analysis of Canadian pre-legislation midwifery as a movement of the well-educated middle class is a typical narrative that was used to advance the social and legal legitimization of midwifery in the early years of the midwifery revival. Following the publication of *Midwifery is Catching*, developments in feminist theory and practice contributed new critical perspectives about the universalizing women's experience that were relevant to midwifery practice revivals (Pierson). Growing recognition of the limitations of the midwifery community's ability to reflect and serve diverse women consolidated a discourse of homogeneity regarding midwives and the women they served. Critics from within and outside the Ontario midwifery movement highlighted the predominance of white, middle-class women as providers and recipients of care. The failure of pre-regulation midwifery to reflect the diversity of Ontario's population was variously used by social scientists, midwives, and their supporters to critique or to forward midwifery's legal recognition. Those who supported legal recognition asserted that midwifery's integration into the Ontario publicly funded health care system would improve accessibility for both childbearing women and midwifery practitioners (Van Wagner, "Why Legislation" 77-78). Others saw legal reform as a means for midwives to consolidate their privilege and reinforce exclusionary practices of the pre-legislation Ontario midwifery movement (see the works of Bourgeault and Nestel).

According to Margaret MacDonald, "resistance to biomedicine" played a key role in identity formation for Ontario midwives, in addition to the dominant narratives of "nature, tradition and home" (*At Work* 52-92). Midwives' engagement in political campaigns for legal reform is interpreted in contradictory and contested ways, reflecting ideological differences about the value of "mainstreaming" versus "disengaging" midwifery (Davis-Floyd and Johnson). Midwifery scholars and practitioners who viewed legislation as strengthening midwifery and improving women's access to childbirth alternatives interpret midwives' political activism favourably (Armstrong and Armstrong 27-28; Van Wagner, "Why Legislation"). Others, who saw midwifery's integration into official health care as undermining midwifery's autonomy and core values, interpret midwives' political involvement as incompatible with midwifery's political stance as an outsider to medicine and the law. Activist midwives' aspirations for "insider" status were interpreted as a move away from the "outsider" maternal counterculture midwife figure and the caring qualities it represented and toward a professional midwifery identity and medical model of childbirth (Davis-Floyd and Johnson, "Renegade Midwives" 447-468; De Vries; De Vries and Barroso; Mason, *Trouble with Licensing Midwives*; Sullivan and Weitz). Ontario midwife and scholar Betty-Anne Daviss, for example, notes that midwives interested in legal reform were more closely aligned with feminism as compared to the "radical fringe" that prioritized "spiritual enlightenment ("Reforming Birth" 81).

The binary of "counterculture midwives" and "state-employed midwives" underlying Mason's critique of midwifery regulation (*Trouble with Licensing* 1-3) mirrors a binary of "elite" and "non-elite" midwives that emerges as a dominant narrative in critical scholarship on the professionalization of Ontario midwifery. Bourgeault portrays the community of Ontario pre-legislation midwives as polarized by tensions about legal reform into a binary of urban political "elite" midwives allied with medicine and the state versus "other" or "non-elite" counterculture midwives working in partnership with childbearing women (Bourgeault and Fynes, "Delivering Midwifery in Ontario" 250; Bourgeault, *Push!* 262-266). Midwives in political leadership positions are portrayed as skilled lobbyists controlling midwifery's "professionalization project," which threatens to undermine midwifery's founding principles and autonomy from medicine and the state. This dichotomy of caring midwives versus political activist or aspiring professional midwives mirrors the gendered dichotomy of midwifery and medicine that infuses Ontario midwifery discourse. Whereas the political implications of midwives' daily work resisting and redefining mainstream maternity care was not seen to disrupt essentialist constructions of midwives and their motivations to practice, elite midwives' pursuit of a relationship with the system is portrayed as a potential threat to caring relationships with childbearing women (Benoit, "Uneasy Partners"; James; Sharpe).

Theories of elite Ontario midwives construct understandings that they were not only less caring, but also less maternal. Some writers suggest that elite midwives were able to devote themselves to midwifery's professionalization project because they had less domestic responsibilities or were childless (Bourgeault, *Push!* 82). Midwives' political activism and sexual orientation were conflated by some writers to bolster arguments about the dangers of midwifery's legal recognition to the essence of Ontario midwifery. *The Compleat Mother* was a grassroots childbirth and parenting magazine in the pre-legislation period. Editor Catherine Young authored a critical commentary on the legalization of midwifery in Ontario that equates regulated midwifery, male medicalized obstetrics, and what she saw as symbols of lesbian identity. Young describes politically engaged midwives as "a small cliquish body of obstetric midwives who now has [the Emperor] wearing hob-nailed boots," with reference to illusory power portrayed in the Hans Christian Andersen fairy tale "The Emperor's New Clothes" and a style of dress she associates with midwives that are not womanly enough. She reflects on midwifery's integration into the hospital system with the statement: "It will be a grim statistic when three Mamas go into a maternity hospital where the issue of control is wrestled from the hands of the female head nurse/male obstetrician into the iron hands of the lesbian midwife-in-charge" (4). Young is suggesting that midwives that are not womanly enough will reproduce the power dynamics of the medicalized system.

Alternative constructs of midwives' engagement in campaigns for legal reform also appear in midwifery literature. Midwives' participation in political work has been interpreted as strengthening midwifery's position in relation to medicine and the state. Some scholars link midwives' commitment to legal-change work to their deeply held beliefs that midwifery's autonomy, accessibility, and diversity would be strengthened by midwifery's integration into the publicly funded health care system (Ford and Van Wagner; Kaufman and Soderstrom; Tyson et al; Van Wagner, "Why Legislation"). As Canadian sociologist Brian Burtch and midwifery scholar Vicki Van Wagner argue, self-regulation was superior to the tenuous legal conditions of pre-legislation practice where midwifery was regulated by the criminal justice system rather than by recipients of care as forwarded by critics of regulation (Burtch 4; Van Wagner, "Why Legislation" 78). The impact of midwifery's legal recognition was also interpreted as enhancing midwifery's core values of caring and respect for normal birth by formalizing midwifery as a primary health care profession and infusing midwifery's values into mainstream maternity care (Kaufman; Van Wagner, "With Women").

Almost 20 years have passed since midwifery's transition from an alegal to legal practice in Ontario. Uncertainty about the future of midwifery that influenced the literature published at the threshold of midwifery's changing status in Ontario has diminished. Scholars, whose work gave voice to concern from both inside and outside midwifery about the loss of midwifery's distinct professional identity by its "incorporation" into the medically dominated health care system, have begun to publish accounts of Ontario midwifery as an international leader in creating a "birth model that works" (for example, MacDonald and Bourgeault 89-117). Scholars have increasingly offered less gendered and more nuanced and optimistic understandings of the ways in which political activism holds meaning for midwives (Daviss, "From Calling"). Midwives' interest in political and social change has been reinterpreted as more than a desire for personal gain and professional status. There is a growing body of literature on Ontario midwives' commitment to social justice and political change through participation in local and structural initiatives to improve health equity (Burton and Ariss). Most scholars have moved away from a simplistic analysis that opposes midwifery and medicine, increasingly using "hybridity" as an analytic tool. Some propose "hybrid" models for effective maternity care, which blends caring and science and blurring stereotypes (Davis-Floyd, "Daughter of Time" 705-710; Davis-Floyd et al., "Conclusion" 454; MacDonald "Postmodern Negotiations" 266-268).

CONCLUSION AND THE CONTRIBUTION OF ORAL HISTORY

Midwifery's interrupted history in Canada over much of the twentieth century means the concept of the midwife was not well understood when midwifery first reappeared in the 1970s. It is not surprising that public and professional reactions to midwives were polarized with midwifery's emergence as a grassroots childbirth reform movement on the margins of official health care. Narratives about midwifery's modern renewal in Ontario as part of a broader North American movement to reclaim midwifery and home birth as natural childbirth alternatives typically characterize midwives and physicians as ideological rivals (Paterson and Marshall). Early accounts of pre-legislation midwifery juxtapose midwifery as a caring female practice supporting normal birth against medicine's modern scientific paradigm and reliance on technology. Representations of midwives as counterculture mothers and as feminist activists both reflect and construct normative gender ideals. While these figures are most often valorized in midwifery literature and popular culture as gendered humanizing figures, their position outside official health care and their basis in tradition were also used by opponents to dismiss midwifery as a regressive practice and to forward the superiority of modern obstetrics. Midwives working outside formal health care and education were vilified in the public and professional press as dangerous practitioners lacking knowledge and skill in modern, scientific methods of managing childbirth.

As midwifery moved closer to legal reform in Ontario, critical perspectives on pre-legislation practice and regulation painted dichotomous portraits of midwives reminiscent of the binary of midwifery and medicine. Politically active midwives are variously portrayed as skilled lobbyists bringing needed reform to the Ontario maternity care system and as a self-interested elite undermining midwifery's foundational principles of women-centred care and normal birth by aligning midwifery with medicine and the state. The pre-legislation period of practice is often romanticized in critical scholarship on midwifery regulation as unmediated by medicine and the law, overlooking the harsh realities of practicing in a model of private practice and payment in tenuous legal conditions (Burtch 159). The social and racial homogeneity of Ontario pre-legislation midwifery as a white, middle-class movement was exposed by social scientists from within and outside the midwifery community. Midwives interested in legal reform are simultaneously represented as seeking to diversify the midwifery profession for recipients and providers of care and as consolidating their privilege by furthering their exclusionary practices. Accounts of tensions about midwifery's relationship to the feminist reproductive rights movement, specifically in relation to abortion rights, further reinforce the image of Ontario pre-legislation midwives as divided along lines of political change.

How midwives are represented is filtered through the lens of the interpreter and reflects social and policy debates about midwifery and about gender norms. The counterculture mother trope embodies a desire for humanizing childbirth through anti-science and technology by reclaiming traditions of female caregiving and support for the normal physiological process of childbirth. This trope is also used to condemn midwifery as unprofessional and marginal to mainstream health care. The feminist activist stereotype betrays ambivalence within the general culture about women's increasing politicization, especially in relation to reproductive justice and autonomy. Within the midwifery community, this figure could be viewed positively as an agent for social change in childbirth and negatively as undermining midwifery's outsider status and traditional roots. Those who supported midwifery and its legal recognition valorized the figure of the aspiring professional midwife, whereas those who opposed regulation vilified this figure as either a sell out or as a strident opportunist.

Another perspective on representations of midwives during the Canadian midwifery revival is emerging from recent work on the oral histories of pre-legislation midwives (Allemang; Davies; Lemay). To gain a fuller understanding of Ontario pre-legislation midwives beyond these counterculture and feminist stereotypes, I conducted oral history interviews with 21 midwives who practiced prior the enactment of midwifery legislation for my Master of Arts thesis research. My goals were to capture this transitory and significant period of Ontario midwifery history and to understand who the midwives were and their motivations to become and practice midwifery in an alegal context. The methods and findings are fully described elsewhere (Allemang). The findings are predominantly but not fully consistent with the portrayals of pre-legislation practitioners as white, middle-class, well-educated mothers. While my oral history research confirms the observation made by midwives and scholars that many who could choose to take on practice outside the protection of legal regulation did so from a relative position of privilege, it also shows how this characterization obscures important nuances and contradictions. The midwives' narratives reveal working-class backgrounds, single-parent families, high school dropouts, and those who faced challenges to fit into the counterculture midwifery movement because they were too young, too old, had no children, were male, or did not identify as heterosexual. Although midwifery discourse valorizes the "outsider" midwife figure, one third of the interviewees were formally trained midwives or nurses first, a proportion consistent with the pre-regulation population of Ontario midwives (Eberts et al. 72).

My oral history findings also reveal significant differences that stem from variation in the social era in which the midwives grew up, as well as their cultural backgrounds and personal ideologies. The ages of the interviewees varied by nearly 40 years, with the majority born in the postwar North American baby boom. Although most were influenced by the social era in which midwifery re-emerged and the counterculture and second-wave feminist movements, some of the interviewees who came of age during the interwar and postwar years recognized the impact of other forces that shaped their educational and professional opportunities. For example, several interviewees spoke of the centrality of their Mennonite cultural and religious heritage in shaping their lives as midwives.

Finding profound meaning and beauty in the normal physiologic process of birth and the caring work of midwifery was a persistent theme in the midwives' oral histories, uniting interviewees who were mothers and non-mothers, nurses and non-nurses, women and men. The strength of the midwives' attraction to the physiologic process of birth, sometimes from a young age, and their sense of the social meaning and importance of birth work infused the midwives' narratives of their inspirations. A strong sense of obligation to provide access to midwifery care for other women was expressed by many of the interviewees. Some recalled wanting to share their experiences of midwifery or home birth with other women, whereas others were motivated by difficult, often medicalized, childbirth experiences. Those who were unable to access the care they wanted for themselves from midwives remembered feeling galvanized to make home birth and midwifery services available to other women. Interviewees also related feelings of moral or ethical responsibility to respond to requests from childbearing women in their communities planning home births, with or without the presence of a reluctant midwife. For those who worked in formal maternity care systems, the desire for childbirth reform was a strong motivator, sometimes flowing from their experiences working as midwives internationally or their exposure to Canadian obstetrical practice in their work as nurses.

The midwives' narratives also challenge stereotypical portraits of pre-legislation midwives and why they did what they did. Rather than simply the rebel-outsiders portrayed in popular and scholarly literature, many sought to improve the safety of birth through alliances with physicians and by increasing their knowledge and skills through formal training. Some crossed continents and oceans to do so. The hesitation in midwifery revival literature about the suitability of formally trained midwives and nurses for the woman-centred care that defined counterculture midwifery is challenged by the experiences of interviewees who were nurses and passionate advocates for women's autonomy and choice in childbearing, both inside and outside health care institutions. The majority of interviewees also blurred the lines of caring work and political work in the pre-legislation Ontario context. Some were inspired through midwifery to become involved in political change projects, whereas others were inspired by politics to get involved in midwifery. But for most, caring and politics were both inherently part of the work of midwifery and they did not describe divisions between "different types" of midwives. These narratives complicate portraits of pre-regulation midwives as either grassroots nurturers or "elite" professionalizing activists.

Representations of midwives as heroes and villains still persist in the process of recognizing and integrating the profession of midwifery in Canada, still a relative newcomer to the maternity care system. These representations are often not fact-based; rather they reflect tensions about how childbirth is valued and conducted and about gender and childbirth. Understanding how and when these kinds of representations are at work is important for practitioners, policymakers, and scholars of midwifery to deconstruct their meanings and their relevance for childbirth reform.

[1]I use the term "alternative birth literature" to refer to popular and scholarly writings that critique the medical model of maternity and promote midwifery as a woman-centred alternative practice.

WORKS CITED

Abel, Emily K. and Margaret K. Nelson, eds. *Circles of Care: Work and Identity in Women's Lives*. Albany: State University of New York Press, 1990. Print.

Adams, Tracey L. and Ivy Lynn Bourgeault. "Feminism and Women's Health Professions in Ontario." *Women & Health* 38.4 (Jan. 2004): 73-90. Print.

Adamson, Nancy, Linda Briskin, and Margaret McPhail, eds. *Feminist Organizing for Change: The Contemporary Women's Movement in Canada*. Toronto: Oxford University Press, 1988. Print.

Allemang, Elizabeth. "Alegal Midwives: Oral History Narratives of Ontario Pre-Legislation Midwives." MA thesis. University of Toronto, 2013. Web. 10 Jan 2015.

Arms, Suzanne. *Immaculate Deception: A New Look at Women and Childbirth in America*. Boston: San Francisco Book Company/Houghton Mifflin Book, 1975. Print.

Armstrong, Pat and Hugh Armstrong. *Women, Privatization and Health Care Reform: The Ontario Case*. Toronto: National Network on Environments and Women's Health, 2006. Print.

Association of Ontario Midwives. *Become a Midwife*. Ontario Midwives, n.d. Web. 9 Jan. 2015.

Baldwin, Rahima. *Special Delivery: The Complete Guide to Informed Birth*. Millbrae, CA: Les Femmes, 1979. Print.

Barrington, Eleanor. *Midwifery is Catching*. Toronto: NC Press, 1985. Print.

Beckett, Katherine and Bruce Hoffman, "Challenging Medicine: Law, Resistance, and the Cultural Politics of Childbirth." *Law & Society Review* 39.1 (Mar. 2005): 125-70.

Benoit, Cecilia. "Midwives & Healers: The Newfoundland Experience." *Healthsharing* (Winter 1983): 22-6. Print.

Benoit, Cecilia. "Professionalizing Canadian Midwifery: Sociological Perspectives." Shroff 93-114.

Benoit, Cecilia. "Uneasy Partners: Midwives and their Clients." *The Canadian Journal of Sociology/Cahiers canadiens de sociologie* 12.3 (1987): 275-84. Print.

Benoit, Cecilia and Dena Carroll. "Aboriginal Midwifery in British

Columbia: A Narrative Untold." *A Persistent Spirit: Towards Understanding Aboriginal Health in British Columbia*. Ed. Peter H. Stephenson, Susan J. Elliott, and Leslie T. Foster. Victoria: Western Geographical Press, 1995. 223-48. Print.

Biggs, C. Lesley. "The Case of the Missing Midwives: A History of Midwifery in Ontario from 1795-1900." *Ontario History* 75.1 (Mar. 1983): 21-35. Print.

Biggs, C. Lesley. "Rethinking the History of Midwifery in Canada." Bourgeault, Benoit, and Davis-Floyd 17-45.

Bourgeault, Ivy Lynn. "Delivering Midwifery: An Examination of the Process and Outcome of the Incorporation of Midwifery in Ontario." Diss., University of Toronto, 1996. Print.

Bourgeault, Ivy Lynn. "The Evolution of the Social Science of Midwifery and Its Canadian Contributions. *Canadian Journal of Midwifery Research and Practice* 1.2 (2002): 4-8. Print.

Bourgeault, Ivy Lynn.*Push!: The Struggle for Midwifery in Ontario*. Montreal: McGill-Queen's University Press, 2006. Print.

Bourgeault, Ivy Lynn and Mary Fynes. "Delivering Midwifery in Ontario: How and Why Midwifery Was Integrated into the Provincial Health Care System." *Health and Canadian Society* 4.2 (1996/1997): 227-62. Print.

Bourgeault, Ivy Lynn and Mary Fynes. "Integrating Lay and Nurse-Midwifery into the U.S. and Canadian Health Care Systems." *Social Science & Medicine* 44.7 (1997): 1051-1063. Print.

Bourgeault, Ivy Lynn, Cecilia Benoit, and Robbie Davis-Floyd, eds. *Reconceiving Midwifery*. Montreal: McGill-Queen's University Press, 2004. Print.

Buckley, Suzann. "Ladies or Midwives? Efforts to Reduce Infant and Maternal Mortality." *A Not Unreasonable Claim: Women and Reform in Canada, 1880s-1920s*. Ed. Linda Kealey. Toronto: The Women's Press, 1979. 131-149. Print.

Burfoot, Annette. "Midwifery: An Appropriate(d) Symbol of Women's Reproductive Rights?" *Issues in Reproductive and Genetic Engineering* 4.2 (1991): 119-127. Print.

Burtch, Brian. *Trials of Labour: The Re-emergence of Midwifery*. Montreal and Kingston: McGill-Queen's University Press, 1994. Print.

Burton, Nadya and Rachel Ariss. "The Critical Social Voice of

Midwifery: Midwives in Ontario." *Canadian Journal of Midwifery Research and Practice* 8.1 (2009): 7-14. Print.

Butter, Irene H. and Bonnie J. Kay. "Self-certification in Lay Midwives' Organizations: A Vehicle for Professional Autonomy." *Social Science & Medicine* 30.12 (Jan. 1990): 1329-339. Print.

Canadian Association of Midwives. *Midwifery Education in Canada*. Canadian Association of Midwives, n.d. Web. 9 Jan. 2015.

Canadian Midwifery Regulators Consortium. *Bridging Education Programs*. Canadian Midwifery Regulators Consortium, 2011. Web 7 Jun. 2015.

College of Physicians and Surgeons of Ontario "Out-of-Hospital-Births." *The College Notes* (March 1983): 5. Print.

Connor, James T. H. "'Larger Fish to Catch Here than Midwives': Midwifery and the Medical Profession in Nineteenth-Century Ontario." *Caring and Curing: Historical Perspectives on Women and Healing in Canada*. Ed. Dianne Dodd and Deborah Graham. Ottawa: University of Ottawa Press, 1994. 103-134. Print.

Couchie, Carol and Herbert Nabigon. "A Path Towards Reclaiming Nishnawbe Birth Culture: Can the Midwifery Exemption Clause for Aboriginal Midwives Make a Difference?" Shroff 41-50.

Davies, Megan J. "Women Unafraid of Blood: Kootenay Midwives 1970-90." *BC Studies* 183 (2014): 11-36, 191. Print.

Davis, Elizabeth. *A Guide to Midwifery: Heart and Hands*. Santa Fe: John Muir Publications, 1981. Print.

Davis-Floyd, Robbie. *Birth as an American Rite of Passage*. Berkeley: University of California Press, 1992. Print.

Davis-Floyd, Robbie. "Daughter of Time: The Postmodern Midwife (Part I)." *Revista da Escola de Enfermagem da USP* 41.4 (2007): 705-710. Web. 20 May 2013.

Davis-Floyd, Robbie and Elizabeth Davis, "Intuition as Authoritative Knowledge in Midwifery and Home Birth." *Childbirth as Authoritative Knowledge: Cross Cultural Perspectives*. Ed. Robbie Davis-Floyd and Carolyn Sargent. Berkeley: University of California Press, 1997. 315-349. Print.

Davis-Floyd, Robbie and Christine Barbara Johnson, eds. *Mainstreaming Midwives: The Politics of Change*. New York: Routledge, 2006. Print.

Davis-Floyd, Robbie and Christine Barbara Johnson. "Renegade

Midwives: Assets or Liabilities?" 447-468.

Davis-Floyd, Robbie, Lesley Barclay, Betty-Anne Daviss, and Jan Tritten, eds. *Birth Models that Work*. Berkley: University of California Press, 2009. Print.

Davis-Floyd, Robbie, Lesley Barclay, Betty-Anne Daviss, and Jan Tritten. Conclusion. 441-462.

Daviss, Betty-Anne. "From Calling to Career: Keeping the Social Movement in the Professional Project." Davis Floyd and Johnson 413-446.

Daviss, Betty-Anne. *From Social Movement to Professional Project: Are We Throwing the Baby Out with the Bathwater*. MA thesis. Carlton University, 1999. Print.

Daviss, Betty-Anne. "Reforming Birth and (Re)Making Midwifery in North America." *Birth by Design: Pregnancy, Maternity Care, and Midwifery in North America and Europe*. Ed. Raymond G. De Vries, Cecilia Benoit, Edwin R. van Teijlingen, and Sirpa Wrede. New York: Routledge, 2001. 70-86. Print.

De Beauvoir, Simone. *The Second Sex*. Trans. and ed. H. M. Parshley. New York: Knopf, 1968. Print.

De Vries, Raymond G. *Regulating Birth: Midwives, Medicine and the Law*. Philadelphia: Temple University Press, 1985. Print.

De Vries, Raymond G. and R. Barroso, "Midwives among the Machines: Recreating Midwifery in the Late Twentieth Century." *Midwives, Society and Childbirth: Debates and Controversies in the Modern Period*. Ed. H. Marland and A. M. Rafferty. London: Routledge, 1996. 248-72. Print.

Eberts, Mary, Alan Schwartz, Rachel Edney, and Karyn Kaufman. *Report of the Task Force on the Implementation of Midwifery in Ontario*. Toronto: Queen's Printer of Ontario, 1987. Print.

Ehrenreich, Barbara and Deirdre English. *Witches, Midwives, and Nurses: A History of Women Healers*. New York: The Feminist Press, 1973. Print.

Epp, Marlene. *Mennonite Women: A History*. Winnipeg: University of Manitoba Press, 2008. Print.

Epp, Marlene. "Midwife-Healers in Canadian Mennonite Immigrant Communities: Women Who 'Made Things Right.'" *Histoire sociale/Social History* 40.80 (2007): 323-44. Print.

Ferguson, Derek. "Inquest was a Political Event from the Outset."

Toronto Star 16 Jul. 1985: G5, G8. Print.

Firestone, Shulamith. *The Dialectic of Sex*. 1970. New York: Bantam Books, 1971. Print.

Foley, Lara and Christopher A. Faircloth. "Medicine as Discursive Resource: Legitimation in the Work Narratives of Midwives." *Sociology of Health & Illness* 25.2 (2003): 165-84. Print.

Ford, Anne Rochon and Vicki Van Wagner. "Access to Midwifery: Reflections of the Ontario Equity Committee Experience." Bourgeault, Benoit, and Floyd 244-62.

Friedan, Betty. *The Feminine Mystique*. 1963. New York: Dell Publishing, 1975. Print.

Fynes, Mary Teresa. "The Legitimation of Midwifery in Ontario, 1960-1987." MA thesis. University of Toronto, 1994. Print.

Gaskin, Ina May. *Spiritual Midwifery*. Rev. ed. Summertown, TN: Book Publishing Company, 1978. Print.

Government of Ontario. Ontario Legislative Assembly. *Bill 56: An Act Respecting the Regulation of the Profession of Midwifery*. 35th Leg., 1st Sess. Toronto: Queen's Printer for Ontario, 1991.

Green, Monica H. "Gendering the History of Women's Healthcare." *Gender & History* 20.3 (November 2008): 487-518. Print.

Hough, Carolyn A. "'I'm Living My Politics': Legalizing and Licensing Direct-Entry Midwives in Iowa." Davis-Floyd and Johnson 347-374.

Hossie, Linda. "Opposing Philosophies at Issue in Midwifery Inquest." *The Globe and Mail* 1 July 1985: 14. Print.

James, Susan Gail. "With Woman: The Nature of the Midwifery Relation." Diss. University of Alberta, 1997. Print.

Jasen, Patricia. "Race, Culture, and the Colonization of Childbirth in Northern Canada," *Social History of Medicine* 10.3 (1997): 383-400. Print.

Karmel, Marjorie. *Thank you, Dr. Lamaze: A Mother's Experiences in Painless Childbirth*. Philadelphia: Lippincott, 1959. Print.

Kaufman, Karyn J. "The Introduction of Midwifery in Ontario, Canada." *Birth* 18.2 (1991): 100-03. Print.

Kaufman, Karyn and Bobbi Soderstrom. "Midwifery Education in Ontario: Its Origins, Operation, and the Impact on the Profession." Bourgeault, Benoit, and Davis-Floyd 188-203.

Kay, Bonnie J., Irene H. Butter, Deborah Chang, and Kathleen

Houlihan, "Women's Health and Social Change: The Case of Lay Midwives." *International Journal of Health Services* 18.2 (1988): 223-36. Print.

Klassen, Pamela E. *Blessed Events: Religion and Home Birth in America.* Princeton, NJ: Princeton University Press, 2001. Print.

Laforce, Hélène. "The Different Stages of Elimination of Midwives in Quebec." *Delivering Motherhood: Maternal Ideologies and Practices in the 19th and 20th Centuries.* Ed. Katherine Arnup, Andrée Lévesque, and Ruth Roach Pierson. New York: Routledge, 1990. 36-50. Print.

Lang, Raven. *Birth Book.* Paolo Alto, CA: Genesis Press, 1972. Print.

Langford, Nanci. "Childbirth on the Canadian Prairies, 1880-1930." *Journal of Historical Sociology* 8.3 (Sept. 1995): 278-302. Print.

Lay, Mary M. and Kerry Dixon. "Minnesota Direct-Entry Midwives: Achieving Legislative Success through Focusing on Families, Safety, and Women's Rights." Davis-Floyd and Johnson 231-87.

Lemay, Céline. *Être là: Étude du phénomène de la pratique sage-femme au Québec dans les années 1970-1980.* Ph.D. diss. Université de Montréal, 2007. Web. 10 Jan 2015.

Lemke-Santangelo, Gretchen. *Daughters of Aquarius: Women of the Sixties Counterculture.* Lawrence, KS: University Press of Kansas, 2009. Print.

Lenskyj, Helen. "A 'Natural' Calling? Issues of Choice and Diversity for Midwives." Unpublished paper. University of Toronto, 1996: 1-15. Print. Used with permission of the author.

MacDonald, Margaret. *At Work in the Field of Birth: Midwifery Narratives of Nature, Tradition, and Home.* Nashville: Vanderbilt University Press, 2007. Print.

MacDonald, Margaret. "Postmodern Negotiations with Medical Technology: The Role of Midwifery Clients in the New Midwifery in Canada," *Medical Anthropology* 20.2/3 (2001): 245-276. Print.

MacDonald, Margaret E. and Ivy Lynn Bourgeault. "The Ontario Midwifery Model of Care." Davis-Floyd, Barclay, Daviss, and Tritten 89-117.

Mason, Jutta. "A History of Midwifery in Canada." Appen. 1 *Report of the Task Force on the Implementation of Midwifery in Ontario.* Eberts, Schwartz, Edney, and Kaufman. 195-232. Print.

Mason, Jutta. "Midwifery in Canada." *The Midwife Challenge*. Ed. Sheila Kitzinger. London: Pandora Press, 1988. 99-129.

Mason, Jutta. *The Trouble with Licensing Midwives*. Ottawa: Canadian Research Institute for the Advancement of Women, 1990. Print.

Mitchinson, Wendy. *Giving Birth in Canada, 1900-1950*. Toronto: University of Toronto Press, 2002. Print.

Neilans, Mary. "Midwifery: From Recognition to Regulation, The Perils of Government Intervention." *Healthsharing* 13.2 (1992): 27-9. Print.

Nelson, Margaret K. "Working-Class Women, Middle-Class Women, and Models of Childbirth." *Social Problems* 30.3 (Feb. 1983): 284-297. Print.

Nestel, Sheryl. "The Boundaries of Professional Belonging: How Race Has Shaped the Re-emergence of Midwifery in Ontario." Bourgeault, Benoit, and Davis-Floyd 287-305.

Nestel, Sheryl. "Delivering Subjects: Race, Space, and the Emergence of Legalized Midwifery in Ontario," *Canadian Journal of Law and Society/Revue canadienne droit et société* 15.2 (2000): 187-215. Print.

Nestel, Sheryl. "A New Profession to the White Population in Canada: Ontario Midwifery and the Politics of Race." *Health and Canadian Society/Santé et société canadienne* 4.2 (1996/97): 315-41. Print.

Nestel, Sheryl. *Obstructed Labour: Race and Gender in the Re-emergence of Midwifery*. Vancouver: UBC Press, 2006. Print.

Nestel, Sheryl. "'Other' Mothers: Race and Representation in Natural Childbirth." *Resources for Feminist Research/Documentation sur la recherche féministe* 23.4 (1994/1995): 5-19. Print.

O'Neil, John and Patricia Kaufert. "Irniktakpunga! Sex Determination and the Inuit Struggle for Birthing Rights in Northern Canada." *Conceiving the New World Order*. Ed. Faye D. Ginsberg and Rayna Rapp. Berkeley: University of California Press, 1995. 59-73. Print.

Oppenheimer, Jo. "Childbirth in Ontario: The Transition from Home to Hospital in the Early Twentieth Century." *Ontario History* 75.1 (Spring 1983): 36-60. Print.

Paterson, Stephanie. "Feminizing Obstetrics or Medicalizing Midwifery? The Discursive Constitution of Midwifery in Ontario, Canada." *Critical Policy Studies* 4.2 (Jul. 2010): 127-45. Print.

Paterson, Stephanie. "Ontario Midwives: Reflections on a Decade of Regulated Midwifery." *Canadian Women's Studies/les cahiers de la femme* 24.1 (2004): 153-57. Print.

Paterson, Stephanie and Cherry Marshall, "Framing the New Midwifery: Media Narratives in Ontario and Quebec during the 1980s and 1990s." *Journal of Canadian Studies/Revue d'études canadiennes* 45.3 (Fall 2011); 82-107. Print.

Pierson, Ruth Roach. "The Mainstream Women's Movement and the Politics of Difference." *Canadian Women's Issues. Volume I: Strong Voices*. Ed. Ruth Roach Pierson, Marjorie Griffin Cohen, Paula Bourne, and Philinda Masters. Toronto: James Lorimer & Company, 1993. 186-214. Print.

Rich, Adrienne. *Of Woman Born: Motherhood as Experience and Institution*. 1976. New York: W. W. Norton, 1986. Print.

Rothman, Barbara Katz. *In Labor: Women and Power in the Birthplace*. 1982. New York: W. W. Norton, 1991. Print.

Rothman, Barbara Katz. *Recreating Motherhood*. New York: W. W. Norton, 1989. Print.

Rushing, Beth. "Ideology in the Reemergence of North American Midwifery." *Work and Occupations* 21.3 (1993): 46-67. Print.

Rushing, Beth. "Market Explanations for Occupational Power: The Decline of Midwifery in Canada." *American Review of Canadian Studies* 21.1 (1991): 7-27. Print.

Ruzek, Sheryl Burt. *The Women's Health Movement: Feminist Alternatives to Medical Control*. New York: Praeger, 1978. Print.

Sharpe, Mary. "*Intimate Business: Woman-Midwife Relationships in Ontario, Canada*." Diss. University of Toronto, 2004. Print.

Shroff, Farah M., ed. *The New Midwifery: Reflections on Renaissance and Regulation*. Toronto: Women's Press, 1997. Print.

Solares, Allan. "The Key to Keeping Midwifery Alive in the 1990s." *Midwifery Today* 14 (1990): 30-1, 39. Print.

Spoel, Philippa and Susan James, "Negotiating Public and Professional Interests: A Rhetorical Analysis of the Debate Concerning the Regulation of Midwifery in Ontario, Canada." *Journal of Medical Humanities* 27.3 (Sept. 2006): 167–86. Print.

Sullivan, Deborah A. and Rose Weitz. *Labor Pains: Modern Midwives and Home Birth*. New Haven, CT: Yale University Press, 1988. Print.

Sweet, Lois. "No Easy Answers for the Political Battle." *Toronto Star* 16 Jul. 1985: G5, G6. Print.

Taylor, D. Wayne and Faith Nesdoly. "Midwifery—From Parasite to Partner in the Ontario Health Care System." *Health Manpower Management* 20.5 (1994): 18-26. Print.

Tedesco, Teresa. "Inquest Called Political, Make Midwifery Legal Coroner's Panel Urges: Inquest Called Political Battleground." *The Globe and Mail* 18 Jul. 1985: 1, 2. Print.

Thomas, M. *Post-War Mothers: Childbirth Letters to Grantly Dick-Read, 1946-56*. Rochester, NY: University of Rochester Press, 1997. Print.

Tyson, Holliday, Anne Nixon, Arlene Vandersloot, and Kate Hughes. "The Re-emergence and Professionalization of Midwifery in Ontario, Canada." *Issues in Midwifery*. Ed. Tricia Murphy-Black. Edinburgh, UK: Churchill Livingstone, 1995. 163-75. Print.

Umansky, Lauri. *Motherhood Reconceived: Feminism and the Legacies of the Sixties*. New York: New York University Press, 1996. Print.

Van Wagner, Vicki. "Why Legislation? Using Regulation to Strengthen Midwifery." Bourgeault, Benoit, and Davis-Floyd 71-90.

Van Wagner, Vicki. "With Women: Community Midwifery in Ontario." MA thesis. York University, 1991. Print.

Van Wagner, Vicki. "Women Organizing for Midwifery in Ontario." *Resources for Feminist Research/Documentation sur la recherche feministe* 17.3 (1988): 115-18. Print.

Van Wagner, Vicki and Bob Lee. "Principles into Practice: An Activist Vision of Feminist Reproductive Health Care." *The Future of Human Reproduction*. Ed. Christine Overall. Toronto: The Women's Press, 1989. 238-58. Print.

Weston, Lisa. "Message from the President: Passion and Perseverance." *Association of Ontario Midwives 2013 Annual Report* Ontario Midwives, n.d. 3. Web. 9 Jan. 2015.

Young, Catherine. no title. *The Compleat Mother* Summer 1994: 4. Print.

Spacemaking and Midwifery

With, Within, Without

Out beyond ideas of wrongdoing and rightdoing, there is a field. I will meet you there. —Rumi (36)

THIS CHAPTER FOCUSES ON A PARTICULAR realm of tocology (the study of birth) expressed through topology (the study of space). It explores some meanings that the phenomenon and treatment of "space" hold for the woman, the midwife, and their relationship during pregnancy, birth, and the postpartum. It navigates the interior and exterior landscape, the interplay between the tangible and intangible. And it describes how midwives and women are co-creators of a "precreative" space in this ambience. Drawing from literature that examines woman-midwife relationships, relational aesthetics, institutional ethnography, and urban and feminist theory, the chapter examines spacemaking from the personal to the community, through the schema of "with," "within," and "without."

We start with a brief overview of Ontario midwifery, the context of our discussion, with notes on the history and the model of midwifery care. We then move to notions of space, place, and spacemaking in places of birth and places where midwifery care is provided: the home, the clinic, the hospital or institution, and the birthing centre. We reflect how actions and representations within these spaces may either underpin or undermine midwifery philosophy and the midwife's promotion and protection of it. And then we consider the effect of the presence of a clinic and a birth centre on its neighbourhood.

LIMITATIONS

This paper emerges from experiences with the Ontario model of midwifery and may not be generalizable to the ways space is experienced in other models of maternity care, locally or globally. We explore "at-homeness" but recognize that many women have no home; their lives are transitional, or they may feel they don't belong to a neighbourhood. Throughout, we speak of "women," yet acknowledge that this language is not inclusive of those who also give birth but do not identify as women. Furthermore, midwives herein have been written as women, though at the time of writing there is one registered midwife in Ontario who is male and perhaps others who do not identify as women. What we put in this paper is partial, reflective and suggestive rather than definitive.

BACKGROUND

There was a long history of many generations of women helping women with their births on this land now called Ontario. Traditionally, neighbour women or lay midwives working within their communities were specially chosen and respected as the primary helpers at births. As well, numerous women in Ontario, over the years, out of choice or necessity, birthed alone.

The agency of lay midwives in Ontario was disturbed by the gradual medical takeover of birth and by the transportation of women to centres where hospital deliveries and the possibility of anaesthesia and instruments existed. (This practice continues to be disruptive and destructive to the personal and family lives of Aboriginal pregnant women in the far north who, weeks before the birth, are transported to medical centres far away.)

Women's options for choice of caregiver at birth were then largely limited to male physicians and the choice of place to the hospital. The work of women involved in birthing and reproduction was considered illegal or dangerous. This framing became a means of suppressing and discrediting midwives, who were occasionally objects of persecutions and inquests. In the late nineteenth century, doctors began attending births in larger numbers; by

1935, half of the births in Ontario took place in hospitals and by 1960, practically all. Home births were occasionally attended by Aboriginal or nurse midwives, especially in the north or in rural areas where physician services were scarce; however, within two or three generations, from 1920–1960, midwife-attended births had almost completely disappeared in Ontario.

Women began to critique the medicalization of childbirth in the 1950s, and by the 1970s the women's movement was strongly involved in education about reproduction and birthing. Women worked alegally and illegally to help one another. They struggled to obtain safe abortions and to empower choice over place of birth. Among the sites of political action were childbirth classes, breastfeeding support groups, and women's health groups. In late 1970s and 1980s Ontario, there was a renaissance of lay midwives who were involved in these activities. Women began to request home births of their physicians.

In the early 1970s, a small number of family physicians were still attending home births, usually assisted by nurses from the Victoria Order of Nurses (VON). Along with the service of the VON at the birth, women planning homebirths were provided with their supplies and with a week's homecare help. In 1976, government funding for the VON and related services were discontinued as an "unnecessary" expense. A group of parents and professionals then created the Home Birth Task Force to protest this action. Home birth had become popular as a reaction to restrictive policies of hospitals, where babies were often delivered with instruments in cold rooms and were immediately separated from their mothers. A growing understanding of the importance to the baby of gentle birthing practices and the infant's need for continuous nurturing contact with his/her mother inspired this group. Without the VON, the new need for assistants to physicians at home births was met by women aspiring to become midwives. These lay midwives had found a gap in the health care system that allowed them to grow and organize, and along with significant consumer support and support of many legislators, regulation of midwifery took place in 1991. Ironically, this process initially excluded many racialized foreign-trained midwives who, in the absence of midwifery regulation, had often found work as labour and delivery nurses (Nestel

24). The *Ontario Midwifery Act* of 1991 supports a model that purportedly allows the midwife the maximum space to work her craft, reflecting what she would wish for the parturient woman: autonomy, funded services, collegial and professional support, respect, and acknowledgement.

This model places the woman and her baby at the centre of care and recognizes that family members and friends important to the woman are her chief supporters. She is cared for by a small number of midwives whom she knows and is offered a choice of birthing place: hospital, home, or birth centre. The midwife is available for long visits and has time for clinical tasks and time to develop a relationship with her client. Ideally, the woman's story—her primary narrative—is allowed to unfold, not dominated by the clinical agenda of the caregiver.

SPACE AND PLACE

The space and place within which midwifery practice occurs inevitably shape the nature of that practice.
—Athena Hammond et al. (277)

The physical nature of place is influenced by the intangible affective quality of space. The notion of space represents both physical and discursive constructions. According to Ivy Bourgeault et al., it "imparts symbolic importance as a site of meaning-making and identity construction" (583). Deborah Davis and Kim Walker describe spaces both as "physical locations such as home or hospital" and as "specific conceptual arrangements such as the discursive fields constituting medicine and the obstetrical hospital" (379). It is the interplay of material and intrinsic value that makes space and imparts meaning: "If place is where experience occurs, then space is where [people] are guided and shaped into the meanings that we create for them" (Rowles 27).

Michel Foucault proposes the multi-layered, liminal spaces of heterotopias, while Norma Tracey describes "precreative space" as the psychic space that precedes new life. "Space" is a geometric variable that may impact activity patterns, whereas "place" is recognized as more than a physical setting—a "container for health and health care activities" and a set of "situated" social dynamics (Poland et al.).

Urban theorist Jane Jacobs (*Dark Age* and *Death and Life*) concerns herself with the ways in which space and place make neighbourhoods languish or thrive. "Placemaking" can be described as philosophy and process, "both an overarching idea and a hands-on tool for improving a neighbourhood, city, or region" (PPS: Project for Public Spaces). This concept, together with the concept of midwives "arranging the setting" (Sharpe *Intimate Business* 128), has inspired the concept of "spacemaking" for this paper. Spacemaking, then, we loosely define as an attention to space as an intention to improve and inspire relationships among individuals or members of a community.

In *The Poetics of Space*, Gaston Bachelard says that a poet needs a safe and secure space where inspirational images are available. As midwives, we wish that the realm of possibilities for the parturient women could be as sacred as poetic space. It is the newness of each woman's pregnancy and birth that midwives wish to support and celebrate, the creation of a new poem on an ancient theme.

In the literature on space and place, the concept of "ontology," the study of the nature of being, appears frequently. Andrew Moore et al. describe "ontological security" as a feeling experienced by patients of trust that they will be cared for as a result of the staff's integrity in their work (155). Bachelard, in deriding the "ontological determination" of fixed adverbs of space such as "here and there," suggests that "the terms 'inside' and 'outside' pose problems of metaphysical anthropology that are not symmetrical" (215). Here we explore some alternative meanings for "with," "within," and "without." We join midwife Susan James in seeing "with" as a companion word, suggestive of being accompanied in a space—"with woman," "with child" (James 20). "With" can be considered philosophically as a container for the co-existence of the micro ("within") and the macro ("without"). "Within" here represents the psychosocial space inside the woman or practitioner or between woman and practitioner. "Without" here infers "outside the clinic" and alludes also to what is unseen and not accessible or experienced (James).

WITH

Begin from where we are located bodily.
—Dorothy E. Smith ("Women's Perspective" 29)

"With" evokes the middle space, a step outside from my "within" space to where I brush, entangle, and merge "with" others—shared space, bringing together the private and the public. This space is negotiated with the particularity of the owners of the space as well as with their construct of the space, whether intentional or not. Tangible objects and images play a part as individuals derive meaning from their personal context. This is the space that midwives endeavour to enter with women; it is a space where the physically constructed place and its representations of birth interact with notions and experiences of birth. The way the midwife arranges the setting where she meets with a woman—the ambience she creates—can bring a subtle and intentionally designed (perhaps even propagandic) influence to bear on the woman's understanding of pregnancy and birth. While the choice of place of birth can be a matter of preference, convenience, or circumstance, it can also be political (Davis and Walker 378). It is also a site where women can assert their autonomy and play out their resistance to the culturally dominant place of birth, the hospital (Bourgeault et al. 585; Difilippo). In the way one uses a space or enters, one can make a choice or resist something else.

The Home

Bachelard sets out to show that the home, *la maison*, is "one of the greatest powers of integration for the thoughts, memories, and dreams of mankind" (6). Bachelard uses the home as a tool for the analysis of the human soul and writes of homes being "in us as much as we are in them" (Bachelard xxxvii). Midwives appreciate attending home births; they are guests in the woman's home, privileged to be there, welcomed into the woman's experience. "Nidation," or "nesting," the process by which new life nestles into the endometrium several days after fertilization, is also evocative of place, of home. The home is where cooking, sleeping, lovemaking, and so much of the contextual and intimate detail of life occurs; it is also the space where economic or social circumstances are reflected through colour, texture, objects, and art—or starkness. Home birth celebrates the particular and is an antidote to the homogenizing, often flattening, effect of an institution setting. Home is usually the woman's space. Nonetheless, when the midwife enters her client's home, she brings her equipment, her physical presence, and also perhaps those of her student and, later, the second midwife. The way they occupy the home space—whether they sit or stand, how they move, closer, farther away, what functions they perform and when, how they might displace or acknowledge others—are all part of a delicate dance that requires attention.

The oxygen, the anti-hemorrhagic drugs, the birth instruments, and other equipment can be comforting reminders of attention to safety and the practical necessities of birth or they could be alarming signs of "what might happen." Some women may quietly resist their caregivers' chosen setting in a spot with light and equipment waiting and choose to give birth in the dark by the stairs or in a closet. Or midwives may follow the woman around with their birth instruments until the woman settles into her chosen space to birth. Niles Newton speaks of the inhibiting effect of disturbances on the birthing hormone, oxytocin (Newton et al. 375). An important role for the midwife is to assist in finding and supporting the woman's preferred spatial conditions that will best allow her body's natural processes to take place.

The Clinic

Midwives pay great attention to the details in their practice setting, developing, creating, and embellishing their clinic spaces to meet their functional needs and the possible needs of a diverse clientele. They express the importance of the setting being homey, comfortable, warm, and inviting—a space where women can feel relaxed and at ease. To address the more conservative elements in a neighbourhood, to help women feel safe during prenatal and postpartum care, the clinic may need to appropriate the landscape of a medical setting—and seem extremely professional. Like any person who comes into a space, consumers of midwifery care "read a room" (Bachelard 38). Settings where women and midwives meet may or may not relate to the woman's context. Representations of women and birthing need to be inclusive of children's rights, disabilities, and diverse sexual identities. The midwife herself is contextualized within the clinic, with its multiplicity of meanings and interpretations of displayed objects and images, and with representations of diversity, inclusion, and perhaps even unintended cultural appropriation present. For example, representations of hill-tribe mothers in an urban midwifery practice may not be appropriate to a user who does not recognize these images as part of her context—"not my community, not my experience." Even well-intentioned images or decor may present as problematic in relation to a diverse clientele and the values, tastes, and sensibilities of women and their supporters. Images that are too explicit can become generalities and, for that reason, block the imagination—"We've seen, we've understood, we've spoken. Everything is settled" (Bachelard 121). We wonder how a space might remain flexible and leave a space in the canvas for each woman to illustrate. It is not the midwives' space; it is a site of interaction, a public space for private matters.

Midwives can further extend the invitation to women. Midwives can engage in strategies such as arranging more home visits for multiparous women who find it difficult to travel; reserving spaces for late-to-care women; and offering clinic births for uninsured women who do not wish to birth at home, but would otherwise face hospital fees, and connecting them with institutions that have supportive policies for their care (Burton and Ariss). Many midwives engage in neighbourhood outreach work (infiltrating other spaces) at community centres, detention centres, teenage centres, immigrant women's centres, educational institutions, and places of religious worship, as well as in the media. These are important features of spacemaking in midwifery—making room for diverse and vulnerable populations, racial or linguistic minorities. Spatial justice is further supported by policies that recruit and educate midwives of diverse cultural backgrounds and linguistic competencies.

The Hospital / Institution

Since approximately 81 percent of midwife-led births in Ontario currently occur in hospital, this setting and the interprofessional relationships developed there are central to the midwife's work.

The hospital was instituted as a birthing space in North America in the early twentieth century to provide access to anesthesia and instrument-assisted births and with an assumption that hospitals offered the space with the safest and best care. Philosopher Paul Ricoeur has suggested that the aim of a just institution is to support "living well" and that this aim is supported by a "bond of common mores and not that of constraining rules" (Ricoeur 32). It would seem, then, that the ideal institutional birthing space would function on the basis of an agreed-upon ethos, principles, and philosophies that would help women and their babies to "live well." The way we define "living well" is of course mitigated by differing perspectives and views of health, safety, and risk: "The fact that the aim of living well encompasses the sense of justice is implied in the very notion of the other" (Ricoeur 32). Welcoming the other has been attempted in the pervasive transformation of sterile hospital delivery rooms to homelike bedroom spaces with curtains, wallpaper, and sofa chairs. Nonetheless, new technical artifacts enter the space, for example, the electronic fetal monitor and the computer.

Foucault is concerned about the effect on personal freedom of surveillance in an institution, the way it affects spatial justice, and the resulting desire to seek out other spaces. He deconstructs the emergence of the institution as an inquiry into the power and knowledge dynamics that accompany medicine into the spaces it governs. Odent, in analysing the geography of birth that surrounds modern obstetrics, goes as far as to express concern for the very future of humanity. He suggests that health is shaped during the primal period of labour and childbirth, and he is concerned that the space for this primal period is being constricted by increasing medical management and intervention. Midwife Brandeis echoes this concern: "I fear that so much of the charting impacts quality of care.... [I]t took up so much space [but now it is becoming] antithetical to care with women, and yet the system is moving more in the direction of 'computer-centred care.'"

The integration of midwives into hospital spaces was a great triumph of midwifery regulation yet it continues to provide significant challenges. Midwives bring the woman-centred model to the hospital and participate in the disruption of institutional habits.

"We have a really pivotal, important role to play in maternity care and we need to get into leadership positions," Carol Cameron says. "A midwife should be the director in a hospital" (qtd. in AOM). As clinical manager at the childbirth centre at a large hospital, she has helped reduce cesarean rates (AOM). Midwives could continue to strive to recognize and mitigate the effect of power relations in institutional settings and work toward resisting being drawn into them.

Texts

The increasing amount of complex and difficult material that midwives need to discuss and explore with their clients, and the items on the prenatal forms, drive the agenda of the prenatal visits.

—Christine Sternberg

Midwifery space is structured with contrasting chronologies of time (Foucault 7). On the one hand, records and charts are an "archiving" of the birth space, with frequent entries and the accumulation of data and evidence. On the other hand, the midwifery space is also temporal, with "immediate knowledge" being discovered during the time with the woman. The medical record is a necessary "legal document" predicated on the potential for lawsuits and litigation. Yet the items on the prenatal forms can crowd out the woman's story. Midwives need to actively listen to women's stories and continue to seek ways to keep pathways open, to try to create spaces for their clients' agendas and for themselves, spaces where strength is built: "A revolution that does not produce a new space has not realized its full potential ... but has merely changed ideological superstructures, institutions or political apparatuses" (Lefebvre 54).

Dorothy Smith ("The Relations") helps us to look at invisible relations of ruling that exist in institutional settings and in textual representations. Special attention is needed, she says, to recover a measure of freedom to coexist with these texts. In *Making Gray Gold*, Timothy Diamond draws attention to the gaps between accounts that are produced textually and off-the-page accounts of the care of elders—the care that is not captured in the text or or does not find a place on the chart. "If it wasn't charted, it didn't happen," he writes. "But much more happened than got charted" (137). Marginalia, writing that occurs outside prescribed spaces, can be considered a rejection of homogenization. Far from diminishing the primacy of the text, marginalia enhance the text with valued stories about interaction with it, as Heather Jackson recounts in her book *Marginalia: Readers Writing in Books* (15). Midwives might add to their notes spontaneous reflections such as: "The siblings tumble over the bed ... searching to grasp the baby's tiny hand, bringing the baby little gifts" or "The grandmother kneels down on her one good knee to deliver the placenta" (Sharpe, *Intimate Business* 367).

Midwives also make space for reproductive justice by attending to whether particular language widens or restricts space. Midwives have worked in their practices to shift language, to resist formulations that are not liberatory for women. Even if the language of texts and medical forms may be somewhat restricting within the medical norm of birth, such forms can be freeing in that they provide order and context and serve to communicate among caregivers information about care needed and care provided. Certainly, they preserve a record or history of care that may be valued by the woman, her child, and their descendants. If the space is infused with medical terms such as "fundus," "umbilicus," or "quadrant," midwives may unwittingly exclude the woman from a sense of sharing or belonging in the clinic space. For a midwife whose mandate it is to explain and inform, is it appropriate to use a "foreign coded language" with her client? (Sharpe, *Intimate Business* 269). If practitioners refer to women as being "high risk," as having "an inadequate pelvis" or a "lazy uterus," "they present a view of the world, and the place of women in it, that imposes a certain set of values and that assumes that they, as scientists, can step back and make judgments separate from the objects and systems they study" (Kitzinger 55). The way midwives refer to the spaces where they work can similarly convey a range of messages related to their inclusiveness. Consider the nuances, for example, of the term "practice" or "community midwives" as compared to "clinic" or "hospital."

Midwives' use of an institution and institutional requirements for obstetrical care could avoid these pitfalls and do as much as possible to foster "living well" for all concerned in the birthing environment. Perhaps a complete paradigm shift is needed: "The struggle [for justice] doesn't just occur in space but also for space.... [O]nce the space of the old political system has been taken over, it becomes necessary to produce a new spatial order" (Dufaux et al.). The institution of midwifery, in whatever physical space it is practiced, whether in a home, hospital, or birthing centre, could be the very institution that we find ourselves seeking. Midwifery, with all it implies, can always follow the woman, sharing and enhancing her space of well-being wherever it may be.

WITHIN

The world is large, but in us it is deep as the sea.
—Rainer Maria Rilke (qtd. in Bachelard 181)

Each woman and practitioner contains within herself a world of particularity and uniqueness. These are the worlds that they bring to the relationship they come to share. This becomes a space of subtlety, care, and nuance. In this context, the space "within" is ethereal, but it is also the inner, intimate space of the woman's biology. This world is experienced also within the clinic space, with its micro-representations of the realms of human anatomy and reproduction, relationships and intimacy, awareness, and being.

Making space within ourselves: relationship with self

In midwifery practice, we see being "with the self" as a form of spacemaking. Midwives are seekers on a journey, travelling often into unknown and unexpected spaces. Serving women is an intention, a wish, and a high call. Sustaining the midwifery model requires moments of courage—staying constantly with women during the long hours of labour and working with the unexpected—and ordinary moments, the repetitive tasks where the terrain is very familiar, taking blood pressure, drawing blood (Sharpe, "Midwifery Practice"). This work could be a kind of alchemy, a work done with the attention that could metaphorically turn ordinary materials into gold. Attentive care can be transformative and the dynamics of inner space can change as woman and midwife reach an increased level of comfort and at-homeness. Midwifery work is often inconvenient; it sometimes puts the midwife in situations beyond her level of comfort. It asks the midwife occasionally to stretch herself, to extend her awareness and patience, to make sacrifices—to participate in transforming the birth space into a space of possibility.

On sharing the space within

Most serious undertakings, spiritual or otherwise, are done with the support of others; the seekers of fairy tale and myth form bands to help support each other in their quest, or solitary seekers find helpers along the way. Midwifery work is generally not solitary; two midwives attend every birth and midwives work in group practices and hold peer review and practice meetings. The support of their midwifery partners is key to their ability to work happily. The availability of physical time and space needs to be matched by an inner space in the midwife so that she can be available ... so that she can listen. If her inner space gets too crowded or constrained by tension, hurry, fear, or anxiety, the ability to listen and make sound judgments is affected. Midwives might consider how to work towards keeping themselves available for this transformative, attentive work. Above all, a sense of proportion is needed—a sense of our place in the immense scale of the universe. Galaxies turn as we sit here, yet we are fixed on our small problems. Time and space and silence are needed for moments of being present to each other. Even during times of quiet, repetitive thoughts, comparisons or worry enter the space. Midwives know the role of relaxation, breathing, and lowering of anxiety for women, but to what extent are they aware of the need to relax tensions in their own bodies when they work? Attunement between the midwife and the woman influences the birth space and is an important feature of the ability to adapt to nuances of cultural sensitivity and merge with one's environment.

Looking for a space within, peace inside

Attention to the quality of the relationship between the midwife and the woman is at the core of spacemaking. Both the midwife and the client bring layers of knowing, at-homeness, and being at home in one's body to the birth space. In the space between caregiver and client, conditions for a third entity of space can be created. What Tracey calls a "precreative space" can appear—an intimate space for being, a space of quiet, still awareness in which the most subtle relationship between the woman and caregiver can find expression. Tracey likens this precreative space to Bachelard's "pre-happiness," as the epicentre of intimacy (25). It is a space that, in proportion to the deepening of the intimacy it allows, opens to a sense of grandeur:

> Daydream undoubtedly feeds on all kinds of sights, but through a sort of natural inclination, it contemplates grandeur. And this contemplation produces an attitude that is so special, an inner state that is so unlike any other that the daydream transports the dreamer outside the immediate world to a world that bears the mark of infinity. (Bachelard 183)

Another expression of this quality of the space is the deep listening that the Australian Aboriginal elders call Dadirri: "It is the place before we were born, before we were in our mother's womb" (Farrelly viii). Through the profound concentration of listening and patience, the midwife becomes a co-creator in this space of intimate encounter.

Liminal Space

Liminality, the quality of not knowing, the transitional place between states of certainty, an ambiguous "in-between" nature, is yet another quality of birth space. For the woman it might be seen as the space of passage between the state of pregnancy and the state of motherhood, the passage from potential to actual parenthood. In the process of birth itself, a liminal inner psychic space of consciousness may exist, which a midwife might intentionally tap into, for example, to help "bring the woman back" to the space of the birth room if she feels the woman is metaphorically moving away. Here again, metaphor is used to speak to the abstract geography of the stage the woman is going through, within the material aspect of the room, that tangible construction of the space. Using a spatial image such as "I need you to come around the corner," the midwife may speak to the woman who is in the liminal space, that space just before pushing, and call her back to the temporal space.

Spacemaking is expansive and transcends the borders of a room, what happens within the space, and among immediate users of the space. In a home, it contains the life that continues outside the birth room. In other settings, it can include impressions from nearby spaces and other life events. Consider how what is happening in one room affects what is happening in another room. For example, recently at the Toronto Birth Centre a woman gave birth in tandem with the sound of a drum circle happening upstairs. The outer space layered onto the birth space. Furthermore, birth is often supported or mirrored by activities that are taking place outside the room, within a partnership or family, within a community, and within a society.

WITHOUT

As recipients of culture, as well as its producers, people attend to countless nuances that are assimilated only through experience.
—Jane Jacobs (*Dark Age Ahead 5*)

We use the subtitle "without" to convey the macrocosm where women, families, and midwives take their experiences and relationships with birth into the wider community and where others brush up against representations of birth as part of the geography of their neighbourhoods. We consider how the influence of birth space follows its users into their communities and, conversely, how communities come to understand birth through the space that is occupied by its architecture and imagery.

It is widely accepted that culture is inherited and assimilated through visual art, song, and story. As well, culture is dynamic and an ongoing response to interpretations and adaptations that people make in their everyday lives. Received representations of birth similarly come to influence the "culture of birth" and our understandings of birthing: "The ways in which birth is managed are profoundly culturally shaped, so much so that it can never be described as a purely physiological or even psychological event" (McCourt 2). While stories of birth as normal and woman-centred are part of the landscape of midwifery, we are concerned about essentialism—for example, about ways in which the "nuances" of midwifery space protect, preserve, and advance normal birth practices, even the way prenatal care is performed. We wonder how midwifery can expand the space for possibilities in birth culture "to become part of creating a better world" (MacDonald 6).

The Neighbourhood

While we take meaning from within a space, we also take meaning from outside the space, for example, how the presence of a midwifery clinic directly or indirectly engages with its neighbourhood and what is still lacking, taking into account factors such as walkability, community development, gentrification, accessibility, and immigrant and refugee health.

Elizabeth Brandeis tells of a midwifery practice moving from an office tower to a street-level space, "from an invisible space to a visible space," being part of the streetscape, and having a recognized address: "Accessibility from the street level is important, but the broader interpretations of accessibility, with midwives as part of the neighbourhood fabric, is really interesting." The presence of the midwifery clinic itself, its signage or name, may provide a certain representation of birth to its immediate neighbours or those who pass by. One of Jacobs' core principles is to make a city a place of hope, a place that challenges conventional thinking and where neighbourhood knowledge is respected. Not unlike the famed Preservers of Intangible Cultural Property in Japan, midwives in Ontario, conscious of what was being lost, worked to reclaim and preserve normal birth (resisting standardization and medicalization and advocating for women's choice of birthplace) and carved out spaces in which to practice their art.

The Toronto Birth Centre, like other midwife-led birth centres, is an extension of the preservation and growth of midwifery, expanding new spaces for birth. Designed and operated by Indigenous midwives, it is a space that is inclusive and representative of Indigenous people, a space where indigeneity is visible. Cheryllee Bourgeois, one of the founders, describes its importance to Indigenous and non-Indigenous culture alike: "The [Toronto Birth Centre] was deliberately designed with 'birth as a community event' as central to the space, and to create opportunities for interactions between families." Though it was designed as an Indigenous space, it was also intended as a space where all midwives would be able to work. Notions of place, space, and biographical continuity for the woman and her family informed the design of the Toronto Birth Centre. Seeking to bring awareness to normal birth and midwifery, the Aboriginal community wanted it located where it would be seen and where neighbourhood parents could walk by and say to their children, "You were born there." Situating the Toronto Birth Centre in the city's Regent Park was a deliberate strategy to reclaim birth in the community and to be located in a neighbourhood that was representative of the Toronto Birth Centre's priority populations. The redevelopment of Regent Park would densify the neighbourhood; housing units were being bought by young families and couples. Thus, the area could support a birth centre (Bourgeois).

The Toronto Birth Centre is a fine expression of the renewal Jane Jacobs presents regarding the notion of "rebirth after decay" (*Dark Age Ahead*). Jacobs saw cities as "organic, spontaneous and untidy" (PPS) and stressed the benefit of mixed use in creating community vitality. It is in pedestrian spaces that expectant or new parents come into contact with children, with the elderly, with people on their way to and fro. Young children learn how to negotiate traffic and strangers; parents boast about their new baby to admiring onlookers. Similarly, passersby come into contact with pregnant women and new parents, as well as with representations of birth by way of the clinic signage. The space outside the Toronto Birth Centre is a space where this "sidewalk ballet" comes to life (Jacobs *Death and Life* 96). Jacobs further identified how cities function as dynamic ecosystems, changing in response to people's interactions with them (*Death and Life*). Some residents may live far from their hometowns and homelands, lacking access to family help and traditional knowledge of birth and motherhood. The incidence of post-partum depression in urban mothers is higher than in rural mothers (Vigod et al.). Community buildings and midwifery clinics may serve as links for displaced and transient mothers.

A feature of the Ontario government's new action plan is to move procedures out of hospitals, where possible, and provide more community-based care: "The right care, at the right time, in the right place" (Ontario's Action Plan). Birth centres support that vision. Midwives already provide, and have always provided, community-based care. In other areas of the health care system, practitioners are more firmly rooted in institutions and don't necessarily have the infrastructure in place to provide care in the community, but midwifery does (Bourgeois).

Comparing the birth centre to a hospital setting, midwife Brandeis describes midwives as being "central" rather than "peripheral." Further, she describes the space at the centre as "a space for normal birth, a midwife-led space, [and] that is significant, our work being the orientation and the focus of the institution, as opposed to a hospital setting where we need to claim space." Preliminary research prior to the opening of the Toronto Birth Centre suggested that some women who were planning a home birth would change these plans to give birth at the centre (Rogers 5). The birth centre may be seen as an improvement on the potential chaos and messiness of home birth. We wonder, however, if a common community birth space reduces the diversity, the particularity, of birth at home. We see examples throughout the world of birth moving from home, small maternity homes, and local hospitals to larger "centres," extinguishing the presence of local and visible places for birth. "Homelike" though it may be, there may be something static about births in a community taking place in the same space, alongside the same mural, the same art. Attending a home birth allows the midwife an opportunity to participate in a woman-led space and might inspire a particular form of deep listening and meaning-making. Perhaps in a home there can be more room for the precreative space to appear.

Without: the absence of with

While we observe that birth space is being "revolutionized" by inside and outside forces, it is also influenced by what is not seen. We speak of the homelike setting, a sense of belonging and familiarity; however, some women experience, rather, a sense of "not belonging," alienation, and being in someone else's space. James is interested in what is "unseen" in a setting. How many women are without support, without a partner, without resources, without choices, without a home—or have notions of home that are not about feeling safe or welcomed?

We wonder if fabricated homelike spaces, like the birth centre, recognize the woman's reality. Birthing women may find themselves remotely situated without access to care that expands their options in birth, or they may be centrally located within a system that, in offering them circumstances alien to them, distances them from finding their inner space.

IMPLICATIONS FOR PRACTICE AND FUTURE RESEARCH

As new birthing centres emerge in Ontario, further exploration of how space is experienced and redefined will offer important discoveries into standpoint theory as part of institutional ethnography (Smith, "Women's Perspective"). For example, an analysis of the reclaiming of birth space among members of the community surrounding the Toronto Birth Centre would function as a measure of community health and well-being. Likewise, there may be implications for city planners, who could measure the impact of dedicated buildings like the Toronto Birth Centre as part of neighbourhood redevelopment. With new "community helpers" on the block, crime rates might be reduced. Perhaps there may be an increase in families as part of the demographics where access to local commerce and services for families has been improved.

The visibility or invisibility of birthplace and space has implications for midwifery and its representation, promotion, and protection of normal birth. Visibility familiarizes and normalizes and allows for the inclusion of birth in neighbourhoods. For example, the disappearance (thus invisibility) of funeral homes from neighbourhoods has minimized society's proximity with death, shrouding undertakers from community view and centralizing and commodifying funeral services somewhere out of view, all of which contributes to a distancing from death. This could be the same for birth. A project for future research might be to use data from birth registries to acknowledge out-of-hospital births. Hospital births are currently recorded by postal code, and home births could easily be included in mapping the geography of birth, rendering the invisible home birth visible. There is a broader geography of privilege in the uneven distribution of resources to rural and remote birthplaces. Transcending this sense of privilege (access to the space of the clinic, control of space, distribution of power) is already central to midwifery. Research is needed into areas where privilege is experienced. Attention is needed to make space for differences.

While this paper focuses on spacemaking among women providers and clients, spacemaking and gender identity on a wider scale would be an important area for future research. Exploring the meaning of space and how it is experienced in midwifery around the world is also an area of needed research, especially considering the wide variety of practice models and cultural variations of at-homeness. With new trends in live-streaming of births and digitized images of children, whereby parents and friends share video-files and photographs online, an area of scholarship around virtual space and lack of private space is timely. The sharing of very personal space as it enters into many homes may arguably violate a child's rights. Spacemaking, on the threshold between the private and the public, demands a review of where one's rights lie.

Midwives all have a stake in the significance and meaning of space. As the home birth movement has softened institutional boundaries, people have begun to see what a huge variance has existed in experiences of spaces and their quality and what the compatibilities for spacemaking in the future may be.

CONCLUDING THOUGHTS

The spaces we are born in and inhabit imprint on us and shape our comprehension of "home." Similarly, the spaces occupied by midwives in their practice or by clients on their journey to parenthood play out in our understanding of wellness, birth, parenthood, family, and community. As Bachelard proposes in his study of homes, the virtues of the birth space are transposed into human virtues and vice versa: "The house remodels the man" (Bachelard 47). The birth space, we suggest, is influenced by how the setting is arranged, where the midwife places herself, and where the birthplace is located geographically. All these factors affect the possibility of experiencing the precreative space in the presence of labour and birth—the quality of what Bachelard touches on as a "nuance of being" (Bachelard 217).

Midwives and women, as co-creators of birth space, can experience intimacy, security, and calmness (Bachelard 229) and, simultaneously, an expansion of space and an opening to new possibilities: more opportunities for spatial justice and more space and visibility for normal birth in city geography. The internal landscape exists in tandem with the external landscape as a "dynamic continuity" (Rilke in Bachelard 230). Midwifery is now integrated in Ontario as part of the health care system, but it remains innovative in providing services outside the institution. The process of midwifery's integration into the community and into the health care system may be seen as analogous to the exploratory process of discovering a city as a walker. In the words of Rebecca Solnit, writer on politics, place, and art:

> Walkers are "practitioners of the city," for the city is made to be walked. A city is a language, a repository of possibilities, and walking is the act of speaking that language, of selecting from those possibilities. Just as language limits what can be said, architecture limits where one can walk, but the walker invents other ways to go. (213)

The model of the Toronto Birth Centre, and midwifery for that matter, are examples of community-based health care that the province of Ontario is aiming to provide. Unlike many other organizations, midwifery happens to have the infrastructure in place to achieve the province's goal. Midwives have created "other ways to go" in the health care system. One might say their political roots and their desire to have out-of-hospital births recognized and supported were originally anti-establishment, or outside ("without") convention. Yet their impulse to practice in a manner then not widely accepted and followed now sees them well-situated and supported as leaders of community change and celebrated as they were during the opening of the Toronto Birth Centre. Their work for change must continue.

WORKS CITED

Association of Ontario Midwifes (AOM). "An Ontario First: A Midwife Who Runs A Hospital Birth Unit." *Newsletter* (Winter 2013). Web. Accessed August 19, 2014.

Bachelard, Gaston. *The Poetics of Space: The Classic Look at How We Experience Intimate Places.* Boston: Beacon Press, 1964. Print.

Bourgeault Ivy L., et al. "Problematising Public and Private Work Spaces: Midwives' Work in Hospitals and in Homes." *Midwifery* 28.5 (2012): 582–590. Print.

Bourgeois, Cheryllee. Personal interview. July 2014.

Brandeis, Elizabeth. Personal interview. July 2014.

Burton, Nadya and Rachel Ariss. *"Diversity in Midwifery Care: Working Toward Social Justice."* AOM Conference presentation, Orangeville, ON. 2014.

Davis, Deborah and Kim Walker. "The Corporeal, the Social and Space/Place: Exploring Intersections from a Midwifery Perspective in New Zealand." *Gender, Place and Culture* 17:3 (2010): 377–391. Print.

Diamond, Timothy. *Making Gray Gold: Narratives of Nursing Home Care.* Chicago: University of Chicago Press, 1995. Print.

Difilippo, Shawna. *"Trust and Transformation: Women's Experiences Choosing Midwifery and Home Birth in Ontario, Canada."* MA Thesis. University of Toronto, 2014. Print.

Dufaux, Frédéric et al. "Justice in the Street?" *Spatial Justice* 3 (2011). Web. Accessed June 1, 2014.

Farrelly, Eileen. *Dadirri: The Spring Within.* Darwin, Australia: Terry Knight and Associates, 2003. Print.

Foucault, Michel. Trans. Jay Miskowiec. "Of Other Spaces: Utopias and Heterotopias." *Architecture/Mouvement/Continuité.* France: Groupe Moniteur, 1984. Print

Hammond, Athena et al. "Space, Place and the Midwife: Exploring the Relationship between the Birth Environment, Neurobiology and Midwifery Practice." *Women and Birth* 26 (2013): 277–281. Print.

Jackson, Heather. *Marginalia: Readers Writing in Books.* New Haven: Yale University Press, 2001. Print.

Jacobs, Jane. *Dark Age Ahead.* Toronto: Vintage Canada, 2005. Print.

Jacobs, Jane. *The Death and Life of Great American Cities.* New York: Vintage, 1992. Print.

James, Susan and Cameron, Brenda. "Researching Intersubjectivity: To be with." Ramapo College, New Jersey. International Human Sciences Research Conference, June 2008. Conference presentation.

Kitzinger, Sheila. "Obstetric Metaphors and Marketing." *Birth* 26.1 (1999). Web. Accessed February 25, 2013.

Lefebvre, Henri. *The Production of Space.* London: Blackwell, 1991. Print.

MacDonald, Margaret. *At Work in the Field of Birth.* Vanderbilt University Publishing, 2008. Print.

McCourt, Christine, ed. *Midwifery and Conceptions of Time. Volume 17, Fertility, Reproduction and Sexuality.* New York: Berghahn Publishing. 2009. Print.

Moore, Andrew, et al. "'I am closer to this place'—Space, Place and Notions of Home in Lived Experiences of Hospice Daycare." *Health and Place* 19 (2013): 151–158. Print.

Nestel, Sheryl. *Obstructed Labour: Race and Gender in the Re-Emergence of Midwifery.* Vancouver: UBC Press, 2007. Print.

Newton, Niles et al. "Experimental Inhibition of Labor through Environmental Disturbance." *Obstetrics & Gynecology* 27.3 (1966): 371–377. Print.

Odent Michel. *Childbirth and the Future of Homo Sapiens.* London: Pinter and Martin, 2013. Print.

Ontario's Action Plan for Health Care. Web.

Poland, Blake et al. "How Place Matters: Unpacking Technology and Power in Health and Social Care." *Health and Social Care in the Community* 13.2 (2005): 170-180. Print.

PPS: Project for Public Spaces. N.d. Web. Accessed August 14, 2014.

Ricoeur, Paul. *Oneself as Another.* Trans. Kathleen Blamey. Chicago: University of Chicago Press, 1995. Print.

Rogers, Judy and Ayesha Haque. *Final Report to the Toronto Community: Midwifery Client Birth Centre Study*. Toronto, Ryerson University Midwifery Department, 2012. Print.

Rowles, Michelle. *Being Well: Environmental Design for Wellbeing*. Diss. Faculty of Environmental Design, University of Calgary. 2006. Print.

Rumi, Jalaludinn, *The Essential Rumi*. Trans. Coleman Barks et al. New York: HarperCollins. 2010. Print.

Sharpe, Mary. *Intimate Business: Woman-Midwife Relationships in Ontario, Canada*. Diss. Ontario Institute for Studies in Education of the University of Toronto. 2004. Print.

Sharpe, Mary. "Midwifery Practice and the Quest for Intention, Attention and Sincerity." AOM Conference Presentation. Orangeville, ON. May 2014.

Smith, Dorothy E. "The Relations of Ruling: A Feminist Inquiry." *Studies in Cultures, Organizations and Societies* 2.2 (1996): 171-190. Print.

Smith, Dorothy E. "Women's Perspective as a Radical Critique of Sociology." *The Feminist Standpoint Theory Reader: Intellectual & Political Controversies*. 1974. New York and London: Routledge, 2004. 21–33. Print.

Solnit, Rebecca. *Wanderlust: A History of Walking*. Penguin Books, 2001. E-book.

Sternberg, Christine. Personal interview, July 2014.

Tracey, Norma. "Precreative Space." *Psychoanalytic Review* 96.6 (2009) 1025-1084. Print.

Vigod, Simone N. et al. "Relation between Place of Residence and Postpartum Depression." *Canadian Medical Association Journal* 185.13 (2013): 1129.-35. Print.

2.
LOOKING AT BIRTH

Refusing Delinquency, Reclaiming Power

Indigenous Women and Childbirth

T HE PREVALENCE OF IMAGERY AND METAPHOR related to pregnancy, birth, and mothering in Indigenous cultures of Turtle Island reveal the significance of these life events within these communities. While negative representations of Indigenous women are used by colonizing forces to legitimize extermination and assimilation projects, Indigenous artistic representations of pregnancy, birth, and mothering continue to be a powerful tool to push back against these efforts. Artwork by contemporary Indigenous artists depicting pregnancy, birth, and mothering present a positive image of contemporary cultures, recognizing the ceremonial value of these experiences and creating powerful narratives of Indigenous women and communities.

The artwork described in this chapter is part of a larger collection of work compiled by Indigenous Registered Midwife Claire Dion Fletcher (Lenape/Potawatomi) as part of a research project to add Indigenous content to the Birth and its Meanings course at the Ryerson University Midwifery Education Program. The aim of the project was to compile artwork and images related to Indigenous people, pregnancy, birth, breastfeeding, and families. Works by both Indigenous and non-Indigenous people were included, as well as both historical and contemporary works. The collection of artwork was put together through Internet research, museum visits, library visits, reading and listening to stories, and discussions with Indigenous mothers, midwives, and artists. Dion Fletcher, a recent graduate of the Midwifery Education Program, currently holds the collection, with the intent that the Midwifery

Association of Indigenous Students will preserve and grow the collection.

PRE-CONTACT SELF-REPRESENTATION

A sense of self, a sense of purpose; a sense of being, a sense of community; you learn that from the womb.
—Mosôm Danny Musqua

Pregnancy, birth, and mothering have never been relegated to private, nuclear family events within Indigenous cultures of Turtle Island. These important life events play a central role in both the daily life and ceremonial cycles of all Indigenous cultures—pregnancy, birth, and breastfeeding play a fundamental role in many Indigenous creation stories, both in symbolism and literal reference. Indigenous Knowledge and stories about pregnancy, birth, and breastfeeding exist in the cycles of the moon, the changing of seasons, plant and animal life, as well as cultural practices such as Haudenasonee planting ceremonies. They can also be seen in the sweatlodge and the Sundance, ceremonies originating from Indigenous nations living in the prairies and now widely practiced by many nations across Turtle Island. Women's bodies are equated to the land, with parallels being drawn in the ability to provide for a family or nation and the care needed to cultivate a strong people. In this way, the physical experience of pregnancy and birth connects us to the cosmology of Indigenous Knowledge, the histories of Indigenous nations, and the continuation of family and clan lines.

Pregnancy and birth are sacred events in Indigenous communities. Pregnant women are to be honoured and cared for in their role in continuing the life of the family and community (Anderson, *Life Stages* 43). Women are considered to have a deeper connection to the spirit world when they are pregnant because of the spirit they are growing and caring for (43). Birth is understood as a ceremony in itself; Katsi Cook, Mohawk and Aboriginal Midwife, teaches that "birth itself is a ceremonial process, accomplishing ritual purification. It expands relationships and establishes identity in relation to kin and the larger cosmic family" (26). Images and representations of pregnancy, birth, and mothering created by Indigenous peoples of Turtle Island in the pre-contact era illustrate the importance of these experiences. On display at the Canadian Museum of History in Gatineau, QC, Canada, are two works of note, both from the West Coast of Canada and both created prior to 1879. The first is an amulet by a Haida artist that shows a pregnant woman curled around to listen to her pregnant belly, evoking thoughts of celebrating the role women take in listening to their bodies and taking care of themselves during pregnancy. The second, a Nuu-chah-nulth statuette, depicts a woman breastfeeding a baby, prominently displaying the nourishing and care giving role of women. These pieces highlight the power of women in the role of pregnancy and breastfeeding. The Smithsonian's National Museum of the American Indian in Washington, DC, is currently home to "The Birthing Pipe," a carved steatite pipe of Cherokee origin. The pipe has a carving of an eagle head on one side and a woman giving birth to a baby on the other. This piece particularly demonstrates how pregnancy and birth straddles physical and spiritual worlds through ceremony. The connection of the baby crowning, at "the threshold of life," a woman in the midst of the ceremony of birth, and the eagle, a symbol of leadership and communication, speaks to the power of women as life-givers during pregnancy, labour, and birth (Cook 26).

Pregnancy, birth, and breastfeeding are present in most Indigenous creation stories. In her work, Paula Gunn Allen investigates the role of women and a multitude of female identities in creation stories from different nations. Gunn Allen calls attention to the sacred identity that women hold in connection to creation: "The ancient ones were empowered by their certain knowledge that the power to make life is the source of all power and that no other power can gainsay it" (27). Many creation stories from different nations across Turtle Island have a female spirit that is responsible for creation. She comes in many different forms and in many different stories, but a common theme is her power and prominent role in creation (Gunn Allen 11-29). Elder Edna Manitowabi is exceptionally eloquent in her explanation of the personal significance of creation stories. Manitowabi draws a deeply powerful link between Anishnawbe history, cosmology, and personal identity when she describes how each birth experience is a physical reliving and reenacting of the Anishnawbe creation story (Simpson, *Dancing* 35-39). The acknowledgement of the relationship between pregnancy, birth, and creation in these teachings demonstrates the significance of these life events for Indigenous families and communities.

Some stories, like the Haudenasonee creation story of Sky Women, have very specific references to birth, while others tell of female beings responsible for creation in other ways: thinking beings into creation, breathing life into beings, infusing beings with life and vitality, speaking to the different female powers of creation, not limiting birth to the physical act (Gunn Allen 14-15). This is a very important point Gunn Allen makes when it comes to discussing women and creation from an Indigenous perspective: while women are recognized for their power in pregnancy and birth, fertility and childbearing are not the only realms of women's worth and jurisdiction. Limiting women's role and value to the physical processes of birth and mothering diminishes women's agency while not recognizing the roles, responsibilities, and contributions of women who are not mothers, or who mother in different ways. Creativity, vitality, planting, and cultivating the personal, familial, and communal interests of a nation are of equal value as women's responsibilities. Countless representations of creation stories and the women who influence them exist among Indigenous nations. These stories continue to be a rich source of imagery, strength, and rebirth for Indigenous peoples today.

In her work *Dancing on our Turtle's Back*, Leanne Simpson, Anishnawbe writer and activist, discusses her experiences of pregnancy, birth, and breastfeeding while critically analyzing how these relationships and experiences teach us about Anishnawbe political culture and governance (*Dancing* 106-109). Simpson writes about her experiences of becoming a mother and the teachings that she received from Elder Edna Manitowabi. On reflection on one of these teachings, Simpson discusses how the experience of breastfeeding is the way that we teach our children about treaties and being in relationships with others. "Nursing is ultimately about a relationship. Treaties are ultimately about a relationship. One is a relationship based on sharing between a mother and a child and the other based on sharing between two sovereign nations" (*Dancing*

107). Using the skills attained while learning to breastfeed as a way to approach political action and responsibilities challenges patriarchal and colonial notions of the public and private spheres being separate. Simpson does this while simultaneously demonstrating the unique ways in which women's roles and responsibilities are relevant beyond the confines of the European understanding of home, making it clear that women's lived experiences hold tangible and applicable lessons for community governance.

COLONIAL IMAGERY

The dirty, easy squaw was invented long before poverty, abuse and oppression beset our peoples.

—Kim Anderson

Colonizing powers, from French and British settlers to the Canadian government, have actively defined and policed Indigenous identity and used it as a tool to legitimize and justify control over and eradication of Indigenous peoples of Turtle Island. Regrettably, some contemporary portrayals of Indigenous identity and peoples continue this colonial project. With some instances being more subtle than their historical counterparts, imagery of Indigenous people continues to promote representations of Indigenous people as inadequate, as savages, and as unfit parents.

Colonial narratives and government policy consistently dehumanized Indigenous women to validate physical and sexual violence, the removal of children from families, and the limiting of Indigenous women's access to resources (Carroll and Benoit 269-270; Anderson, *Recognition* 99-112; Smith). The image of the Indian princess, the innocent and young yet highly sexualized girl, was common among early colonizers. This narrative promoted the idea of Indigenous women as "available and willing for the white man" (*Recognition* 100) while conflating the idea of accessibility of Indigenous women's bodies with the availability of the land for the taking by the colonizers (*Recognition* 100-101; Smith).

When colonial actors met resistance from Indigenous women, the image of the "squaw drudge" was used. The description of Indigenous women as violent, unclean, and "beasts of burden" was in direct opposition to the European notion of femininity, serving as justification for the civilizing actions of settlers and the Canadian government (Deiter and Otway 3; Anderson, *Recognition* 102-10). The introduction of European models of a male-dominated nuclear family, the Ideology of Separate Spheres, and European definitions of femininity were promoted as a means of civilizing the savage people of the so-called New World. Historic art pieces such as *Treaty of Penn with Indians* by Benjamin West, 1771-1772, (figure 1) and *The Creek Indians* by Benjamin Hawkins, 1805, are examples of artwork from this time that demonstrate these ideals. The Leni-Lenape and Creek peoples in these works are depicted in stark contrast to the civilized white settlers. In both paintings, an Indigenous woman is shown breastfeeding a baby. The woman's breasts are exposed in the midst of a scene depicting what would have been considered, by settlers, exclusively male activities. Having a woman present during trade or treaty signing, let alone a woman breastfeeding her baby, exposing her body in a public sphere, is simultaneously an affront to European ideas of women's place in society at the time as well as affirming and forwarding the story of Indigenous women as both animal-like and sexually provocative. These images depict Indigenous nations, and in particular women, through a colonial lens and use the opportunity to further the settler agenda of civilizing Turtle Island's original inhabitants. While Indigenous cultures often considered men and women's work in the family and greater community of equal value, European family ideology placed importance on male work in the public sphere and deemphasized the importance of women's work. These images uphold a colonial agenda by placing these Indigenous women in stark contrast to proper European women, undermining the role and jurisdiction of Indigenous women within their own communities (Deiter and Otway 3; Anderson, *Recognition* 102-103). Colonizers used racist and sexist imagery of Indigenous women to confirm base narratives of Indigeneity while advancing their objective of undermining Indigenous family and community structures.

Representations that dehumanize Indigenous women were, and continue to be, commonplace in settler society. The narrative of immoral and carnal behaviour is particularly persistent in historical

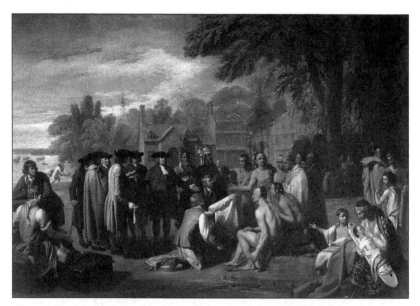

Figure 1. West, Benjamin. *Treaty of Penn with Indians.* 1771-1772. Pennsylvania Academy of the Fine Arts, Philadelphia. The State Museum of Pennsylvania. Web. Sept 2013..

accounts and depictions of pregnancy and birth. In line with the narrative of Indigenous women as "beasts of burden," their birth is often portrayed as easy, sexualized, and / or animal-like due to closeness with nature compared to the civilized European women. Images from the book *Labor among Primitive Peoples* (1883) by George J. Engelmann, an obstetrician, clearly demonstrate this perspective (figure 2). The women in the images are naked or barely covered and many of the images and descriptions have a clearly sexual nature to them. Nearly naked and ragged looking Indigenous men also make several appearances in these images, highlighting the uncivilized nature of a people who would let "untrained men" participate in a women's practice. Indigenous knowledge and practices surrounding labour and birth were dismissed as rudimentary, often being compared to witchcraft.

The positioning of Indigenous women as lazy, immoral, and ignorant contributed to the devastation of Indigenous midwifery and birth practices. When it suited their purpose and policies, settlers and government officials actively undermined the practice of Indigenous midwifery and midwives, using negative representations and narratives of Indigenous women to justify

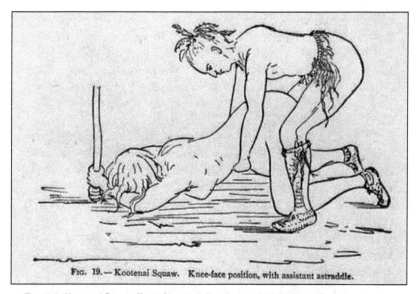

Figure 2. *Kootenai Squaw.* From George J. Engelmann, *Labor among Primitive Peoples.*
2nd ed. St. Louis: J. H. Chambers & Co., 1883. Web. June 2014.

limiting their role in childbirth (Carroll and Benoit 269; Native Women's Association of Canada 5). Indigenous birth knowledge, practices, and midwives were dismissed as primitive, uneducated, and unsafe. Doctor-attended births at hospitals were promoted as the civilized way (Carroll and Benoit 269; NWAC 5). The destruction of traditional birth knowledge and practices further contributed to the disempowerment of Indigenous women and communities. The violent assault on women's sacred and powerful role in community through imagery, narrative, and policy undermined Indigenous women's identity as strong, capable, crucial community members.

After the formation of Canada as a nation, the government continued to promote an image of Indigenous women that would both line up with and justify their policy decisions. The intent of destroying Indigenous identity, social structures, and nationhood is clearly articulated in the Deputy Superintendent of Indian Affairs mid-nineteenth-century enfranchisement policy: "Our object is to continue until there is not a single Indian in Canada that has not been absorbed into the body politic, and there is no Indian question, and no Indian department" (Lawrence 75). The portrayal of

Indigenous women as unfit parents justified the forcible removal of children from their homes to residential schools. Later, this same narrative contributed to the broadening of government intrusion into Indigenous people's lives to include a culture of increased policing of Indigenous mothers and families and placement of children into the foster care system. Cheryl Gosselin argues, "Only certain women are thought to embody the ideals of the imagined community and have public and private support to bear and raise children. Other women are either policed or punished for reproducing" (202). Images of Indigenous women as dirty squaws, as poor and lazy people, were used to perpetuate the idea that Indigenous women were inherently bad mothers. Indigenous mothering was contrasted against the "ideal of motherhood," thereby justifying the removal of children from Indigenous families to be properly cared for and civilized by the church, the state, or non-Indigenous families (Anderson *Recognition* 104; Cull 141; Hunting and Browne 38; Gosselin). The widespread physical, emotional, and sexual abuse that Indigenous children endured in the residential school system is a well-documented fact (Deiter and Otway 4). Residential schools were designed to extinguish Indigenous culture, with the ambition of assimilating Indigenous people into civilized society (Deiter and Otway 4; Lawrence 70). Forcible removal of children from their families disrupted transmission of cultural practices and norms. Disconnection from family not only denied children access to their mothers' and extended kin's maternal knowledge (Gosselin 199), but the system was also meant to teach Indigenous children that their parents and parenting practices were abnormal and inferior. The intergenerational trauma of forcible removal of Indigenous children from their families has resulted in a loss of Indigenous identity for thousands of individuals and families while continuing to undermine the crucial role that Indigenous women play in the family and community (Gosselin 199; Deiter and Otway 4; Lawrence 75).

The image of Indigenous women as unfit mothers is perpetuated in contemporary health education and promotion posters, in particular those representing pregnancy. There is still a widely held misconception that Fetal Alcohol Spectrum Disorder (FASD) disproportionately affects Indigenous populations when there is

growing evidence that FASD is equally represented in non-Indigenous populations (Hunting and Browne 36). While FASD is not
solely an Indigenous issue, the only health promotion posters
available from the Health Canada website relating to Indigenous
pregnancy are posters listing the dangers of using drugs or alcohol while pregnant and the effects of FASD. Furthermore, these
posters are also the only posters available from Health Canada
in Indigenous languages. The association of substance abuse
during pregnancy with Indigenous women perpetuates the image
of Indigenous women as incapable of being successful mothers.
Health education as a primary prevention method for FASD assumes that Indigenous women are uneducated or ignorant of the
effects of substance use during pregnancy (Hunting and Browne
40-43). This prevention method not only ignores the complex,
intersecting social issues associated with substance use, it positions
addiction as a rational decision that Indigenous mothers choose
(Cull 150). If substance use is a choice that Indigenous mothers
make within the context of being educated by the government
and healthcare system, then those women are bad mothers, a
harm to their children and society as a whole. Excessive scrutiny
and intervention by the state in Indigenous women's ability to
mother is then justified (Hunting and Browne 43-44; Cull 150).
Discourse surrounding substance use in pregnancy and mothering
is another tool used to perpetuate the idea of Indigenous women
as delinquent mothers.

RESURGENCE – PREGNANCY, BIRTH AND
ABORIGINAL MOTHERING

> By reclaiming our responsibilities as carriers of our cul-
> tures, we resist, we revitalize, and we teach another way
> is possible.
> —Leanne Simpson

Imagery of Indigenous pregnancy, birth, and mothering has always
been ripe with metaphor and significance. It is not surprising then
that this imagery and subject matter was distorted while being put

to use as an assimilationist tool. However, the profound meaning of pregnancy, birth, and mothering continues to resonate with Indigenous people today, people who have taken up its use as a form of resistance and pride. Contemporary art works created by Indigenous artists are drawing on the prominent role of women as understood and explained within Indigenous cosmologies. Women's role in the creation/recreation of worlds or the creation and mothering of individual beings is being used as a metaphor, a symbol, and a powerful example of cultural resurgence that promotes a positive representation of Indigenous women. Visual art is being used as a site of resistance, a method for decolonizing everyday lives. Art that promotes a cultural resurgence, and with it a resistance to the trauma of colonization, is a way for individuals, families, and communities to begin healing from the effects of colonization.

Contemporary Indigenous art often focuses on pregnancy and birth as an act of resistance to colonialism, government policies, or historic narratives of Indigenous womanhood. Some images clearly call on individuals to actively oppose and challenge government policies of assimilation, in particular those that threaten land and Indigenous bodies. More subtle imagery evokes the power of Indigenous women as creators and carriers of our culture. All these works remind Indigenous people that Indigenous culture has not been lost and that living an Indigenous existence despite extreme assimilationist impositions is, in itself, an act of resistance.

The Native Youth Sexual Health Network is an Indigenous organization that "works across issues of sexual and reproductive health, rights and justice." #MediaArtsJustice is one of their initiatives that raise public awareness of the connection between environmental violence and reproductive rights. The artwork in this initiative by Métis/Cree artist Erin Marie Konsmo combines images and symbolism of reproduction—women's bellies, uteri, strawberries—with images and symbolism of environmental violence, corporations, and the State—oil pump jacks, factories, nuclear symbols, gas masks (figure 3). The artwork calls on the viewer to make connections between environmental degradation, reproductive rights, and sovereignty over both Indigenous land and Indigenous bodies. The provocative images are a powerful call to action confidently rooted in Indigenous identity and politics urging Indigenous peoples and allies to resist corporate and government policies that seek to harm lands and ecologies and, in doing so, harm Indigenous bodies and restrict reproductive rights.

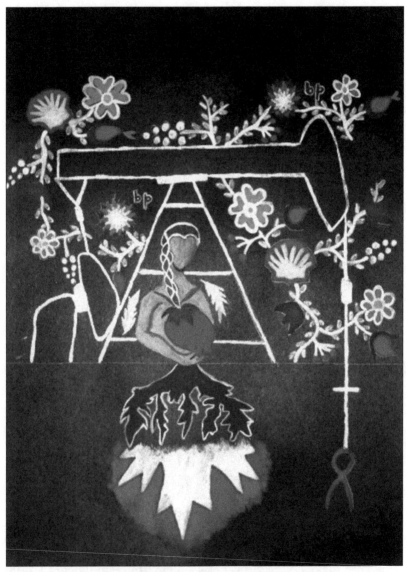

Figure 3. *Reproductive/Environment Justice.* Erin Marie Konsmao, *Reproductive/Environmental Justice*, 2010. Erin Marie Konsmo Art Through a Birch Bark Heart. Web. 10 June 2014.

In discussing the history of resistance among Aboriginal people Leanne Simpson writes:

> The Ancestors not only fought, blockaded, protested and mobilized against these forces on every Indigenous territory in Turtle Island, they also engaged in countless acts of hidden resistance and kitchen table resistance aimed at ensuring their children and grandchildren could live as *Indigenous* Peoples. The Grandmothers, Mothers and Aunties were particularly adept at keeping us alive, and passing down whatever traditions they could so we would have warmth in our hearts and warmth in our bellies. (*Dancing* 102)

Seemingly simple acts, such as choosing to have a baby or raise children in adherence to Indigenous culture, are acts of resistance. Propagating Indigenous peoples, especially confidant, educated, self-actualized Indigenous people, is in direct opposition to assimilation policies. Contemporary art that depicts positive images of pregnancy and birth, drawing from cultural symbolism and realistic representations, not only contradicts the notion that Indigenous women and people have disappeared from North America but also celebrates and honours the roles of women that colonizers have tried so violently to destroy. Work such as the sculptures of Inuit artists Silas Kavakiuak and Mary Oashutsiaq depict Inuit women giving birth—babies quite literally at the threshold of new life with their heads born while the rest of their body is not yet out. These birth scenes with women helping other women place the experience and control of that moment in the hands of Inuit women. Paintings by Potawatomi artist Daphne Odjig and Metis artist Leah Dorian depict pregnancy, motherhood, and birth scenes firmly rooted in Indigenous perspectives, including physical and spiritual understandings of these experiences. *Earth Mother*, a painting by Daphne Odjig depicting an image of a woman or female being with a baby in her womb, emphasizes the connection between pregnancy, birth, and creation. *Givers of Life* by Leah Dorion is a painting depicting various women in different stages of motherhood: women with children, women pregnant, women with new babies, and midwives/Grandmothers/Aunties helping these mothers. The women are all under a tree with its roots visible under the ground interspersed with medicine wheels and turtles. The system of roots calls on images of placentas with the system of veins and arteries that nourish a growing fetus and connect woman and child. The interspersed medicine wheels and turtles remind us that through our mothers we are connected to the land and our people. These are some examples of contemporary art that does not try to hide pregnancy and birth or shame Indigenous mothers. This art celebrates the role of Indigenous women in the creation process, and brings this ceremony into the everyday.

The *Nindinawemaaganidok/All My Relations*-Mural Project is a community-based public art project at Allen Gardens in Toronto. Lead artists Tannis Nielson (Cree/Metis) and Phillip Cote (Shawnee/Lakota/Potawatomi/Ojibway) along with twenty-one community artists created this mural that spans the length of two football fields. The south wall of the mural is the Water Wall (figure 4). The mural done by graffiti artists demonstrates the importance of water to all creation. The imagery of the Water Wall was a collaborative effort, which included input and participation from Indigenous midwives; it is full of imagery and symbolism related to pregnancy and birth. The cycles of the moon are depicted, as is a woman in the throes of labour, plant life blooming, and animals caring for their young. The meaning of this project goes beyond the pride that comes with displaying Indigenous-conceived and created art so prominently in a park in downtown Toronto: it is Indigenous people claiming public space.

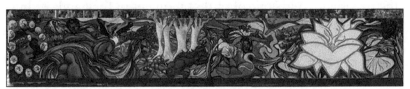

Figure 4. Detail.
Water Wall. Lickers, Lindsey, Nyle Johnston, Issac Weber, Honey Smith, and Shelby Rain. *Nindinawemaaganidok/All My Relations - Water Wall.* 2014. Toronto. Mural.

Cree/Métis scholar Kim Anderson argues that for Indigenous communities to heal from the effects of colonization women must reclaim their identity as strong and powerful women (*Recognition* 238). One of the ways she and others suggest this can be accomplished is through reclaiming the authority and power that women once had (Anderson, *Recognition*; Simpson, "Birthing"; Carroll and Benoit). Katsi Cook teaches that the "production and reproduction of human beings is integral to sovereignty and that this sovereignty falls in the domain of the female universe ... that women are the base of generations, the carriers of culture" (Simpson, "Birthing" 29). Indigenous women across Turtle Island are reclaiming birth practices and knowledge, resisting the colonial narrative of bad mother, and fighting against assimilation by taking part in the ceremony of birth. Indigenous midwives working closely with women, their families, and communities are helping to reclaim this knowledge and ensure the continuation of Indigenous birth practices. The National Aboriginal Council of Midwives (NACM) brings together Indigenous midwives from across Canada to promote excellence in reproductive health for Indigenous people and to advocate for Indigenous midwifery services for all Indigenous families (*Our Mission*). NACM strives for Indigenous midwives to have access to cultural and traditional knowledge and for the recognition of the importance of this knowledge in reproductive care.

While the work of reclaiming traditional birth practices and knowledge often happens at an individual level—lone or small groups of Indigenous midwives, doulas, mothers, grandmothers, and aunties providing culturally safe care that promotes Indigenous birth customs—there are a growing number of larger scale projects that are also contributing to this work. The Inuulitsivik Health Centre in Nunavik Quebec is a community-led initiative that serves communities along the Hudson Bay coast. The first birth centre opened in 1986 in Puvirnituq. The centre has a midwifery-led collaborative model of care and is a direct result of community activism and organization by Inuit women (Van Wagner et al. 384). Elders, traditional midwives, childbearing women, and young women were all involved in the consultation for the birth centre, and the women were selected from the community to be midwifery students. The program has grown to serve seven communities and has dramatically reduced the number of women being transferred to the south to have their babies. The commitment to care that is rooted in the community, training community members as mid-wives, has contributed greatly to the success of the program and has promoted the return of birth to these Indigenous communities (Van Wagner et al.).

Tsi Non:we Ionnakeratstha Ona:grahsta', the child and maternal care centre located on the Six Nations of the Grand River Reserve in southern Ontario, is a current initiative providing traditionally informed care to Aboriginal women and their families. Staffed by fulltime Aboriginal Midwives, the centre offers a variety of services, including complete prenatal, intrapartum, and postpartum care, and also includes an Aboriginal Midwifery training program. The training program and the centre combine western medicine, obstetrical practice, standards of the Ontario College of Midwives, and traditional Aboriginal knowledge and practices (National Aboriginal Health Organization 34). The centre is recognized by a variety of organizations as an example of best practice for Aboriginal midwifery in Canada (NAHO 34, NWAC 7).

In 2005, after working for many years in private practice, midwives in Fort Smith, Northwest Territories, were officially integrated into the local health care system. Indigenous midwife Lesley Paulette credits the success of their model of care to its roots in the community. Midwives started caring for women within their homes and communities; after re-establishing this connection, midwifery has now been integrated into the local health care system (NACM, *Aboriginal Midwifery*).

The Toronto Birth Centre (TBC) is one of the more recent examples of Indigenous-led midwifery initiatives. The TBC, located in downtown Toronto, opened in January 2014. The TBC is part of the Ontario Government's birth centre pilot project. It is a midwife-led and Indigenous-governed facility, guided by an Indigenous framework. The TBC offers both Indigenous and non-Indigenous women a site within the urban centre where they may access culturally safe care and where traditional birth knowledge and practices are celebrated. While the work of recovering birth knowledge and practices is at times challenging, midwives, women, and families across Turtle Island are taking on this work and revitalizing Indigenous birth culture.

While demeaning imagery of Indigenous women has been used as colonial and assimilation tools in an attempt to destroy Indigenous culture, it is simultaneously a crucial site of cultural resurgence. Metis leader Louis Riel said, "My people will sleep for a hundred years, and when they awake, it is the artists who will give them back their spirit." True to this prophecy, these contemporary artists create works that celebrate and promote the role of women in creation and bring the ceremony of pregnancy, birth, and motherhood into our everyday lives. When we see representations of Indigenous pregnancy, birth, and motherhood all around us, it is a strong reminder that assimilation policies did not succeed; Indigenous people and culture are still very much alive and thriving. The work of these artists reasserts the importance of Indigenous birth knowledge and customs, re-establishing the self-determined narrative of Indigenous women and families as vital, healthy, and connecting us to vast Indigenous cosmologies.

WORKS CITED

Anderson, Kim. *A Recognition of Being: Reconstructing Native Womanhood.* Toronto: Second Story Press, 2000. Print.

Anderson, Kim. *Life Stages and Native Women: Memory, Teachings, and Story Medicine.* Winnipeg: University of Manitoba Press, 2011. Print.

Carroll, Dena and Cecilia Benoit. "Aboriginal Midwifery in Canada: Merging Traditional Practices and Modern Science." *Reconceiving Midwifery.* Ed. Ivy Lynn Bourgeault, Cecilia Benoit and Robbie Davis-Floyd. Montreal: McGill-Queen's University Press, 2004. 263-286. Print.

Cook, Katsi. "Protecting the Child in the First Environment: Preconception Health to Save the Native Future." *National Museum of the American Indian,* Winter 2011. 24-27. Pdf.

Cull, Randi. "Aboriginal Mothering Under the State's Gaze." Lavell-Harvard and Lavell 141-156.

Deiter C., and Otway L. *Sharing Our Stories on Promoting Health and Community Healing: An Aboriginal Women's Health Project.* Winnipeg: The Prairie Women's Health Centre of Excellence, 2001. Project No. 31. Pdf.

Gosselin, Cheryl. "'They Let Their Kids Run Wild': The Policing of Aboriginal Mothering in Quebec." Lavell-Harvard and Lavell 196-206.

Gunn Allen, Paula. *The Sacred Hoop: Recovering the Feminine in American Indian Traditions*. Boston: Beacon Press, 1986. Print.

Hunting, Gemma and Annette J. Browne. "Decolonizing Policy Discourse: Reframing the 'Problem' of Fetal Alcohol Spectrum Disorder." *Women's Health and Urban Life* 11.1 (2012): 35-53. Pdf.

Lavell-Harvard, D. Memme, and Jeannette Corbiere Lavell, eds. *"Until Our Hearts Are On the Ground" Aboriginal Mothering, Oppression, Resistance and Rebirth*. Toronto: Demeter Press, 2006. Print.

Lawrence, Bonita. "Mixed-Race Urban Native People: Surviving a Legacy of Policies of Genocide." *Expressions in Canadian Native Studies*. Ed. Ron F. Laliberte, Priscilla Settee, James B Waldram, Rob Innes, Brenda Macdougall, Lesley McBain and F. Laurie Barron. Saskatoon: University Extension Press, 2000. 69-94. Print.

National Aboriginal Council of Midwives (NACM). *Aboriginal Midwifery*. National Aboriginal Council of Midwives, 2012. Web Video. 5 Jun. 2015.

National Aboriginal Council of Midwives (NACM). *Our Mission*. National Aboriginal Council of Midwives, 2012. Web. 5 Jun. 2015.

National Aboriginal Health Organization (NAHO). "Celebrating Birth—Aboriginal Midwifery in Canada." Ottawa: National Aboriginal Health Organization, 2008. Pdf.

Native Women's Association of Canada (NWAC). "Aboriginal Women and Reproductive Health, Midwifery, and Birthing Centres." *National Aboriginal Women's Summit*. June 20-22, 2007. Corner Brook, Newfoundland. Pdf.

Native Youth Sexual Health Network. *Native Youth Sexual Health Network*. N.d. Web. 6 Jun. 2014.

Simpson, Leanne. "Birthing an Indigenous Resurgence: Decoloniz-ing Our Pregnancy and Birthing Ceremonies." Lavell-Harvard and Lavell 25-33.

Simpson, Leanne. *Dancing On Our Turtle's Back: Stories of*

Nishnaabeg Re-Creation, Resurgence and a New Emergence. Winnipeg: Arbeiter Ring Publishing, 2011. Print.

Smith, Andrea. *Conquest: Sexual Violence and American Indian Genocide.* Cambridge: South End Press, 2005. Print.

Van Wagner, Vicki, Brenda Epoo, Julie Nastapoka, and Evelyn Harney. "Reclaiming Birth, Health, and Community: Midwifery in the Inuit Villages of Nunavik, Canada." *Journal of Midwifery & Women's Health* 52.4 (2007): 384-391. Pdf.

Resistance and Submission

A Critique of Representations of Birth

THIS PAPER EMERGED FROM MY WORK for a Ph.D. in Creative Writing. Motivated by a desire to analyse women's life stories, and informed by many years as a midwife, I took on the task of retelling a life story revolving around the centrality of the character's bodily experience of womanhood, manifested through her experiences of rape, intimate violence, birth, and mothering. This enterprise opened the door to a critical understanding of the nature of subjectivity as represented and re-presented in fiction and non-fiction in the form of birth narratives. As a midwife and a feminist, I had long been aware of severe deficits in the linguistic and narrative framing of birth but had not been at leisure to analyse these in any detail. Engaging with the dynamics of women's life writing and narrative theory allowed me to critically appraise the nature of dominant birth narratives in Western culture utilising some key referents from fiction and so-called "reality TV" as points of analysis.

A critique and comparison of narratives representing birth identifies motifs of resistance and submission that mirror feminist and other discourses locating women as oppressed and responding to oppression in the same way as they respond to other uniquely female experiences, including rape and sexual violence. In this chapter, I use textual narratives from fiction as an initial reference point to analyse visual narratives from television "reality" shows which constitute, it could be argued, powerful and defining narratives that affect people's knowledge, cognition, and even their identity formation (Ryan and Macey 2). This critical discussion emerges

172

from work carried out within critical studies on women's life writing and fiction, which engendered a new appreciation of the impact of culturally derived and defining narratives found in populist media (most specifically, "reality TV"). These narratives include the BBC Television series *The Midwives* (series one and two), a reality television show that shows the work of midwives in a number of different obstetric units across the UK; a similar show produced by the UK's Channel 4 entitled *One Born Every Minute* (series one), which again focuses on the work of midwives and doctors in busy UK maternity units;[1] and the literary narratives of birth and sexual violence found in Margaret Atwood's *The Handmaid's Tale* and the rape narrative in Sarah Dunant's *Transgressions*.[2]

The creative element of my Ph.D. was a fictional text entitled *Inshallah* (Einion 2). The novel centres around a woman's experiences of rape and childbearing, which are the causal elements precipitating the emplotment of life events that characterise the main character's life story. The juxtaposition of these two essentially female bodily experiences brought about a strange mimesis between one and the other that was derived from an almost subconscious melding of my own experiences of birth and of supporting birthing mothers and my imagined creation of narratives of rape and intimate violence. The aim was to expose a subjective experience that is viewed entirely through the lens of the woman's bodily experience. "All novels require us to uncover some hidden design" (Mullan 169), and my work focused on uncovering the inevitable design of the woman's life experience as it is mediated by the fact of her being physically and socially female. As Pilar Villar-Argaiz suggests, "Women's representations of rape and domestic violence can exert a forcible social critique of women's victimization by patriarchal social structures that confine and silence them" (134).

It was only *after* the creation of micro-narratives of birth and of continued intimate violence within my novel that I became aware of the similarities between the two bodily experiences, one mediated by my imagination and intellectual knowledge, the other by my personal, professional, and theoretical knowledge. I found myself "suspended between material and semiotic worlds" as author, negotiating my own position relative to victim and to violators, and with an authorial position that I realised was defined by the encoding of representations of birth and of intimate violence (Tanner 3). Tanner argues that "it is the materiality of the body which defines its susceptibility to violence, it is the vulnerability of the subject accessible through that body that renders the victim susceptible to violation" (3). To rephrase this in terms of the representation of birth, I could say, "It is the materiality of the reproducing body which defines its susceptibility to intervention, it is the vulnerability of the subject accessible through that body that renders the woman susceptible to medical control."

The relationship between the materiality of the body and the power dynamics of social and institutional structures that affect the body is thus made clear and provided the first indication of the answer to my question of how it could be that narratives of birth echoed narratives of rape. It has been argued that "the dynamics of violence often involve a violator who appropriates the victim's subjectivity as an extension of his own power, turning the force of consciousness against a victim for whom sentience becomes pain, consciousness no more than an agonizing awareness of the inability to escape embodiment" (Tanner 3). In narratives of birth, as shown below, inescapable embodiment and pain feature strongly.

If this is the case for violence, its mirror image can be found in the subjection of the female body to the institution of medicine as a representation of social structures that define the appropriate behaviours of womanhood. Christina Mazzoni, for example, highlights how the institution of medicine may have moved away from "asserting women's biological inferiority and weakness" but argues that the negative regard of medicine continues in the ways that "contemporary obstetricians subject healthy women to a systematic clinical gaze even as they reject a vocabulary of outright domination" (8). Thus, Mazzoni begs the question, "Can we distinguish between women's concerns and those that society imposes on us, between our corporeal bodies and the culturally inscribed bodies of social representation?" (8). If we accept this critical relationship among the culturally inscribed and ascribed female body, the semantics and dynamics of power and control, and the struggle for these in representations of the female as much as in representations of the birthing mother, then it comes as no surprise to see similarities in representations of intimate or sexual violence and representations of birth. It is also no surprise to find that the representation of birth within the terms of more dominant narratives of violence against the female body is partly due to the relevant absence of empowered, powerful, or meaningful birth narratives in mainstream media. As Carol H. Poston shows in *Childbirth in Literature,* the female voice in representations of the childbirth experience is largely absent (20) and this means that male voices—male perspectives—dominate such narratives. Sears and Godderis make a similar argument, stating that in their analysis of an American childbirth "reality" series, the "construction of the birthing woman is grounded in a patriarchal framework where ideas of powerful groups in society are given space and airtime" (192).

Oakley emphasises the trope of the passive female—the representation of women as naturally passive—manifested in art and in writing. Oakley (71) blames two ideological constructs for this positioning of the female as passive, including religious (Christian) ideology and the effects of industrialisation on women's roles in society. It is not news to us that the evolution of a society founded in the ideals of the Church has relegated women to an inferior position, with masculine authority dominating and defining the role of the "proper wife" (Oakley 71). However, Oakley also equates this to a capitalist patriarchal society in which women are relegated to a particular form of production, that of wives, mothers, and homemakers (71). Barbara Katz Rothman relates this strongly to the commodification of motherhood as a form of production (5-6). She refers to the mechanisation of the female reproductive body as a product of Cartesian dualism in which the mind-body divide assumes the ability to have absolute control over the "natural" body (32-33). This can be extended along lines that define the demarcations of power in our society today in which women as childbearing machines are subject to the power of science and medicine.

The key feature of this subject role in representations of birth is that it not only places the woman in a position of having less power than the institution which surrounds her but that she has no voice in this institution: "The passive victim lacks a voice of her own—inarticulateness is the mark of an oppressed group"

(Oakley 72). When examining birth narratives, the lack of women's agency in expression of that experience, in the exercise of true choice and autonomy, is clear. Yet this should not be the case—too much has been written in the last two decades about the issues of choice and control in childbearing, arguing that all providers of maternity care should be fostering and supporting women's control over the birthing experience and choice in who provides care and in what way (Sandall 206; Snowden et al. 1). It is shocking to see that in the twenty-first century, women are so successfully disempowered in this one arena where their power should reign supreme.

Only women can bear and birth children. In this essential fact lies our power and such a singular fact should afford women the highest status in the reproductive arena.[3] Yet what we see in many of the narratives of birth found in mainstream media spaces is a continued reinforcement of the woman as passive, as subject, as lacking the ability to give birth safely without assistance from the technology of science and the hegemonic knowledge of medicine. There is no doubt that there is a trope of motherhood in our society, and that that trope is variously defined through the ideological structures of our society. Mothers enjoy a paradoxical position of glorification, such that the "ideal mother" is placed on a pedestal, and of denigration, in which the mothering role is relegated to that of production of the next generation *regardless of the cost to the mother.*

As a midwife writing in such a critical manner about birth practices and their representations, I find myself in an invidious position, a position in which I am forced to criticise my own profession for its part in this great machine that is medicine. I occupy a paradoxical position as a midwife subject to the rules and regulations of my profession, teaching other women how to be midwives within this inherently flawed system, and a midwife and feminist arguing for the recognition of the power and wonder of women's ability to birth naturally and without fear and interference. It is from this position that I have attempted to observe the shape of the birth scripts that are repeatedly represented in the media today.

What we see is a paradoxical representation of mothers as beatific, as capable, as nurturing, and self-sacrificing, with the cult of the child dominating the discourses surrounding childbearing, alongside mothers represented as incapable of birthing their children without medical intervention. This cult of the child places children as the highest priority in society and, as such, women's productivity as mothers is limited to her physiological capacity to reproduce, with the "end product" being the most important part of the whole process (Katz Rothman 32-33). Therefore, any means is acceptable to ensure the woman is "delivered of" the child successfully.[4]

Fictional and quasi-fictional narratives of birth seem, in their narrative arcs, characterisation, and representation, to mimic narratives of rape and sexual violence in positioning the birthing woman as subject, where resistance is overcome by threat. Positioning women during "normative" birth narratives represents woman as inferior and subject to threat and control, often by multiple perpetrators at once. In the birth narrative, the threat is of harm to or death of the baby. The birthing woman, particularly the woman with defined high risk, controls the level of risk to self by submitting to the authority of the institution. The birth script transforms a human experience into struggle for power in which the victim is stripped of the ability to define and control his or her participation.

This analysis does not equate the *experience* of birth with sexual violence. It equates the *representation* of birth with the *representation* of sexual violence. Both representations show women in various stages of resistance and submission. I argue that representations of birth in the media and in literature show birth as something that the woman suffers in order to fulfill her role as producing mother. Poston (23) equates this to a representation of birth as something savage and animalistic, something that the woman has no control over, which then places them as external observers of their own experiences. Thus, representations of women's bodies through the lens of patriarchal and technocratic tropes of femininity, physiology, biology, and helplessness have been accepted and even perpetuated by women themselves. This creates a cycle of expectation in which women themselves buy into the dominant trope of subject/object, passive recipient or deviance, through the act of resistance.

Tanner states that "acts of intimate violence, then, transform human interaction into a struggle for power in which the victim is stripped of the ability to define and control his or her participation" (3). Again, I would like to transpose this into birth narratives and state that the act of birth transforms a human experience into struggle for power in which the victim is stripped of the ability to define and control his or her participation. Sears and Godderis (181-182), in their analysis of reality television and specifically one "birth" series, suggest that they can identify specific discourses that occur within these particular visual narratives, discourses which include the birthing story being framed in such a way as to present a particular kind of narrative representation, the role of medical practitioners, and agency and resistance associated with women's loss of control within the childbearing experience. And just as pain and vulnerability allow a perpetrator to exercise control over the "victim," so does vulnerability to pain and "dysfunction" allow the institution of the state, and the institution of medicine, to exercise control over the childbearing woman:

> The body's susceptibility to pain lends the violator power over a victim whom he attacks not just as a body but as subject: the victim's body becomes the material extension of vulnerability, its susceptibility to pain rendering it the locus of attention for a victim for whom subjectivity and materiality become hopelessly entangled." (Tanner 5)

Reality television narratives of birth seem to reinforce "cultural beliefs about the fundamental role of medicine in childbirth" (Sears and Godderis 189). Thus, such narratives contribute to the fundamental meanings attributed to childbearing by those who consume them and reinforce negative stereotypes of women and of the institution of medicine (192).

This process of meaning making cannot be rendered into simplistic dimensions either, as being gendered male versus female, because the creators of the systems that have resulted in these representations of birth are both female and male. Thus, when we explore such narratives, we explore the roles of significant actors or characters who have, in the case of birth narratives, become essentially genderless, except for the birthing woman herself. The understanding of these representations is achieved through the application of narrative theory in which the plot and characters are viewed in the context of "style, viewpoint, pace and so on," which can be understood as the "whole 'packaging' of the narrative which creates the overall effect" (Barry 223).

In the BBC 2 series *Midwives* (2014), the narrative arcs show a typical representation of the power of the institution, manifested by the behaviours and language of the midwives. The focus of all births is the product of the birth process—the baby—and all actions, in the trope of the childbirth narrative, are justifiable for that noble cause. Midwives speak in patronising tones, infantilising women and utilising language and other communications markers that disempower and diminish women and inflate and authenticate the power of the institution. The plot focuses on the same structured flow: woman as subject/quester, midwife/doctors as hero, obstacles/antagonists in the form of the woman's body failing to perform as required (i.e. to give birth), heroic intervention, and happy resolution in which the subject must sacrifice something in order to achieve their final goal.[5] An alternative version sees the midwives/doctors as protagonists and the woman as antagonist, with protagonist doing battle with the antagonist until they have subdued the uncontrollable beast. This can be seen in the micro-narratives, in particular where women argue against the institution and its representatives. In such narratives, the woman is represented in a negative light, as someone who steps outside the system (as deviant), as an anti-hero, as the villain of the piece. In these narratives, doctors and midwives, as the representatives of science, reason, and knowledge, act in a heroic manner to engage with the "bestial" force of the resisting woman, grappling with her ignorance and wilfulness in order to coerce her into a more seemly and proper acceptance of their authority. And the greatest weapon wielded by these heroic proponents of science and medicine is the fetus. It is disturbing to find such narratives dominating in a social context in which midwifery holds a strong professional position. Sears and Godderis (190) cite a similar observation, suggesting in their analysis of similar types of narratives that women who were active in labour could be viewed as displaying resistance because they have not adopted the accepted, recumbent and passive, position on the birthing bed.

It was my work analysing narratives in fiction that sharply illuminated this idea of the subject female occupying a specific position within the wider societal construct that is the fictional world. This analysis underlines both the connection between fictional narrative creation and the "framing" and construction of so-called reality TV and what appears to be the deliberate perpetuation of divisive constructs and characterisations which serve to keep women oppressed. For example, in Margaret Atwood's *The Handmaid's Tale*, a futuristic, dystopian narrative, women are commodified within strict social roles: Marthas, who do housework and menial tasks; Wives, who are married to the men with power, the Commanders; and Handmaids, who produce babies for the infertile Wives. The "sex" scene in Atwood's book can be seen as a powerful signifier, what Barthes would describe as a "cardinal function," something that is both consecutive and consequential within the narrative (Barthes and Duisit 248).[6] I have been fascinated for many years with Offred's story (Offred is the narrator of Atwood's novel) and the paradoxical responses of admiration and discomfort it evokes. The scene of "the ceremony," an act of ritualised rape, is important in terms of explaining the meaning behind Offred's current situation and in explicating the religious and societal codes within which she is forced to exist. Although the reader has been already prepared by the preceding narrative for what exactly Offred's role is, it is never made explicit until this scene unfolds and the symbolic nature of the circumstances is made clear, along with Offred's reaction to what is occurring. I argue that this mimics the ways that birth scenes in "reality" television present the symbolic nature of the birthing woman's circumstances.

The birth scene in Attwood's novel is a parody of a natural birth: surrounded by a crowd of women, the Handmaid, who has submitted to enforced penetration and fertilisation by the Commander in the presence of his Wife, gives birth in a subject position in a specially designed chair in which the Wife sits above her, and the product of the Handmaid's womb is handed to the Wife. The entire narrative structure focuses on the outcome, the fetus, and its viability. The entire social system described in this novel is created to address decreasing fertility and to provide babies for the social elite. This reflects "reality" narratives that focus entirely on the primacy of the fetus as a justification for the subjugation and, at times, physical violation of a woman's body. This text, written more than three decades ago, is defined as fiction, yet it is through this lens that we can view a relationship between culturally fabricated concepts of birth (deliberate in Atwood's fictional narrative) and the assimilation of those concepts into normative behaviour and belief as represented in current media. Atwood's novel in particular raises the status of the fetus and child above that of the mother, a significant conceptualisation which, while viewed as extreme, is also culturally relevant.

Christina Mazzoni suggests that "the constraints imposed on the pregnant body by a society seen to increasingly valorize the fetus as subject at the expense and objectification of the expectant woman are now a topos in feminist considerations of pregnancy" (15). In current lexicon, we have witnessed the elevation of the fetus and fetal wellbeing to a status above that of the mother, "accusing contemporary culture of reading the woman's body as being 'in the service of the fetus' and in need therefore of external constraints and regulations" (Mazzoni 15). It is most disturbing to me to note that there is little resistance to the increasing medical pressure for all individuals to behave in state-defined "healthy" ways and little critique or questioning of the increasing state control of the personal as manifest in the body. This is where I can draw the closest relationship between narratives of birth and narratives of rape or sexual violence. As Tanner argues:

> The mimetic qualities of fiction function through a series of complex mediations involving not only the gap between sign and referent but between the text and an empirical subtext drawn from the reader's assumptions about violence—an understanding of its impact, dynamics, and consequences drawn from experience in the empirical world as well as from fictional and nonfictional representations." (6-7)

In order to critique this relationship, it was necessary to make some critical distinctions, the first of which is "the distinction between violence itself—which exists outside that symbolic order—and its conceptualization and expression, which exist inside it" (Tanner 8). Thus, it is possible to draw a direct comparison between the narrative structures (textual and visual) that represent women as victims of physical and sexual violence and those that represent women as "victims" of the birth process. It is my argument that such representations of birth, as with representations of rape and sexual violence, serve to reinforce the legitimacy of a system in which the framing of birth in such terms becomes accepted. In both rape narratives and birth narratives, "the victim's sense of powerlessness reduces her to a violable body that is not only the literal site of physical violence but the figurative doorway to a subject that the body renders vulnerable to assault" (Tanner 6). Thus, if we continue to represent birth utilising particular narrative conventions—such as those that ascribe character roles to specific actors (birthing mother, midwife, father, doctor)—we then re-define people's real expectations of birth and their anticipation of how they will both experience birth and be expected to behave within it.

This is most problematic when considering visual narratives: "In exposing the conventions associated with the representation and viewing of woman as body or spectacle, film renders visible many of the dynamics that also underlie acts of representing and reading violence, especially violence against women" (Tanner 11). The editing and photography of the television programmes I studied create narratives in which the typical arc is of the woman in need, the intervention of the institution (wielding their knowledge and power), and the result of a baby.

I wrote this paper because I wanted to question the very fact that I, as a feminist and a midwife, had represented what I felt was a realistic birth narrative in a manner that identified the mother as dominated, violated, and complicit in that violation. I came to the realisation that the framing of birth narratives, fictional and non-fictional, may define how women see, anticipate, and behave during their own births: "Only through an understanding of the way in which narrative force is constituted can a reader hope to resist a narrative that both represents and enacts violence" (Tanner 14).

I would argue further that those who create birth narratives are also subject to the conventions that restrict such narratives. The power of the birth machine to control the animalistic nature of birth is continually represented in the media, particularly in programmes from the UK and America. As Kutulas states, birth stories

> are ... told against a larger social backdrop. They are necessarily about how society contextualizes women's events, how men receive and react to babies, and how the culture talks about men's and women's responsibilities vis-a-vis babies. Maternity stories are a perfect example of the hegemonic dialect between culture and ideology, reinforcing culturally dominant ideas about motherhood.... Stories about pregnant women titillate viewers with subversive gender acts, but finally contain that behaviour in socially acceptable ways.... Television both echoes and contributes to a female experience where pervasive social guilt about never being good enough turns liberation back onto women and makes its limitations their fault." (15, 30)

A prime example of this is found in the popular British programme *One Born Every Minute*. The first episode of the first season demonstrates a narrative that places women as subject. The introductory sequence shows multiple, swiftly changing shots of women lying on beds, on their backs, subject to machinery, with partners, midwives, and doctors standing over them, or peering down at them, staring between their open legs to see what is happening and how the birth process is progressing. The language used when interacting with these women is directive: "Push now" and "You've got to." The titles and the music then move to a more emotive, positive note, focusing on how fathers are made and then on the faces of the newborn babies. This narrative progression discounts any agency on the part of the women giving birth. Women are represented in limited roles. The receptionist is filmed typing and putting on her lipstick. A woman is birthing on her back on a bed, with two midwives on one side, one of whom is entirely focused on her vagina, and her husband on the other side with his hand on top of her head in a dominant position. The receptionist speaks in a baby-ish, patronising tone, stating, "Hello

... there's a lady that's just walked in and she's contracting at my desk." At no point does the tone or content of her words convey the experience of the woman, who is largely invisible behind the high wooden desk. Instead, she speaks patronisingly to her asking if she is finished yet as the woman is almost on the floor with the intensity of a contraction.

The scene cuts to midwives in the office, with one midwife saying, "Today's agenda—get through it." This emphasises the concept of midwifery work as a production line, a system. There is laughter. There is no mention of the women and no sense of the women's voices. The women are completely depersonalised. The head of midwifery states that the midwife's job is privileged, but then talks about the woman being pregnant and "the moment that baby comes out." This language removes any sense of agency on the part of the birthing mother. The woman does not give birth, does not labour herself, but instead, the baby comes out. The focus is on the baby, as something precious and miraculous. A woman called Tracey, who is having her fourth baby, cries out and her husband laughs, sitting relaxed on a chair and observing her. It is not a loving laugh. They are accompanied by their eighteen-year-old son who makes fun of the noises his mother is making—those primal, animal noises that women make naturally when labouring naturally. The mother asks her husband to pass her coffee and be ready to take it from her when the contraction starts, and the husband reluctantly rises to do so, saying, "What, you want me to actually hold the cup while you drink it?" as if this is an excessive demand. The woman denies this, but the sardonic look on his face and the continued laughter frames her as someone who is making excessive demands upon her husband.

Here we see the worst kinds of gender stereotypes and gender roles being played out, without any challenge. It is crucial to re-member that these are created narratives, carefully edited along a specific narrative arc with the aim of representing births in a specific way. The focus is not directed by the mother herself, but by the programme maker and, as can be seen, this results in the validation of a narrative trope of male superiority (and rational-ism) and the inferiority of the woman in the throes of biological inevitability. She is debased by her animal nature.

In the programme, Steve, the husband, mocks Tracey's behaviour during contractions. This could be viewed as light-hearted banter but is also indicative of the way that the woman's experience is minimalized by the two men in the room. Tracey cries out in pain but her husband is too busy playing around with a stethoscope to really pay attention to her, and even though she has told him not to give her coffee during a contraction, he tries to do so as soon as her next contraction comes. He has paid no attention to her experience or her needs. Father and son laugh together while the mother labours in pain. The husband then mocks his wife saying in a baby voice, "I'm going to do it all naturally." As the pain intensifies, the husband blows up a glove and tries to tease his wife with it. The overall effect is to undermine the status and power of the experience for this woman by telling the narrative through the eyes of the men in the room. The voice-over element of the narrative, functioning much as the back story in a novel, allows the woman to talk about her pregnancy experience—but much of this focuses on the husband and his vasectomy. Meanwhile, the shot cuts to the son who is laughing constantly, finding his mother's pain and labour hilarious. Soon enough, the husband tells his wife to "stop getting nobby and aggressive," removing any power from her and labelling her as deviant.

Later on, Tracey is in the toilet and Steve uses a coin to unlock the door from the outside. Tracey's protests are met with more laughter. When she asks Steve for a glass of water, she apologises for asking and he reacts as if it is an unreasonable request. This birthing mother, in significant pain, then asks her midwife for an epidural but is told the anaesthetist is busy; she backtracks, saying that's fine, that's ok, retaining her passive position, not demanding, not acting with any sense of power. The next scene sees this woman on her back, a midwife connecting a fetal monitor, but instead of focusing on the mother, the midwife talks to the son about his parenting plans and his career choices. They talk across the birthing woman as if she is inconsequential.

In the background, Tracey continues to labour and cry out as she tries to cope with her pain. The camera keeps cutting to the reactions of the men in the room. As the midwife carries out a vaginal examination, the birthing mother cries out that it hurts, but the midwife responds by saying how well she is doing, not acknowledging her pain or discomfort. She then discusses Steve's job with him, again with the camera focusing on him rather than on the birthing woman. When the midwife asks Tracey to move because there are some changes on the fetal monitor, the camera cuts to the husband leaving the room and walking down the corridor.

Tracey struggles on the bed with her pain; the midwife doesn't touch her, but tells her to breathe the Entonox and hurries off to get some gloves. Her son sits and watches; her Steve remains out of the room. No one is supporting or really caring for her. Tracey begins to push and the midwife says in another babying voice, "Not little pushes, big long pushes," as if she is talking to a child. Steve hovers by the door and when asked to help keep the CTG monitor in place, does so, though apparently reluctantly. Tracey doesn't want to push but is told she must. As a midwife observing this and hearing the fetal heart decelerating, I know that urgency is needed to encourage the mother to push, but she is framed as someone to whom this is happening, rather than someone in control of the birth experience. Then comes the use of coercion: "I don't care," the midwife says, "but your baby's had enough. You need to push now, otherwise I'm going to have to go and get the doctors in a minute, and they're going to have to pull it out." The needs of the infant as paramount, and the definition of the mother as subservient to the infant, are framed forcefully: "Your baby really would like to be born now." The midwife sits the woman up. "Oh but that hurts," the woman says. "I know," says the midwife, but I want you to push. I want it to hurt." Eventually another midwife enters, and at last the baby is born. Tracey says, "Oh, I've done it." But, at this moment when she should be supremely proud and powerful, she follows this immediately with, "I do apologise for all the noises."

Another pregnant mother in the same episode is shown being placed on a CTG monitor and given a button to press when she feels the baby move. The woman is disempowered and discounted as a birthing mother; the machine will pick up movements even if she fails to do so. Her agency again is removed by being placed as a passive rather than main actor in this birthing narrative. The machine is focused upon, showing decelerations of the fetal heart; the machine is what has made the decision for her to have an emergency caesarean section. A knowledgeable person such as a midwife would understand that it is the risk to the fetus that prompts this decision, but to the uninitiated, the technology features as a character in its own right in this birth narrative, as the representative of a heroic system in which the woman (who has failed to bear a healthy child—her infant has gastroschisis) must be operated upon to save her child. The woman herself seems lost under the machinery and her confusion and lack of knowledge is clearly evident. The focus in this narrative is on the medical process—time is spent listening to the anaesthetist explaining the anaesthetic procedure. This narrative culminates in the typical medical scene of the operating theatre and a caesarean section. I am not arguing against the need for such obstetric intervention. Indeed, it has been the blessing of my career to work with skilled, proactive obstetricians and to know that I can rely on them to intervene when women truly need help. Without obstetrics, women and children's lives would be in far greater danger. But I take issue with the framing of this procedure with the woman as subject, as passive, and birth as something that is done to her.

The midwives in this programme discuss women in terms of their demands on the midwives' time and the resources of the hospital. The music used and the voice-over emphasise the role of the midwives, doctors, and institution in saving the lives of the babies and caring for women when their biology appears to render them inert, powerless, and useless. And yet, every proponent of natural childbirth, every ounce of research, underlines the fact that women should be fully engaged in the birth experience, and that empowered women are more likely to birth naturally, without fear, without drugs, without the need for intervention (Donna 11-13). Nowhere in these narratives is reference made to the single, unalienable fact of women's physiology, that *our bodies are perfectly designed to carry and give birth to babies*.

Furthermore, while I expected American narratives such as *Deliver Me* (which are not analysed here) to represent medicalised birth because of the way obstetrics dominates birth in the US, I was not prepared for how medicalised the British programmes would be, or how it would be possible to observe so many women adopting various strategies to cope with their subjugation. Sears and God-deris take this critique further in their analysis of the American reality TV series *A Baby Story* (190-191). These researchers suggest that, while they could not identify examples of women display-ing agency and resistance in the programmes they viewed, these scenes had been removed during the editing process to create the visual narratives as they appeared in the programmes. Sears and Godderis draw a critical distinction between "reality" and the deliberate representation of women as passive subjects under the dominance of the medical institution (191).

However, this does not mean that there is no evidence of women exercising resistance and agency in the narratives I studied; indeed, the correlation between fiction and the so-called reality narratives re-emerges at this point. The novel *Transgressions* by Sarah Dunant is a first-person narrative of a woman who lives alone and becomes aware of a growing sense of threat, which culminates in an intruder raping her. Dunant's rape chapter starts with instant alertness—a good sense of realism—and this is given a sense of difference, that these circumstances are not normal. Dunant immediately warns the reader that something "unusual" is going to happen. The rightness and wrongness of the situation is highlighted, effectively building a sense of menace. In the central chapter and scene of the book (155), the rape victim appears to "take control" of the experience of rape by submitting, rather than resisting, as a means of trying to control the level of risk and avoid the threat of death. In the birth narratives I studied, similar precursors highlight the sense of impending danger, and the birthing woman submits in a similar manner, controlling the level of risk to self by submitting to the authority of the institution.

For example, in *Midwives*, a non-compliant woman who re-sists that authority, aiming for control over her own pregnancy and birth, is systematically subjected to coercion and threat and framed in ways that generate a negative characterisation of her. This includes brief interviews with a midwife who indicates that her behaviours are irresponsible and that the wellbeing of the fetus transcends the wishes of the woman. The mother eventually submits to the threats and is tearfully defiant at the end, stating stubbornly that she knew the baby would be all right. The loss of her ability to retain control over her own body is evident, but that control is represented as of secondary importance to the potential threat to the wellbeing of the baby. Her voice is represented in such a way as to limit the capacity of the observer to empathise with her position. This is underlined by the use of voice-over and the use of music to create the dynamic and emotional tension in the scene. We can argue that this is a form of narrative force, a creative act which represents birth according to the dominant ideological tropes of woman/mother as subject.

This critical analysis has also raised another problematic issue, the fact that "feminist discourse often contributes to maintaining the very same unequal relations it seeks to undermine. ... We are told, for instance, that in representing women as victims, feminism often entrenches powerlessness as an identity" (Mardorossian, 766). My argument here is that it is not the discourse of critical discussion that represents the birthing woman as powerless, but the discourse of the maternity services, the media, and the state that serves to locate women in specific roles during representations of birth. And rather than associating the stance of the birthing woman as victim with passivity (Mardrossian 766), I would argue rather that the birthing woman is exerting agency in adopting the role ascribed to her by the dominant narratives of birth. Karin Martin equates some of these roles to gendered definitions, arguing that "gender plays a role in disciplining women and their bodies during childbirth" (54). Martin relates these to "normative gendered in-teractions" (58) in which women fulfill social obligations around behaviour which results in "them not to ask for what they need while giving birth and/or not to put themselves at the centre of the birth experience" (58). Martin also relates these to a "mechanism of power and discipline" that places a great deal of control over how women experience birth (58). Yet women opt to adopt such positions in order to be compliant in the false assumption that this will bring about better birth outcomes. As shown above, those who display resistance are characterised as deviant and selfish.

By articulating the ways in which representations of intimate violence and birth share common narrative structures, I have attempted to provide a critical stance which enables the reader/ observer and the writer to resist the kinds of power dynamics that certain narratives perpetuate through the act of representation. This analysis raises significant issues around conceptualisations of childbearing in which it is experienced as an act of violence or bodily violation met by submission or by resistance. This has been an opportunity for me to interrogate the mechanisms and conventions of narrative through which the material dynamics and symbolic framing of birth are depicted.

I have argued that the representation of the subjectivity of women's bodies in narratives is often associated with narratives of sexual violence. Analysis of such narratives identifies women in the roles of subject/object and in various guises of resistance, submission, or passivity. This paper has presented such an analysis with reference to the process of creation of a woman's life narrative, exploring the questions raised by apparent similarities between representations of the woman's experience of birth and representations of women's experiences of intimate violence. The discussion has attempted to "rearticulate the very terms of symbolic legitimacy and intelligibility" (Butler 3) of acts that are played out upon the body but that are representative of a much greater symbolism within narratives and for women's lives in general. I would therefore conclude, as does Jane Maher, that "appropriate adult femininity, heterosexuality, and women's place in a patriarchal society come together in the future of the pregnant woman and seem to suggest its inertia and compliance" (21).

I posit that the act of representing birth both reflects and serves to define the experiences of birthing women in terms of resistance and submission, generating expectations for many women about their role, power, agency, and position. It is therefore imperative that those experiencing birth and those working within social institutions, including the media and healthcare, generate, contribute to, and are exposed to alternative narrative forms that create a different kind of "reality," generating empowering narratives which place the locus of control fully with the birthing woman. Aminatta Forna states that "the myths around motherhood are seductive traps which set up women in the cruellest way" (23). What is most disturbing is that the majority of women fail to challenge these myths and have little understanding of the ways in which such birth narratives serve the interests of those who wish to control birth and all its aspects. Mary O'Brien argues that the typical trope of womanhood and motherhood defines women as "naturally trapped in the childbearing function" and argues strongly against this, stating that what is needed is a "change in the underlying dialectics of reproductive consciousness" (49-51). I agree. These tropes are wrong. Women are not trapped, and they do not need rescuing from the physiological reality of pregnancy and birth—far from it. They need rescuing from the self-perpetuating hegemonic narratives of birth that generate negative myths of women's helplessness. It is time to overturn the "mother script" and create a new typography of birth in which birthing women are the dynamic heroes of the tale, and to redefine the very parameters of birth narratives, including how they are created and disseminated.

[1] Both the programmes analysed take place within obstetric units, where women are cared for by midwives and doctors. In the UK, midwives are the lead professional for women defined as "low risk" and birth often takes place at home and in midwife-led birth centres as well as in obstetric units. However, a significant number of women who are "low risk" give birth in obstetric units where medical intervention in normal labour is routine.

[2] I have deliberately avoided analysing the fictional BBC Television drama *Call the Midwife* because the focus in this discussion is on the impact of birth stories presented in the media as "real."

[3] I do not argue here that this is the only way that women can achieve status and power, that there is any supremacy in women having children. Women should have as much status and power as men, regardless of whether they choose to or are able to have children.

[4] I use the passive voice deliberately here as this reinforces my experience of the lexicon of birth which dominates normative discourses.

[5] This narrative shape reflects a number of definitions of typical or classical narrative arcs (Barry 222-223).

[6] Barthes distinguishes between consecutive functions, which are merely chronological, and cardinal or consequential functions. He states that "what makes them [cardinal functions] crucial is not their spectacular quality (the importance, the volume, the unusual

nature, or the impact of the enunciated action), but rather the risk involved: the cardinal functions are the risk-laden moments of narrative" (Barthes and Duisit 248).

WORKS CITED

Atwood, Margaret. *The Handmaid's Tale*. London: Vintage Press, 1996. Print.

Barry, Peter. *Beginning Theory: An Introduction to Literary and Cultural Theory*. Manchester: Manchester University Press. 2002. Print.

Barthes, Roland and Lionel Duisit. "An Introduction to the Structural Analysis of Narrative." *New Literary History* 6.2 (1975): 237-272. Print.

Butler, Judith. *Bodies That Matter: On the Discursive Limits of Sex*. London: Routledge, 1993. Print.

Donna, Sylvie. *Optimal Birth: What, Why & How*. Chester le Street, UK: Fresh Heart Publishing. 2011. Print.

Dunant, Sarah. *Transgressions*. London: Hachette. 1997. Print.

Einion, Alys. *Inshallah*. Aberystwyth, UK: Honno. 2014. Print.

Forna, Aminatta. *Mother of All Myths: How Society Moulds and Constrains Mothers*. London: Harper Collins. 1991. Print.

Katz Rothman, Barbara. *Recreating Motherhood*. London: Rutgers University Press, 2000. Print.

Kutulas, Judy. "'Do I look like a chick?' Men, Women and Babies on Sitcom Maternity Stories. *American Studies* 39.2 (1998): 13-32. Print.

Maher, Jane M. "Prone to Pregnancy: Orlando, Virginia Woolf and Sally Potter Represent the Gestating Body." *Journal of Medical Humanities* 28 (2007): 19-30. Print.

Mardorossian, Carine M. "Toward a New Feminist Theory of Rape." *Signs* 27.4 (2002): 743-775. Print.

Martin, Karin. A. "Giving Birth Like a Girl." *Gender & Society* 17.1 (2003): 54-72. Print.

Mazzoni, Cristina. *Maternal Impressions: Pregnancy and Childbirth in Literature and Theory*. Ithaca: Cornell University Press, 2002. Print.

Mullan, John. *How Novels Work*. Oxford: Oxford University

Press, 2006. Print.

Oakley, Ann. *Subject Women*. Oxford: Martin Robertson, 1981. Print.

O'Brien, Mary. "The Dialectics of Reproduction." *Maternal Theory: Essential Readings*. Ed. Andrea O'Reilly. Bradford: Demeter Press, 2007. 49-87. Print.

Poston, Carol H. "Childbirth in Literature." *Feminist Studies* 4.2 (1978): 18-31. Print.

Ryan, Kathleen M. and Deborah A. Macey. *Television and the Self: Knowledge, Identity and Media Representation*. Maryland: Lexington Books. 2015. Print.

Sandall, Jane. "Choice, Continuity and Control: Changing Midwifery, towards a Sociological Perspective." *Midwifery* 11 (1995): 201-209. Print.

Sears, Camilla A. and Rebeca Godderis. "Roar like a Tiger on TV?" *Feminist Media Studies* 11.2 (2011): 181-195. Print.

Snowden, Austyn, Colin Martin, Julie Jomeen, Caroline Hollins Martin. "Concurrent Analysis of Choice and Control in Childbirth." BMC *Pregnancy and Childbirth* 11.40 (2011). Web. 29 May 2015.

Tanner, Laura E. *Intimate Violence: Reading Rape and Torture in Twentieth-Century Fiction*. Indiana: Indiana University Press, 1994. Print.

Villar-Argaiz, Pilar. "The Female Body in Pain: Feminist Re-enactments of Sexual and Physical Violence in Dorothy Molloy's Poetry." *Contemporary Women's Writing* 4.2 (2010): 134-153. Print.

ANNA HENNESSEY

Representations of Birth and Motherhood as Contemporary Forms of the Sacred

THIS PAPER EXAMINES WAYS IN WHICH images of birth and the maternal body are contemporary forms of the sacred, and, controversially, how their production represents a renewed interest in birth and mothering as primary sources of empowerment for many women. Through research in art history, religious studies, philosophy, medical anthropology, and feminism, I first show how members of an international movement devoted to birth and art are actively using religious, secular, and re-sacralized art imagery in the visualization of labour and birth and as a ritualistic part of birth as a rite of passage. While this process of ritualizing art objects is interesting in itself, the focus of the paper then shifts to explore how these images communicate a celebration of birthing and maternal bodies. Emerging from this celebration is a renewed model of feminism that considers physiology, acts of childbirth, and mothering as foundational for the empowerment of many women. This model diverges from dominant forms of feminism that point to the problem of birth and motherhood as negatively related to biological essentialism. Anti-essentialism in feminism grew in part as a reaction to the alternative birth movement of the late twentieth century, and it has been highly influential not only within women's studies and feminist discourse but across the humanities. I contend that a logical fallacy is at the heart of these critiques and examine how they have played a part in silencing academic discourse on childbirth, female physiology, and maternal experiences.[1] Contemporary representations of birth and motherhood act as

194

a powerful material means of reinvigorating these discussions.[2]

A contemporary art movement devoted to images of birth has developed rapidly in the United States and abroad over the past two decades. It has gained international presence through online image sharing and networking and through small exhibitions, including a permanent collection, the Birth Rites Collection, which opened in 2008 at Goldsmiths University in London.[3] The movement has a wide reach, and its members include artists who create artwork about birth, as well as others interested in using the artwork for personal or professional reasons. Such members include writers, pregnant women, fathers, partners, doulas, midwives, doctors, childbirth educators, yoga instructors, and acupuncturists, among others.[4] Many of those involved are interested in ways to facilitate labour and birth, often with a focus on natural or alternative methods of birth. However, the movement cannot be defined as a natural birth movement since its focus is not on natural birth but on how objects and representations of birth are associated more broadly with birth as an important rite of passage. This paper theorizes a particular way in which images are used during birth as a rite of passage.

I begin with a discussion of religious birth art. The particular images that I have chosen show crowning or aspects of birth in an overt way and they are also actively used within the birth community. Appropriated in the context of birth in the twenty-first century, these images are stripped of their religious ontologies and propagated as simple, secular tools used in labour and birth as a rite of passage.

The first image is that of a divine figure giving birth (figure 1).[5] It is a wood carving from India, likely dating to eighteenth-century Southern India (Mookerjee 44). Little is known of this image, although popular sources suggest that the figure represented is the Goddess Kali, one of the most important figures in Hinduism. This identification with Kali is erroneous, however. Kali does not have these markings and always has at least two pairs of arms (and usually more).[6] Other sources suggest the figure is an image of feminine divinity found in the contexts of Tantra and Shaktism.[7]

In its online context, however, interest does not focus on the figure as that of a goddess. In fact, almost all of the websites in

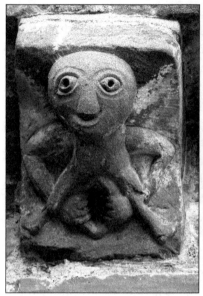 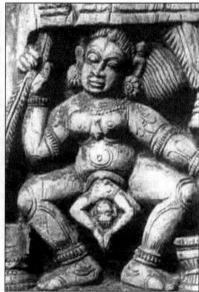

From left to right, Fig. 1:Wood carving of a divine figure. Fig. 2: A 12th century Sheela-na-gig giving birth (detail) India, 18th century Church at Kilpeck, Herefordshire, England.© Mookerjee and Khanna © Copyright Zorba the Geek and licensed for reuse under this Creative Commons License.

which she appears have stripped her entirely of her religious and cultural identities, providing viewers only with the image of her body. On these websites, which are of a non-religious nature and come from around the world, the image is associated with and promoted for the act that she portrays—that of a woman squatting powerfully to give birth—and information provided on the figure is often minimal or not included at all.[8] An example of one such website is lotusfertility.com, whose author is Mary Ceallaigh, a certified yoga teacher and midwifery consultant with an academic background in human development. Ceallaigh's page titled, "Kali Asana—The Yogic Position for Birth" shows the tantric image alongside photos of actual women squatting in the yogic position. The page goes into significant detail about the benefits of birthing while squatting, but it says nothing about the image itself. The figure is displayed less for its relationship to the divine or sacred than it is for its secular aspects, which show birth positioning and the emergence of a baby.[9] The art image also accentuates the birth process through its unabashed depiction of the vulva, which stretches enormously to facilitate delivery. In this contemporary context, the tantric figure helps its viewers on a practical level and not on a sacred one.

Another image with similar purposes is the well-known *Sheela-na-gig,* a stone figure carving identifiable by the figure's large vulva, which opens widely, some say grotesquely, while others claim it to represent the act of birth (figure 2).[10] Originally found in Ireland, Britain and on mainland Europe, the figures, also known simply as "sheelas," measure between nine and ninety centimeters and are still present in old churches, churchyards, and other fortifications.[11] Scholars generally agree that the figures date from the twelfth to the sixteenth centuries, although some have suggested dating as early as the sixth and seventh centuries.[12] The figures are bald with an upper bony body suggestive of old age. Much of the literature describes them as "crones" or "hags." Aside from these features associated with old age, however, the *Sheela-na-gig*'s most distinctive characteristic is its full and enlarged vulva, which is suggestive of vitality and youth. Centered on the body and typically held open by the sheela's own hands, the vulva is the focal point of the object. The original meaning and purpose of the sheelas remain unknown, and contesting theories as to their origins have circulated since the objects first came to scholarly attention in Ireland during the mid-nineteenth century. Speculation and interest in the figure and its meaning have surged in various disciplines over the past two decades. Although a diverse range of theories exist on the subject, they tend to split in three general directions: (1) sheelas represent female divinity and motifs of birth and fertility stemming from pagan understandings of female power; (2) they are connected to Christian warnings against lust and sin as propagated by the medieval Catholic Church; or (3) they are associated with apotropaic devices used within the Church to ward off evil. Within these divisions, scholars have effectively perceived of the *Sheela-na-gig* and its representation of the female body as either sacred, profane, or a combination of the two. In all cases, a common thread emerges to interpret the object's historical meaning: the *Sheela-na-gig*'s ontology is bound to the sacred-profane dichotomy present in modern concepts of religion.[13]

As in the case of the tantric wood carving described earlier, the *Sheela-na-gig* is today used by many who view it as a secular tool to help women during birth. Renowned American midwife, Ina May Gaskin, for example, has written prolifically on the topic of birth for over four decades and has described the practical utility of the *Sheela-na-gig*:

> My idea is that this figure was probably meant to reassure young women about the capabilities of their bodies in birth. Ellen Predergast, in an article written for an Irish journal, remarked, "After a lifetime's awareness of such figures I am convinced their significance lies in the sphere of fertility, and that is what is depicted ... is the act of giving birth." Whether Ms. Predergast and I are right or not, I can testify that a sheela-na-gig figure can be a great help at a birth. As you can see, the vulva of the crouching figure is open enough to accommodate her own head. Such a sight is quite encouraging to a woman in labor. (*Guide* 253)

Gaskin, a highly influential midwife, writer, and proponent of natural birth who has a wide readership and popular presence in the United States and abroad, highlights the object's basic utility as an aid to laboring women.[14] Yet although such focus on the *Sheela-na-gig* and others like it appears to revolve around the secular aspects of birth, the utilization of these images in the visualization of birth also takes part ritualistically in birth as a rite of passage; thus, the ritualistic role that these images may play in this rite cannot be ignored. These images, originally used in contexts associated with religion, are now being transplanted in a trans-religious, transnational, and trans-historical way such that they are not only secularized but are also re-sacralized during contemporary rituals of birth. To understand this process between the sacred and the secular, this paper now turns to an exploration of ritual in birth as a rite of passage. I contend that the use of images like the two just mentioned plays an integral part in how some women are today preparing ritualistically, as well as practically, for birth.

In her comprehensive work on ritual, *Ritual: Perspectives and Dimensions,* Catherine Bell describes birth and birth rituals as providing some of the most foundational models for the ritual processes of most traditional or religious societies. From her theories, it follows that how societies experience birth ritualistically is highly influential in the way that those societies develop other ritualistic traditions. However, in her discussion of secular cultures and the rituals of birth, Bell also states that these societies only mark birth with a few rites. In accord with Bell's thinking here, one finds that birth functions differently or in a lesser capacity as a rite of passage when viewed within its secular context. Yet the secular, claim other scholars, provides rich ground for the rituals of birth. For example, Robbie Davis-Floyd describes in her classic cultural study of birth *Birth as an American Rite of Passage* (1992) a highly ritualistic nature as inherent in the technocratic model of an American hospital birth (see also Klassen). Technological medical procedures in the United States have been standardized in such a way, Davis-Floyd maintains, so as to resemble the standardized rituals at the heart of rites of passage attached to birth in traditional societies. In fact, the rituals attached to the secular tradition of a hospital birth have become so elaborate that their complexity surpasses that found in religious societies (1-2). As such, the birthing woman within this secular context undergoes a cognitive transformation in which she is socialized through the ritual of birth, incorporated as an individual into a shared belief system whereby she joins others to uphold the authority of the technocratic model of birth in her society (2-7). Davis-Floyd also emphasizes the crucial role that symbols play in transmitting the message of the ritual—both to the performers and to the receivers of that ritual (9-10).[15] Based on her examination of neurophysiological research, she finds that symbols are not processed intellectually, which typically happens when a message is verbally decoded in the left hemisphere of the brain. Instead, they are *felt* in a totality of body and emotion, often received unconsciously and filtered through the brain's right hemisphere (9). Davis-Floyd contends that this absorption of symbols is extremely powerful in the shaping of a subject's conformity to the larger social order, giving as an example that of a Marine ordered to sleep with his rifle, repetitively and ritualistically, as a way by which the Marine's superiors reorganize his or her belief patterns to match those of fellow Marines (20).

According to Davis-Floyd, symbols integral to these rituals of birth include everything from a woman's dress in hospital gown and placement in a hospital bed to obstetrical procedures such as electronic monitoring, intravenous feeding, use of pain drugs, epidural analgesia, episiotomies, and c-section. Davis-Floyd's focus is on how the rituals surrounding birth in America are frequently of an obstetrical nature, connected to a different and often conflicting rite of passage, which is that of obstetric training. Within the powerful space of the hospital, she claims, the technocratic model of birth usually replaces the natural model, having the effect of transforming both the rituals attached to the woman's delivery of her baby and to the cognitive transformation that the woman undergoes during her rite of passage. Paralleling Davis-Floyd's work on the secular ritual of birth as it occurs in the hospital setting is the influential research of Melissa Cheyney, a professor, medical anthropologist, and midwife who has examined the rituals of birth as they occur in the case of natural births in the home.[16]

I contend that art images of birth, similar in fashion to the material objects that Cheyney and Davis-Floyd discuss, act as powerful symbols that have the capacity to act ritualistically in both home and hospital births. More significant to my study, however, is the way in which these material objects play a part in revering birth as a sacred event. It is in this reverence for birth, and for motherhood as well, that the secularized art image becomes re-sacralized and treated as a devotional object to be used in birth as a sacred rite of passage. The role that the art object plays here opens up a broader philosophical discussion related to the extent to which objects as a whole may function on an ideological level between the sacred and the secular, for the objects' users negotiate between these two spheres (the sacred and the secular) on three levels: in the first, the object is sacred and religious; in the second, the object is transformed into a secular and practical tool; and in the third, the object is re-sacralized, becoming sacred primarily in its ritualistic function as attached to birth as a rite of passage. Although the material of the object remains unchanged, its ideological import shifts between levels.

The research of Davis-Floyd and Cheyney underscores how material objects involved in birth become emotionally charged

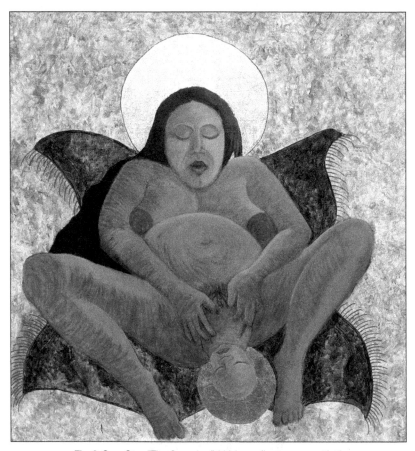

Fig. 3. Sara Star, "The Crowning," 2004, acrylic on canvas, 5'x5'.

and ritualistically meaningful to women before and after their pregnancies. Expanding on this assessment, I propose that religious birth art has the capacity to become sacred of its own accord, even when secularized and detached from its original religious context.

Turning to an examination of contemporary art related to birth and motherhood, I now suggest that the dialectic mentioned above extends even further: artists are representing the secular events of birth and motherhood as divine acts in themselves, inviting their viewers to enter the work with an understanding that the events depicted are sacred. In these works, the sacred and the secular merge, creating a new visual form of sacred secularity in art.

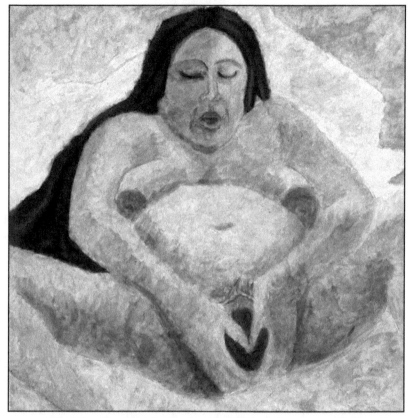

Fig. 4. Sara Star, "Study for The Crowning," 2004, acrylic on canvas, 3'x3'.

Using acrylic on a large 5'x5' hand-built canvas, Sara Star completed her monumental work "The Crowning" (figure 3), which depicts the Virgin Mary giving birth to Baby Jesus. While preparing her subject matter, Star researched the topic of Mary giving birth extensively, but she found no images in all of art history that depicted the event.[17] At the time that she was painting the piece, Star was also unable to find any other paintings of natural birth and so referred to photos in a birthing manual.[18] She then studied traditional iconography with a focus on the style of strokes, verdaccio underpainting, and gold leaf halos, ultimately using modern archival materials. She also completed her *Study for The Crowning* (figure 4) before embarking on her painting of the final piece.[19]

In Star's image of the Virgin Mary, the figures shown are sacred, and yet the focus of the painting is on "the crowning," the act of birth itself, which is shared by Mary and Jesus as mother and child. Whereas this is the only image I know of that depicts the actual birth of Jesus Christ, the emphasis in the birth scene is on the secular act of birth—an event shared by women and children across time, culture, and history. By focusing on *crowning* and not on the Virgin, Star's painting provides for a powerful inversion of art's historical representations of Jesus and the Virgin Mary. Canonical depictions often represent the Virgin as a mythical symbol of motherhood, which some art historians have described as problematically related to a "patriarchal motherhood" or a "sacrificial motherhood" (see Buller). As opposed to emphasizing the Virgin as an archetypal, sacrificial, or divine mother, however, Star highlights the Virgin's characteristics as both a human and a woman.

Sacred secularity is similarly present in Canadian artist Kate Hansen's "Tiara and Eve Marie," which is part of Hansen's *Madonna and Child* series (figure 5). As with other paintings in this series, Hansen depicts an unknown mother and her baby as adorned by the sacred symbol of the halo. Here, the simple union between mother and child is that which represents the sacred.

In Star's and Hansen's paintings, religious imagery is not extracted in order to provide viewers with a practical tool used in birth and labour or to re-sacralize a secularized image. Instead, they have depicted birth and motherhood as sacred events. One might say that paintings such as these therefore rest on the other side of the dialectic in that they offer an understanding of the secular acts of birth and motherhood as sacred acts. And for many women from around the world who examine these images as they prepare for birth, the objects also partake in birth as a rite of passage.

It is within the context of art related to birth and motherhood that a celebration of female physiology emerges as a major source of empowerment. Understanding a woman's own body as connected to her sense of empowerment is controversial, however, in the context of feminism. Essentialism in this context refers to the generalization of a woman's identity based on biological or social properties. In her influential 2004 article "Essentialism and Anti-Essentialism in Feminist Philosophy," Alison Stone provides a definition of essentialism and the feminist debate surrounding it:

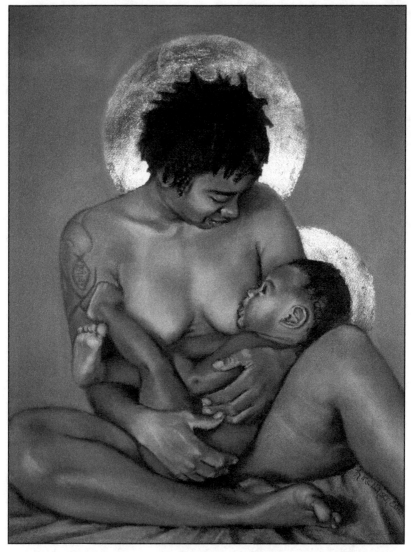

Fig. 5, Kate Hansen, "Tiara and Eve Marie," 2011, conte crayon and gold leaf on paper.
© 2011, Kate Hansen. All rights reserved.

Philosophically, essentialism is the belief that things have essential properties, properties that are necessary to those things being what they are. Recontextualized within feminism, essentialism becomes the view that there are properties essential to women, in that any woman must necessarily have those properties to be a woman at all. So defined, essentialism entails a closely related view, universalism: that there are some properties shared by, or common to, all women—since without those properties they could not be women in the first place. Essential properties, then, are also universal. "Essentialism" as generally debated in feminist circles embraces this composite view: that there are properties essential to women and which all women (therefore) share. (138)

Stone explains that the problem of essentialism has many different strands in feminism, and it is therefore difficult to locate any central themes when discussing anti-essentialism and feminism (137). A prominent strand, however, refers to biological essentialism and the generalization of a woman's identity as based on her physical body, or her capacity or desire to birth and mother children. Critics of this type of essentialism saw its presence in the ideology of the alternative birth movement—a movement that flourished especially during the 1970s and early 1980s—as well as in feminist approaches to reproduction more broadly.[20] Feminist critics of the natural birth movement include Ellen Annandale, Naomi Cahn, Judith Clark, Helena Michie, and Paula Triechler, among others. Natural birth proponents were criticized for promoting an understanding of a male/female binary of gender difference at work by emphasizing the importance of reproduction in the lives of women. One of the main problems with such a duality, the critics asserted, was that it played into a hegemonic male-dominated ideology already inherent in our culture (Beckett 258). In other words, men had always promoted an understanding of womanhood as bound to an identity of birthing and mothering. We see this in canonical western philosophy, as found for example in works by Plato, who categorizes pregnancy and childbirth as mere bodily functions and motherhood as a sub-rational activity; Aristotle, who diminishes and ignores motherhood's import beyond its connection to biology; and Immanuel Kant and Jean-Jacques Rousseau, who naturalize motherhood and describe it as a romantic or naturalistic endeavour as opposed to a philosophical one (Lintott and Sander-Staudt 3).

Criticism of feminist approaches to reproduction is clear in the 1996 article "What Is Gender? Feminist Theory and the Sociology of Human Reproduction," written by Ellen Annendale and Judith Clark. Utilizing the theories of postmodern heavy hitters such as Jacques Derrida, Francois Lyotard, Fredric Jameson, Michel Foucault, and Jacques Lacan, the authors map out a "deconstruction of gender in the context of human reproduction" (17).[21] The authors' primary concerns revolve around the work of radical feminists and sociologists of reproduction (18). Annendale and Clark first describe the feminist position that they oppose, concentrating on how the female body is celebrated for its capacity to create, nurture, and mother:

> In its *strongest* form there is a celebration of women's bodies and the capacity to nurture and create ... and motherhood is celebrated.... There is a sense of a pure and original femininity, a female essence outside of the social and untainted by patriarchy.... The work of Nancy Chodorow (1978) exemplifies this. For Chodorow, a distinct self is formed out of the process of mothering which creates women as different from men through the formation of an essentially *relational* form of interaction with others. In these terms, women must reclaim their bodies from men. (26)

The problem with such a celebration, claim Annendale and Clark, is that it results in essentialism of the female experience and an ideological clumping together of all women into one group and a stifling of individual subjectivities. This same form of essentialism, they assert, is seen in the work of sociologists of reproduction who have pointed to problems of patriarchy in the modern healthcare system and advocated for women to reclaim their bodies through acts such as childbirth:

> Central to the post-structuralist line of argument, then, is the point that duality can become more enslaving than liberating. Reproduction is centred in universal discourses in sociological work on health care; in reclaiming birth (from male obstetrics), it can become the province of all women. [Zillah] Eisenstein, ... referring to women and the

law, expresses this well; she writes: "When the 'difference' of childbearing homogenizes females as mothers, mothers are denied their individuality: all women become the same—mothers—which immediately characterises them as 'different' from men...." Thus in an attempt to create what we can term a "reverse privilege," reproduction is still *centred* for women and put on the agenda as if it were central to all women's lives. This may serve to lock women *into* reproductive roles which may be politically problematic since the centrality of reproduction, contraception and childbirth to *biomedicine* is transferred to women's experiences. (29)

The concerns expressed here, similar to concerns about the universalism of any aspect of history or culture, are an integral part of postmodern ideology. By the end of the twentieth century, postmodernism was the most influential movement in academic discourse of the humanities, and many would argue that it is still dominates that discourse today. Postmodernists believe that the human experience, including the experiences of women, should be deconstructed and described as diverse and subjective, as opposed to universal, essential, or objective. There is, however, an unfortunate irony that results from the postmodern focus on diversification and subjectivity in the context of birth and motherhood, and that is that anything construed as "normative" becomes marginalized. Birth and motherhood, topics already suppressed within academia, and culture more broadly, are further suppressed through postmodern fragmentation and a void therefore perpetuates in studying and describing them.[22]

The experience of giving birth is monumental and transformative for many women from around the world, although certainly not for all of them. It is a simple fallacy, a straw man's argument, to say that acknowledging birth and motherhood as foundations for the empowerment of many women who experience them must also entail biological essentialism and the defining of empowerment for *all* women in the same way. As for being born, it is an experience unarguably universal to the human condition, and although there is variety in the way that birth and mothering happens, it is equally

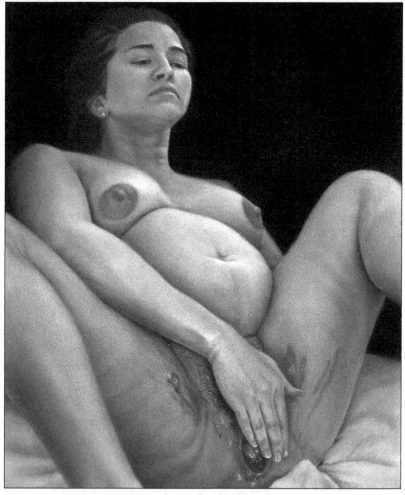

Fig. 6: Jessica D. Clements, "Heather and Daisy," 2009, oil on linen, 25" x 30".

fallacious to claim that the presence of such variety should override celebration of the act itself.

In her theories on how a woman's experience of the phenomenology of pregnancy involves significant social, psychological, and physical metamorphosis, having the capacity to transform a woman's fears of death, Brooke Schueneman acknowledges the complexity of these issues. She addresses, for example, Sara Ruddick's distinction between "birth-giver" and mother in which Ruddick explains how a mother need be neither the birth-giver

nor a woman; and yet Schueneman also carves out space for philosophical discussion of what it is to experience embodiment as
a birth-giver, or what she terms the *becoming-mother* (166-167).
Pregnancy and birth often involve issues that are philosophically
complex, such as the phenomenology of pregnant embodiment, or
the sublime in gestation and birth. Schueneman's work is part of a
new academic wave of interest in embodiment and its philosophical implications during pregnancy, labour, and birth, an interest
manifest in two recent volumes devoted to these topics (see Lintott
and Sander-Staudt; Adams and Lundquist).

In the same vein, artists are creating new expressions and representations of birth that depict birth as a sacred event and re-examine
birth as a topic connected to empowerment. Contemporary artist
Jessica Moore has, in her writing, theorized a feminist aesthetic
of childbirth while also painting works that make manifest her
ideas ("The Act"; see also Butler). In her 2009 painting *Heather
and Daisy*, Moore shows this aesthetic in a crowning woman who
reaches down, unassisted, to feel the head of her emerging baby
(figure 6). As she undergoes physiological transformation, the
subject appears calm and empowered. This painting, like others by
Moore, is realistic and does not hide the visceral and fleshly aspects
of birth. In addition to her work on the aesthetics of childbirth,
the artist has also written about how the advocacy of medicalized
birth procedures often includes a propagation of a myth that birth
is inherently painful and dangerous for women (*Origin of the World*
32). Although birth may involve pain, our culture upholds and
encourages a general understanding that pain and fear are focal
and primary to birth.[23] Moore's artwork and writing about birth
resist these culturally accepted understandings and offer viewers
a different look at how birth may be beautiful and empowering
and how, for some women, a profound connection exists between
birth, mother, woman, and feminist.

In conclusion, the research of this paper has shown that birth,
religion, and art emerge as integral components to birth as a rite
of passage, and that this rite is intimately connected to new feminist understandings of birth. When women re-sacralize religious
and secular objects during pregnancy, labour, and birth, they are
performing an ontological transition of these objects between *the*

religious, the secular, and *the re-sacralized.* Contemporary artists are creating new art about birth and motherhood, representing the events as divine acts in themselves, which suggests that the birth art object is resident to a fourth ontological status devoted exclusively to *the sacred.* The paper has addressed how the postmodern focus on essentialism results in the marginalization of birth and motherhood within academic discourse. In the case of birth, studies of it both as a physiological process and as a rite of passage are deserving of much more scholarly attention and will open up new avenues of research in the fields of religious studies, philosophy, and art history, and have large implications for women's studies and feminist theory.

[1]The silencing of these topics in academia is complex and has many causes. In this paper, I do not map out all of these causes but will do so in a talk ("Uncovering the Topic of Childbirth in Art, Religion, and Philosophy") at the XXI World Congress of the International Association for the History of Religion (August 2015).

[2]As a note to the introduction, this paper's interests in childbirth are not related to the pro-life movement and make no claims about the reproductive rights of women.

[3]I also maintain a website, visualizingbirth.org, which is an archive of art objects used in birth. In terms of art history, two important twentieth-century predecessors to the movement include American artist Judy Chicago and British artist Jonathan Waller. Chicago's *The Birth Project* (1980-1985), a series of monumental needlepoint tapestries depicting birth, represents a critical development in the history of contemporary birth art. As a central figure of the feminist art movement that developed during the 1970s, Chicago investigated art history and soon noted a void in the production of childbirth imagery. From her perspective, the void stemmed directly from a patriarchal history in the arts: "If men had babies, there would be thousands of images of the crowning" (DeBiaso 8). *The Birth Project* represents a five-year artistic commitment during which time Chicago collaborated with 130 needleworkers to produce the show's tapestries. Whereas Chicago's images of birth are abstract, Jonathan Waller's London exhibit *Birth*

(1997) marks a significant move towards realistic depiction of birth. The exhibition was devoted entirely to paintings of his wife giving birth to their first child, and the curators withdrew some of Waller's work based on the reaction of viewers who found it offensive. Waller has since shown his work elsewhere. He is also a faculty member at Coventry University and has a permanent affiliation with the Birth Rites Collection.

[4]I utilize online data sources such as Google Analytics to demonstrate the traceability of the movement as a worldwide phenomenon, and I also look at the types of audiences that some of the websites utilizing the images are geared to. I describe the method and results in more detail in note 8.

[5]The image is now part of an extensive art collection begun by the late Bengali scholar of tantric art Ajit Mookerjee (1915-1990).

[6]In 2013, I wrote to Dr. David Gordon White about this image. White, a specialist in the history of South Asian Religions, noted these aspects and confirmed that the figure could not be Kali. In her work on images found on the *gopuras* (gateway entrance of a Hindu temple in South India), Yuko Fukuroi compares this image to others of her study, finding similarities between the birthing figure and that of Maya, Buddha's mother, although the Buddha was famously born from Maya's side and not vaginally: "Like Maya, this mother seizes a branch of a tree with her right hand. Her left hand and arm are extended downward, and both her feet are turned outward with the knees thrown out sideways" (Fukuroi 273). However, Fukuroi does not indicate the architectural origin of the figure. See also Fowler.

[7]In his work, Mookerjee lists the image as "human birth symbolizing the universal phase of creation. South India, c. 18th century, wood" (44) and the placement of the image occurs in a section of Mookerjee's book devoted to representations of feminine power as found in Tantra and Saktism.

[8]These findings are based on research I conducted in February 2013 and May 2015. In 2013, I used Google's reverse image lookup and found twelve websites that displayed this image. The content of every website pertained to natural birth and was of a non-religious nature. I also used Posterous, a data tracking program connected to my website, visualizingbirth.org. In a two-year

period (2/6/2011- 2/6/2013), Posterous tracked 10,621 visits to the webpage devoted to this figure. During this same time frame, Google Analytics tracked the visits to the image as coming from 56 different countries from around the world (6 continents: North America, South America, Europe, Asia, Africa, Australia). Using Google's reverse lookup again in 2015, the program returned 159 results, many of which were multiple listings from the same page. Broken down, the total listings amounted to 83 individual sites, showing a large increase in usage of the image from 2013; however, the findings were similar in that most of the websites related to birth. The birth-related websites include: 45 individual websites, 26 Pinterest pages, and one Facebook page. The other 11 sites relate either to sacred art, the Goddess Kali, or goddesses in general, although none of these sites provided history of the object. Languages of the birth-related sites include Chinese, Danish, Dutch, English, German, Indonesian, Italian, Portuguese, Russian, and Spanish, with one site devoted to nude figures found in Telugu. I used Google Translate to determine the content of the sites for which I did not know the language.

[9]Based on the research discussed in note 4, I cannot say with any certainty that the emerging form is a baby. But for all intents and purposes in terms of its secular usage, it resembles a baby being born in a fantastical way.

[10]The term *Sheela-na-gig* is the anglicised form of the Irish term *Sigla na gćioch*, which is often translated as "Sheela of the Breasts." For a detailed discussion of the problem of meaning in the name Sheela-na-gig, including alternative meanings, see Freitag or Rhoades.

[11]The majority (at least 110) of extant figures are in Ireland. Approximately 40 others are in England, and a handful more are in Scotland, Wales, Denmark, Germany, and France (Freitag 3-4).

[12]Roberts and McMahon believe some of the sheelas to date back to as early as the sixth century CE, and early-twentieth-century folklorist Edith Guest also suggests dates as early as the seventh century CE (Rhoades 167-168).

[13]This basic division between the sacred and profane stems from Emile Durkheim's discussion of the dichotomy in his *Elementary Forms of the Religious Life*.

[14]Gaskin has lectured all over the world to numerous audiences,

including medical schools. With the translation of her work into numerous languages, she has an international readership and has received numerous awards. She has also appeared in widely seen films such as Ricki Lake's *The Business of Being Born* (2008) and the TEDx series. For a complete biography, see Ina May Gaskins' website: inamay.com.

[15]Davis-Floyd's ideas here agree with the symbolic anthropology of Clifford Geertz.

[16]Cheyney's primary focus is on how women who birth their babies at home use rituals to develop ideals about birth that differ significantly from the dominant ideologies of birth as attached to technocratic society. She describes the way in which rituals that are part of the natural birth model act to transform women during birth: "As the structure and content of ritual carries participants into new representational spaces, the physical body is transformed along with the participant's social status and sense of self. The performance of birth at home enables women to map their own individual experiences onto a collective, mythic, world—in this case, the mythic world of 'natural,' 'alternative,' 'empowered,' or 'woman-centered' childbirth. Emotionally charged symbols (birth tubs, home and reinterpreted technologies like the Doppler) allow social worlds to be manipulated, and it is this manipulation that facilitates a corresponding transformation of the mother's embodied, birthing experience" (535-536).

[17]Star provides scripture as evidence that Mary gave birth in a peaceful way: "After bringing forth her Son, Mary 'wrapped Him up in swaddling clothes, and laid Him in a manger' (Luke 2:7), a sign that she did not suffer from the pain and weakness of childbirth. This inference agrees with the teaching of some of the principal Fathers and theologians. ... It was not becoming that the Mother of God should be subject to the punishment pronounced in Genesis 3:16 against Eve and her sinful daughters. Shortly after the birth of the child, the shepherds, obedient to the angelic invitation, arrived in the grotto, 'and they found Mary and Joseph, and the infant lying in the manger' (Luke 2:16). We may suppose that the shepherds spread the glad tidings they had received during the night among their friends in Bethlehem and that the Holy Family was received by one of its pious inhabitants

into more suitable lodgings."

[18]American artist Judy Chicago encountered the same problem. Unable to locate images of childbirth in all the history of art, she embarked on her monumental *The Birth Project* (1980-1985), in part so as to create images of the act. See note 3.

[19]Correspondence with Sara Star, January 2012.

[20]For excellent overviews of these two movements (twentieth-century natural birth advocacy and later feminist criticism of this advocacy), see Beckett and Moore (Clements), *The Origin of the World*. In her writing, sociologist Katherine Beckett also critiques the natural birth movement by pointing to instances in which medical technology may serve a woman's own interests. She rejects that which she sees as the birth movement's understanding that the pain of childbirth can be empowering for women.

[21]Michel Foucault did not consider himself to be either a postmodernist or poststructuralist. His work and ideas, however, have been appropriated by postmodern scholars across the humanities.

[22]A deep void persists in scholarly and theoretical approaches to the topic of childbirth. In the case of Religious Studies, for example, research overwhelmingly prioritizes the topic of death over that of birth. A review of library and journal resources or any academic press catalogues on religion reveals that the literature available on religion and death greatly outnumbers that on religion and birth. The American Academy of Religion devotes conference sessions exclusively to research on death and yet none are devoted to birth. As for teaching resources, the situation is no different. The Wabash Center for Teaching and Learning in Theology and Religion, a major resource for scholars of religion, dedicates an entire category of its *Internet Guide to Religion* to "Death and Dying," providing its visitors with various syllabi, course listings, and reading materials on death; yet, there is no such category or materials listed for birth. I also noticed this imbalance on a personal level at the University of California, Santa Barbara, while working as one of eight teaching assistants for the very popular undergraduate class "Religious Approaches to Death," which regularly draws over 800 students. Like most other institutions of higher education, UCSB offers no class on "Religious Approaches to Birth" or anything like it. In the fields

of philosophy, fine arts, and art history, the same lack of focus on birth exists.

[23]Renowned natural birth advocates such as American midwife Ina May Gaskin and British obstetrician Grantley Dick-Reed (1890-1959) have written extensively on this topic.

WORKS CITED

Adams, Sarah LaChance, and Caroline R. Lundquist. *Coming to Life: Philosophies of Pregnancy, Childbirth, and Mothering.* New York: Fordham University Press, 2013. Print.

Annandale, Ellen, and Judith Clark. "What is Gender? Feminist Theory and the Sociology of Human Reproduction." *Sociology of Health & Wellness* 18.1 (1996): 17-44. Print.

Beckett, Katherine. "Choosing Cesarean: Feminism and the Politics of Childbirth in the United States." *Feminist Theory* 6 (2005) 251-275. Pdf.

Bell, Catherine. *Ritual: Perspectives and Dimensions.* New York, Oxford: Oxford University Press, 1997. Print.

Buller, Rachel Epp. *Reconciling Art and Mothering.* Burlington, Vermont: Ashgate, 2012. Print.

Butler, Sharon. "Neo-Maternalism: Contemporary Artists' Approach to Motherhood." *The Brooklyn Rail: Critical Perspectives on Arts, Politics, and Culture.* 12 Dec 2008. Web. 15 March 2014.

Ceallaigh, Mary. "Kali Asana—The Yogic Position for Birth." Lotus Fertility. n.d. Web. 10 April 2015.

Cheyney, Melissa. "Reinscribing the Birthing Body: Homebirth as Ritual Performace." *Medical Anthropology Quarterly* 25.4 (2011): 519-542. Print.

Davis-Floyd, Robbie. *Birth as an American Rite of Passage.* Berkeley, Los Angeles, London: University of California Press, 1992. Print.

Durkheim, Émile. *The Elementary Forms of Religious Life.* Durkheim. Trans. Joseph Ward Swain. New York: The Free Press, 1915. Print.

Fowler, David. "Kali." *Encyclopedia of Global Religion.* Eds. Mark Juergensmeyer and Wade Clark Roof. New York: Sage Publications, 2011. 650-651. Web. 15 April 2015.

DeBiaso, Francesca S. "Judy Chicago: The Birth Project." *Schumucker Art Catalogs.* Book 3. 2013. Web. 15 April 2015.

Freitag, Barbara. *Sheela-Na-Gigs: Unravelling an Enigma*. New York: Routledge, 2004. Print.

Fukuroi, Yuko. "Dancing Images in the Gopuras: A New Perspective on Dance Sculptures in South Indian Temples." *Music and Society in South Asia: Perspectives from Japan, Senri Ethnological Studies* 71 (2008): 255-279. Print.

Gaskin, Ina May. "Ina May Gaskin Biography." *InaMay.com*. Web. 12 April 2014.

Gaskin, Ina May. *Ina May's Guide to Childbirth*. New York: Bantam Books, 2003. Print.

Geertz, Clifford. *The Interpretation of Culture*. New York: Basic Books, 1973. Print.

Hansen, Kate. "Madonna and Child Project." n.d. Web. 20 March 2013.

Hennessey, Anna. "Visualizing Birth." 2010-2015. Web. 15 April 2015.

Klassen, Pamela E. *Blessed Events—Religion and Home Birth in America*. Princeton and Oxford: Princeton University Press, 2001. Print.

Lintott, Sheila, and Maureen Sander-Staudt. *Philosophical Inquiries into Pregnancy, Childbirth, and Mothering*. London: Routledge, 2012. Print.

Mookerjee, Ajit. *Kali, The Feminine Force*. London: Thames and Hudson Ltd., 1988. Print.

Moore, Jessica (formerly Jessica Clements). "The Act with No Image: Creating a Feminist Aesthetic of Childbirth." Buller 177-181.

Moore, Jessica (formerly Jessica Clements). *The Origin of the World: Women's Bodies and Agency in Childbirth*. MA Thesis. George Mason University, 2009. Pdf.

Moore, Jessica (formerly Jessica Clements). "Painting Portfolio." n.d. Web. 12 May 2014.

Rhoades, Georgia. "Decoding the Sheela-na-gig." *Feminist Formations* 22.2 (2010): 167-194. Print.

Roberts, Jack and Joanne McMahon. *An Illustrated Map of the Sheela-na-Gigs of Britain and Ireland*. Ireland: Bandia Publishing, 1997. Print.

Schueneman, Brooke. "Creating Life, Giving Birth, and Learning to Die." *Philosophical Inquiries into Pregnancy, Childbirth, and*

Mothering. Eds. Sheila Lintott and Maureen Sander-Staudt. New York: Routledge, 2012. 165-177. Print.

Star, Sara. "Birth Art." *Schnelle Studios Online.* n.d. Web. 12 May 2014.

Stone, Alison. "Essentialism and Anti-Essentialism." *Journal of Moral Philosophy* 1.2 (2004): 135-153. Print.

White, David Gordon. Email communication. 14 February 2013.

NATALIE JOLLY

Does Labour Mean Work?

A Look at the Meaning of Birth in Amish and Non-Amish Society

The bodies of ... women in this way offer themselves as an aggressively graphic text for the interpreter—a text that insists, actually demands, that it be read as a cultural statement, a statement about gender.

—Susan Bordo (169)

IN THIS CHAPTER, I EXAMINE the social landscape of femininity to contextualize women's fear of pain in childbirth. For many women, vaginal delivery has become something to avoid. Trends in medicalization and surgical intervention (including increased rates of elective cesarean section) suggest that childbirth need not involve labour (both generally, in terms of effortful work, and specifically, in terms of the three stages of the birth process). In this chapter, I consider what has motivated this trend towards increased medicalization of birth, with an eye towards the cultural features of our social world. In particular, I suggest that the components of normative femininity devalue a woman's ability to endure pain, to work hard, and to prevail in the face of adversity. Instead, normative gender expectations celebrate a woman's rescue from difficult situations and I suggest that this has material consequences for her conceptualization of pain, her understanding of labour, and her bodily experience of birth. That women might see pain, work, and the indignities of vaginal birth as distasteful and unfeminine should be of little surprise in a culture of femininity that inoculates women against a sense of body- and self-confidence. As a counterpoint, I present data from an ethnography of Amish birth. In a society where both women's bodies and their minds were cast as capable, the strength and the pain tolerance necessitated by unmedicated homebirth did not exist in opposition to an Amish conception of femininity but instead became emblematic of it. The aim here is not to champion pain as a necessary vehicle for women's empowerment during birth but to instead surface the underlying social and cultural features that create an environment where medicated (and increasingly surgical) birth has such wide appeal, and to explore what an alternative conception of femininity might engender.

BORN IN THE USA

When Britney Spears famously confessed in a 2005 *Elle* magazine interview that she "[didn't] want to go through the pain" (Millea) of vaginal childbirth, her words served to illuminate a cultural shift in the meaning of birth in the United States. Spears gave voice to a growing sentiment: the pain associated with labour and vaginal delivery was frightening, hence her decision to electively schedule a cesarean section to surgically deliver her son. Spears is certainly not the first, nor the only, pop star opting for a *celebrity cesarean* delivery (Jolly "Cesarean"). This trend has moved off the red carpet, and now one in three babies in America is being surgically delivered (Quinlan). And while not all cesarean sections are patient choice, new research is suggesting that "fear of giving birth vaginally [has] emerged as the primary reason to request a caesarean section" (Fenwick et al. 395). From where does this fear of birth originate, and what consequences does it have for women's experience of birth? "During the last ten years the wish to avoid a vaginal delivery has resulted in an increased group of women approaching midwives and obstetricians to ask for an elective CS" (Wiklund, Edman and Andolf 451). Many have offered opinions on what has motivated this surgical trend (cesarean section deliveries have risen sixty percent in the last fifteen years)[1] but there has been less interest in inquiring into the source of women's fear of pain in relation to labour and vaginal delivery.

Approximately eight percent of low-risk pregnant women experience fear of childbirth, with about twenty percent of those experiencing "clinical fear of childbirth" severe enough to complicate their pregnancy and/or delivery (Saisto and Halmesmäki 202). Termed "tokophobia" by Western medical practitioners, this growing anxiety "has been associated with pregnancy complications, emergency caesarean section in labour, postnatal depression, and impaired bonding" (Bewley and Cockburn 2128). Increasingly, this has been seen as a psychological disorder attributed to "the general anxiety of the woman" (Saisto and Halmesmäki 204), much like conditions ranging from hysteria to depression. My claim is that tokophobia may in fact be an emblem of a society that subtly undermines women's body confidence. I suggest that conventional psychological analyses may benefit from a sociological examination of femininity to provide context for women's fear of pain in labour. Doing so allows the conversation to wander away from the conventional psychological frame that individualizes women's experience and instead encourages us to consider women's fear of labour pain as illustrative of the problematic nature of normative femininity. Operating within the dictates of gender norms, women are expected (and expect themselves) to *give birth like a girl* (K. Martin) and "bring their socially interpellated selves" (70) to the experience of birth. Meanings of childbirth, then, cannot be fully appreciated without also considering the ways in which gender norms bear on women's understandings of labour and their experiences of pain.

NORMATIVE FEMININITY AND THE MEANING OF LABOUR

Much ink has been spilled in an effort to explore the consequences of gender socialization. From a young age, girls learn the importance of conforming to the edicts of femininity, particularly those surrounding appearance, demeanor, and values (Bordo). Normative femininity, then, is reinforced through a variety of media and gender socialization begins at a young age. Fairy tales celebrate female passivity while championing male heroism (Haase), and cultural products ranging from children's toys (Klugman) to their Halloween costumes (Nelson) instruct girls to be pretty and to be good. Termed the *tyranny of nice and kind* (Gilligan), these gender norms reinforce and reward docility and weakness in girls and women, and leave strength and hard work to boys and men. Goffman reminds us that "boys have to push their way into manhood, and problematic effort is involved, while girls merely have to unfold" ([add page number]). Interleaved is a romanticization of girls and women being rescued, further informing a passivity that celebrates a damsel in distress while chivalrously rewarding men's action, effort, and strength. Martin terms these gendered ways of being our *internalized technologies of gender* and argues that "they discipline and control from the inside, [and] compel us to act in gendered ways from within" (K. Martin 57). Normative gender expectations not only shape others' perceptions of and expectations for our behaviour, but we, too, align ourselves with the dictates of gender. The consequences of this are far-reaching, but the way that the idea of *work* becomes gendered as masculine is of particular interest with regards to women's relationship to the concept of *labour*.[2]

Because femininity is constructed in opposition to physical exertion, the strength and endurance to engage in bodily work is coded as a masculine attribute. And because "women tend to want what the society values" (Klein 249), women then face a paradox when confronting the physicality of vaginal birth: do they embark on the messy, intense, possibly painful, and decidedly physically exertive experience of labour and vaginal delivery, or do they adhere more closely to the politics of passivity prescribed by normative femininity? This notion of *choice* may mischaracterize the situation within which women find themselves, as the voluntary nature of the decision masks the social retribution that often attends gender noncompliance—for many women, the sole *choice* is gender conformity (Bordo). Understanding this may help clarify why so many women "described being 'mortified' at the thought of natural [i.e. vaginal] birth, which left them with a sense of 'sheer terror'"(Fenwick et al. 396). It may also shed light on why "most women expressed a sense of trust and faith in their doctor.... 'I trusted them. I handed control of myself over to them. I was completely in their hands'" (Fenwick et al. 398). That normative femininity devalues a woman's ability to endure pain, to work hard, and to prevail in the face of adversity and instead celebrates a woman's rescue from difficult situations [and] has material consequences for her bodily experience of birth.

So, too, does her immersion into a culture that promotes skepticism about and distrust of female bodies. Beginning with menarche and continuing through menopause, the biological processes of the female body are seen as shameful and disgusting: "Shame, as what we might call a primary structure of a woman's lived experience, extends far beyond her relationship to menstruation, and it becomes integral to a generalized sense of inferiority of the feminine body-subject" (Kruks 64-65). Technologies of gender necessarily incorporate the fraught relationship women have with their bodies, and issues ranging from disordered body image (Bessenoff and Snow) to reductions in academic competencies (Fredrickson et al.) to concern over establishing a significant relationship (Sanchez et al.) to a hindered ability to achieve sexual satisfaction (Schooler et al.) are mediated by a sense of body shame that pervades women's lives. Body shame unsurprisingly colours women's experience of and behaviours during birth, with numerous consequences. To quote Fenwick et al. in their analysis of women's birth fear:

> Enmeshed within the women's narratives of birth fear is a sense of ambivalence, if not distaste, for the value of vaginal birth as a natural, important and significant life process. This is combined with what appears to be a distrust of the body's ability to undertake labour and safely birth a baby. Constructing the pregnant body as a vessel and birth as "getting" a baby, that holds no intrinsic value and necessitates no active participation, reflects a disconnection between the self and the body, and places control outside the self. (398)

For many women, body shame manifests as ambivalence about and distrust of the birthing body. "Bodies of women ... are inevitably entangled in the operations of power" (E. Martin xxviii) and, as such, the body becomes "a medium of culture" (Bordo 165) even during events such as birth, which we may think of as being purely physiological or pre-social. The meanings that a woman attaches to events such as childbirth percolate in the pervasive body shame circulating in society and the choices she makes about her birth practices cannot be separated from this social context.

Femininity shapes women, body and mind. The contradictory nature of female embodiment creates a moment of paradox during childbirth—how do women negotiate and reconcile the social expectations surrounding femininity with the effortful work of labour and the bodily experience of vaginal birth? There is no doubt that the pernicious elements of the culture of femininity position women as apt patients and construct medicated birth and/ or surgical delivery as an appealing option for a growing number of women. This is not to "valorize the experience of natural (i.e. painful) childbirth" (Beckett 260) or to create an environment where women feel constrained against and/or guilty about request- ing pain relief (Brubaker and Dillaway) or to equate pain, labour, and vaginal birth with "Amazonian empowerment" (Crossley 559). Feminist scholars have been wary of claims that celebrate an outdated understanding of an authentic natural female self in order to impose a tyrannical model of unmedicated birth (Beckett). The aim here is not to champion pain as a necessary vehicle for women's empowerment during birth, but to instead surface the underlying social and cultural features that create an environment where medicated (and increasingly surgical) birth has such wide appeal [already stated on page 2]. That women might see pain, work, and the indignities of vaginal birth as distasteful, unfeminine and horrifying (Chadwick and Foster) should be of little surprise in a culture of femininity that inoculates women against a sense of body- and self-confidence [stated on page 1].

AMISH FEMININITY AND THE POLITICS OF LABOUR

It appears, then, that women maintain their commitment to nor- mative femininity, even during childbirth. It's worth considering: what might shift if the norms governing appropriate feminine behaviour were conceived in such a way as to encourage wom- en's body- and self-confidence? Here it is useful to introduce the experience of Amish women, for whom normative femininity is cast in radically different terms.

Below, I draw on material culled from an ethnographic study of birth in Amish society. Spending two-and-a-half years as an apprentice midwife and volunteer healthcare worker in several Old Order Amish communities afforded me a unique vantage point from which to consider the practice of birth within Amish society. Together with a senior midwife in the community (who was not herself Amish),[3] we attended forty Amish homebirths and conducted several hundred prenatal and postpartum visits. For thirty months, I provided prenatal and postpartum care as well as labour support to birthing women and their families. My goal was to draw on local phenomena to understand broader social processes (Eisenhardt), particularly those that involved how Amish women's experience of birth was shaped by their social world.

For Amish women, the dictates of femininity are structured not by *the tyranny of nice and kind*, but are instead shaped by a politics of labour (read: work). Amish femininity was undergirded by an ethic of work, and an Amish woman's identity was realized through her ongoing engagement with and mastery of physical tasks. Within the context of Amish society, femininity was equated with physicality and stoicism, both specifically during childbirth and more widely in daily life. An Amish woman's mettle was measured by a variety of physically demanding and labour-intensive domestic tasks. Labour (both general work and the specific work of childbirth) was the central organizing principle for Amish women's lives.

When I met Lydia, she was a young woman of twenty, newly married and about to become a mother. Her labour, like that of many first-time mothers, was particularly grueling, and her husband, her midwife, and I worked through the day and into the early morning of the next day to help her deliver her son. She walked up and down the stairs to intensify her contractions, and she moved from the bathtub to the birth stool[4] to a hands and knees position on the floor and worked for hours, unmedicated, through a visibly difficult delivery. "You can do this," repeated the midwife until Lydia finally delivered her baby on her back in the middle of a vast living room intended for the much bigger family to come. After the midwife situated Lydia and her new baby in bed together and congratulated her on the work she did, Lydia—while beaming with a new baby in her arms—asked if we've ever seen a labour so difficult. The midwife responded that we had never seen one borne so stoically, as Lydia had hardly uttered a sound through the ordeal. As the midwife prepared to fetch Lydia's mother from her house down the lane, Lydia said, "Tell my mother how strong I was. And how quiet. Tell her how good I did."

Because the details of pregnancy, labour, and delivery are rarely discussed in Amish society,[5] Lydia's desire to have the midwife share this with her mother was profound. And after her mother arrived, Lydia returned to the topic and reminded the midwife to vouch for Lydia's ability to endure the hard work of labour. For Lydia, and for the many other Amish women I attended, mitigating the pain or masking the work inherent in labour undermined the very nature of what it meant to be an Amish woman. Lydia relished the midwife's confirmation of her fortitude. Birth was often recounted through stories of endurance, and these were commonly shared with other women when a mother returned to her church to introduce the new baby into her community.[6] The public nature of these retellings not only awarded a sort of prestige to the new mother, they also calcified Amish femininity in terms of strength. This is not to suggest that Amish women possessed a bald enthusiasm for pain, exhaustion, and bodily discomfort but is intended to remind us that "the construction of femininity is written in disturbingly concrete, hyperbolic terms: exaggerated, extremely literal, at times virtually caricatured presentations of the ruling feminine mystique" (Bordo 169). For Amish women, narratives of hard work in the face of intense physicality supplanted mainstream conceptions of femininity as weakness or passivity.

Configured as such, Amish femininity necessitated a strong body. Slim bodies held little cultural currency in a society where bodies did not serve as ornament. And because labour (read: work) was so intricately threaded through an Amish conception of femininity, Amish women had little doubt of their success in labour (read: birth). As a result, the physicality associated with unmedicated home delivery aligned with the dictates governing Amish femininity. Homebirth provided yet another moment to authenticate her Amish identity; labour (read: childbirth) provided her with an opportunity to labour (read: work). In this context, the pain associated with delivery was not something to fear or avoid, nor was the effort something from which Amish women wished to be rescued. A woman took satisfaction in her ability to accomplish this very physically demanding task, unmedicated and in her own home.

In this particular regard, the patriarchal contours of Amish society nonetheless allowed Amish women a conception of self predicated on strength, tenacity, and bravery: "Amish women approached childbirth without fear of pain and instead equated the noun *labor* with the verb *labor*; they likened it to hard work rather than to agony and suffering" (Jolly, "Amish Femininity" 83). As a result, Amish women saw homebirth as neither a fearful nor risky endeavour; bearing the pain associated with an unmedicated delivery was a source of fulfillment rather than dread. In conceiving of womanhood through a lens of competency, Amish femininity provided Amish women the opportunity to be physically dexterous and intrepid. The result was a strikingly different experience of birth, one where a woman could revel in the strength of her body and in her ability to labour as a seamless part of her femininity. Amish society cast women's bodies as capable, and as a result the strength and the pain tolerance that unmedicated birth necessitated did not exist in opposition to femininity but instead became emblematic of it.

NEW LESSONS FROM THE OLD ORDER

For both Amish and mainstream society, birth is a "socially embedded experience" (Behruzi et al. 206) and one that is partially constituted by the prevailing norms of femininity: "The choices women make in relation to birth and the ways in which they experience (and narrate) childbirth are intertwined with gendered technologies of power" (Chadwick and Foster 325). Such recognition of the role that technologies of femininity play in shaping the meaning of birth has particular relevance to current birth research, as it offers a much needed sociological response to the often individualized and therapeutic approach currently deployed. The creation of "fear of childbirth medical teams"[7] and other such practices that focus attention on the personality vulnerabilities of pregnant woman (Ryding et al.) or on specific caregiving practices to support a birthing woman's self-esteem and personal development (Lyberg and Severinsson) miss an opportunity to consider the zeitgeist shaping a woman's understanding of pain, labour, and childbirth and how those understandings are situated within the social construction of gender.

A sociological reckoning of birth must also consider that femininity is not monolithic but is instead culturally specific and contextual. For Amish women, conforming to the normative parameters of femininity meant that labour and vaginal delivery became an opportunity to showcase the physicality of their bodies. For non-Amish women, femininity makes a pageant of the fragility and weakness of the body, and fear stubbornly speckles women's bodily experiences of birth. This fear of labour and vaginal delivery has very real consequences for women, since "it has been sufficiently established that childbirth-related fear not only poses emotional distress to the birthing woman, but it also has been associated with a longer labor, increased pain and anxiety during labor, and puts a woman at an increased risk for emergency cesarean section" (Eriksson, Jansson and Hamberg 241). As the international healthcare community continues to express concern over medicalized birth and the rising rate of cesarean section (WHO), it is worth investigating whether the growing appeal of these practices relates in part to mainstream American gender norms.

"Meaning plays a causal role in the experience of pain" (Arntz and Claassens 24). I argue that the meaning of childbirth pain is bound up in culturally-specific notions of femininity. Thirty years of research have demonstrated that birth meanings differ across cultures (Jordan and Davis-Floyd) and further research is needed to establish whether such variance stems in part from variations in gender norms and social constructions of gender. In neglecting the relationship between a woman's gender socialization and her experience of birth, we risk seeing childbirth as pre-social and innate. Doing so threatens to fix a social reality into a natural phenomenon. Women's experiences of pain, of labour, and of childbirth are deeply informed by their gendered selves: "As such, it is necessary to constantly interrogate and problematise the milieu in which birthing decisions are made so to avoid slipping into a sensibility that birth is socially decontextualized and that all caesareans [or medical interventions into birth] are freely chosen" (Bryant et al. 1200). Birth does not exist beyond the bounds of normative femininity but is instead enmeshed within it. What might mainstream birth look like if "doing normative femininity" (Chadwick and Foster) allowed for a positive relationship to the physicality and work of labour, rather than a pernicious one?

[1]See, for example, ACOG.
[2]Labour here is meant to refer to both work, generally, and the specific work of childbirth.
[3]Amish women often seek out non-Amish midwives. See Jolly ("In This World") for more on the details that motivate that decision.
[4]The midwife used a three-legged stool in the shape of a horseshoe to position birthing women in a supported squat. The birthing woman would sit on the stool (about fifteen inches off the ground) and her husband would sit behind her (in a chair or on the sofa) to offer her support and help her stay balanced. The midwife would often deliver the baby in this position, as the squatting position often allowed the baby to descend more effectively.
[5]See Jolly ("Amish Feminity") for more on what motivates Amish secrecy surrounding pregnancy and childbirth.
[6]Because church services are held in someone's residence rather than in a dedicated church building, the upstairs bedrooms often serve as gathering spaces for women nursing babies and for mothers with small children, and birth stories were often discussed in this space.
[7]These consist of specially trained midwives, obstetricians, and psychologists.

WORKS CITED

American Congress of Obstetricians and Gynecologists (ACOG). "Nation's Ob-Gyns Take Aim at Preventing Cesareans." ACOG 19 Feb 2014. Web.

Arntz, Arnoud and Lily Claassens. "The Meaning of Pain Influences Its Experienced Intensity." *Pain* 109.1–2 (2004): 20-25. Print.

Beckett, Katherine. "Choosing Cesarean." *Feminist Theory* 6.3 (2005): 251-75. Print.

Behruzi, Roxana, et al. "Understanding Childbirth Practices as an Organizational Cultural Phenomenon: A Conceptual Framework." *BMC Pregnancy and Childbirth* 13.1 (2013): 205. Print.

Bessenoff, Gayle R., and Daniel Snow. "Absorbing Society's Influence: Body Image Self-Discrepancy and Internalized Shame." *Sex Roles* 54.9/10 (2006): 727-31. Print.

Bewley, Susan, and Jayne Cockburn. "Responding to Fear of Childbirth." *The Lancet* 359.9324 (2002): 2128-29. Print.

Bordo, Susan. *Unbearable Weight: Feminism, Western Culture, and the Body.* Berkeley: University of California Press, 1993. Print.

Brubaker, Sarah Jane, and Heather E. Dillaway. "Medicalization, Natural Childbirth and Birthing Experiences." *Sociology Compass* 3.1 (2009): 17. Print.

Bryant, Joanne, et al. "Caesarean Birth: Consumption, Safety, Order, and Good Mothering." *Social Science & Medicine* 65.6 (2007): 1192-201. Print.

Chadwick, Rachelle Joy, and Don Foster. "Technologies of Gender and Childbirth Choices: Home Birth, Elective Caesarean and White Femininities in South Africa." *Feminism & Psychology* 23.3 (2013): 317-38. Print.

Crossley, Michele L. "Childbirth, Complications and the Illusion of 'Choice': A Case Study." *Feminism & Psychology* 17.4 (2007): 543-63. Print.

Eisenhardt, K. "Building Theories from Case Study Research." *The Qualitative Researcher's Companion.* Eds. Huberman, A and M. Miles. Thousand Oaks, CA: Sage Publications, 2002. 5-36. Print.

Eriksson, Carola, Lilian Jansson, and Katarina Hamberg. "Women's Experiences of Intense Fear Related to Childbirth Investigated in a Swedish Qualitative Study." *Midwifery* 22.3 (2006): 240-48. Print.

Fenwick, Jennifer, et al. "Why Do Women Request Caesarean Section in a Normal, Healthy First Pregnancy?" *Midwifery* 26.4 (2010): 394-400. Print.

Fredrickson, Barbara L., et al. "That Swimsuit Becomes You: Sex Differences in Self-Objectification, Restrained Eating, and Math Performance." *Journal of Personality and Social Psychology* 75.1 (1998): 269-84. Print.

Gilligan, Carol. *In a Different Voice.* Cambridge, MA: Harvard University Press, 1982. Print.

Goffman, Erving. *Gender Advertisements.* New York: Harper

Collins, 1979. Print.

Haase, Donald. *Fairy Tales and Feminism: New Approaches.* Detroit: Wayne State University Press, 2004. Print.

Jolly, Natalie. "Amish Femininity: New Lessons from the Old Order." *Journal of the Motherhood Initiative* 5.2 (2014): 15. Print.

Jolly, Natalie. "Cesarean, Celebrity and Childbirth: Students Encoutner Modern Birth and the Question of Female Embodiment." *Curriculum and the Cultural Body.* Vol. 20. Ed. Springgay, Stephanie and Debra Freedman. New York: Peter Lang, 2007. 175-87. Print.

Jolly, Natalie. "In This World, but Not of It: Midwives, Amish, and the Politics of Power." *Sociological Research* 19.2 (2014). Print.

Jordan, B., and R. Davis-Floyd. *Birth in Four Cultures.* 4th ed. Prospect Heights, Ill.: Waveland Press, 1993. Print.

Klein, M. "Why Do Women Go Along with This Stuff?" *Birth* 33.3 (2006): 245-250. Print.

Klugman, Karen. "A Bad Hair Day for G. I. Joe." *Girls, Boys, Books, Toys: Gender in Children's Literature and Culture.* Ed. Beverly Lyon Clark and Margaret R Higonnet. Baltimore: Johns Hopkins University Press, 1999. Print.

Kruks, Sonia. *Retrieving Experience: Subjectivity and Recognition in Feminist Politics.* Ithica, NY: Cornell University Press, 2001. Print.

Lyberg, A., and E. Severinsson. "Fear of Childbirth: Mothers' Experiences of Team-Midwifery Care—A Follow-up Study." *Journal of Nursing Management* 18.4 (2010): 383-90. Print.

Martin, Emily. *The Woman in the Body: A Cultural Analysis of Reproduction.* New York: Beacon Press, 2001. Print.

Martin, Karin. "Giving Birth Like a Girl." *Gender & Society* 17.1 (2003): 54-72. Print.

Millea, H. "Britney's Big Adventure." *Elle Magazine* (2005): 388-94. Print.

Nelson, Adie. "Halloween Costumes and Gender Markers." *Psychology of Women Quarterly* 24.2 (2000): 137-44. Print.

Quinlan, J. and N. Murphy. "Cesarean Delivery: Counseling Issues and Complicaiton Management." *American Family Physician* 91.3 (2015): 6. Print.

Ryding, Elsa Lena, et al. "Personality and Fear of Childbirth."

Acta Obstetricia et Gynecologica Scandinavica 86.7 (2007): 814-20. Print.

Saisto, Terhi, and Erja Halmesmäki. "Fear of Childbirth: A Neglected Dilemma." *Acta Obstetricia et Gynecologica Scandinavica* 82.3 (2003): 201-08. Print.

Sanchez, Diana T., et al. "When Finding a Mate Feels Urgent: Why Relationship Contingency Predicts Men's and Women's Body Shame." *Social Psychology* 39.2 (2008): 90-102. Print.

Schooler, Deborah, et al. "Cycles of Shame: Menstrual Shame, Body Shame, and Sexual Decision-Making." *Journal of Sex Research* 42.4 (2005): 324-34. Print.

World Health Organization (WHO). "Caesarean Sections Should Only Be Performed When Medically Necessary." 2015. Print.

Wiklund, Ingela, Gunnar Edman, and Ellika Andolf. "Cesarean Section on Maternal Request: Reasons for the Request, Self-Estimated Health, Expectations, Experience of Birth and Signs of Depression among First-Time Mothers." *Acta Obstetricia et Gynecologica Scandinavica* 86.4 (2007): 451-56. Print.

Representing Birth

An Inquiry into Art Making and Birth Giving: Implications for Teaching Student Midwives

A S A MIDWIFE AND AN ARTIST, I see many commonalities between art making, midwifery, and birth giving. As a midwifery educator I find value in representing the point of view that birth is a work of art that we are privileged to participate in. As well, I find value in using artistic modalities to explore and teach the art of midwifery. How birth is represented can leave long-term and powerful impressions. How do we, as midwives, present birth to the families we serve? What impressions are left on midwifery students as they traverse our educational systems, and in turn what impressions do they pass on to the families they serve? In this chapter I will draw correlations between art making, birth giving, and midwifery. The question of how to support student midwives in being effective co-creators in the creative process of birth will be explored. Given that in general our educational systems emphasize left-brain thinking, the value of education which supports the ability to intentionally access both left- and right-brain functioning and increase linkages between them, in service of developing practitioners who can practice holistically, will be discussed. Practical applications of incorporating this type of education will be shared through work being done in *Birth and Its Meaning*, a course in the Midwifery Program at the University of British Columbia.

ART MAKING, BIRTH GIVING, AND MIDWIFERY

Art making and birth giving are both highly creative processes.

Looking through an artistic lens can be of value in recapturing the essence of a process that has become routinely medicalized. It can help us remember the fierce creativity that is the heart of the birth process. Both are dynamic unfoldings into the unknown, which some may call "flow experiences" (Kirkam 89-90). To function optimally they both require great presence from all involved (Kennedy; Kennedy, Anderson and Leap). Trust is a key factor for an optimal process. Art making and birth giving have enormous potential to reveal beauty born of deep authenticity and truth. Both have the potential to be transformational and involve working with forces that can be perceived as "larger than oneself" and at the same time as being extremely personal in how they work through any individual. The ability to be in touch with one's internal landscape (self-awareness) is of great value. When transcendence is experienced, oneness with the power of the process may also be experienced. An element of surrender can be optimal in both processes: surrender into the journey as an active participant. Each birth/creative process is unique as it expresses itself through an individual, greatly influenced by all that affects her.

If birth is a work of art that we are privileged to participate in how can we be effective co-creators in the process? How do we practice the art of midwifery? Components to the answer might include (but not be limited to) the ability to be a present caring practitioner, draw on in-depth knowledge and excellent clinical skills, operate in a holistic context, be a guardian of normal birth, recognize and support the truth, negotiate political climates with skillful means, advocate for clients, inspire clients to recognize the opportunity of birth, support women and families in the process of informed decision making, design and carry out excellent and needed research, integrate new knowledge with traditional ways of knowing and practicing, and share knowledge with others in an empowering way.

By definition, midwives provide holistic care (College of Midwives of British Columbia). There are many approaches to expanding one's ability to be a holistic practitioner. I believe recognition / information about the way our brains function can enhance and expand our ability to practice holistically and provide holistic education. Generally, our educational systems emphasize left-brain thinking (Siegel, *The Mindful Brain* 259). The right side of the brain is what gives us our ability to perceive holistically (*Mindsight* 108; Edwards 12). Siegel speaks of the right side of the brain as the "interior specialist, exploring our own and others' internal worlds" (*Mindsight* 113). The right hemisphere has an integrated map of the whole body and receives information via sensing from various parts of the body (*Mindsight* 108). This is key in our ability to know our inner landscape, as well as that of others, and makes attunement and resonance, both valuable skills for midwifery practice, a possibility (Siegel, *The Mindful Therapist* 40-2, 58-60).

The right brain develops earlier than the left brain and is the basis of non-verbal communication as non-verbal signals are created and perceived by the right side of the brain, playing a key role in attachment between baby and parents (Schore; Siegel, *Mindsight* 107). Right-mode functioning incorporates images, metaphors, raw emotion, and autobiographical memory (Siegel, *Mindsight* 108). It "sees a world of interconnecting possibilities... For the left only one view can accurately reflect reality" (Siegel, *Mindsight* 109).

The left brain "loves linear, linguistic, logical and literal communication.... It specializes in syllogistic reasoning, using chains of logic and identifying cause-effect relationships" (Siegel, *Mindsight* 108). These functions of the left side of the brain are essential for our existence, including many of the activities undertaken during pregnancy, birth, and the postpartum period. However, given that the work of birthing is not primarily a left-brain activity (Odent 132; Gaskin, *Ina May's Guide* 167-182), I believe that having an ability to intentionally access both sides of our brain and further develop our capacities will be of great value to ourselves and those we work with. We can see that both sides of the brain have much to offer. Optimally we want to increase linkages between the left and right modes for integrated functioning (Siegel, *Mindsight* 72). The qualities of "flexible thinking, avoidance of premature cognitive commitments, intelligent ignorance, creative uncertainty ... can be seen as the addition of the right mode of processing onto the usually dominant left mode's attempt to create intelligent sureness, clearly defined routes of analysis, categorical clarity, and a sense of certainty and predictability" (Siegel, *The Mindful Brain* 234).

APPLICATION

I have the good fortune to teach *Birth and Its Meaning*, which is a first year course in the University of British Columbia Midwifery Program. Pregnancy, birth, postpartum, and motherhood are explored through a variety of lenses including philosophy, anthropology, sociology, cultural studies, women's studies, history, geography, technology, religion, spirituality, and art. Central questions I have used in the ongoing development of this course include: How do we support student midwives in developing a holistic view of their role as a midwife? As birth is a highly creative process, what supports access to creative energy in the student and what skills will she need to support access to this creative energy in her clients? I believe it is important to support awareness in students of themselves as creative participants in a dynamic creative process and teach skills that will support them in this endeavour. This course weaves together threads that present a holistic view of the midwife's role, nurtures an awareness of the art of midwifery, and introduces the possibility for "other ways of seeing" (Edwards; Downe; Downe and McCourt; McNiff, "Art-Based Research"; Siegel, *Mindsight*) into our curriculum. These goals are achieved in a variety of ways within the course, including the inclusion of course work that acknowledges and fosters artistic expressions of the meaning of birth. There is a growing movement to incorporate the arts into health care education (Elder et al; Reilly, Ring and Duke; McLean; Hall and Mitchell; Naghshineh et al; Davies). Medical humanities programs exist at Dalhousie University, the University of Alberta, Columbia University, the University of Cincinnati, Stanford, Cornell, Brown, Mt. Sinai School of Medicine, Yale, and Harvard, to name a few (Banaszek; McLean). Reasons cited for incorporation of medical humanities include: increasing communication, description, and observational skills; increasing compassion and empathy; improving the wellbeing of students; and increasing awareness of the art of medicine (Banaszek; Reilly, Ring and Duke 251; Eisenberg, Rosenthal and Schlussel 1; Schaff, Isken and Taylor 1272). Kumangi supports the inclusion of medical humanities for the improvement of critical thinking, as a means of self-care and as a "medium for reflecting on the meaning of illness and the nature of doctoring" (1138). She also asserts the function of art as an "expression of identity, a form of social critique and as a means to develop a sense of community of shared values" (1138). Klugman, Peel and Beckmann-Mendez note an increased tolerance for ambiguity as well as increased interest in communication (1268).

Key findings from the 2010 Carnegie Foundation Report *Educating Physicians: a Call for Reform of Medical Schools and Residency* led to the recommendation of four main goals for the improvement of medical education. The development of habits of inquiry and innovation is one of the four goals cited (Cooke, Irby and O'Brien 6). I encourage the practice of inquiry in class based on an open curiosity, which includes a willingness not to know with a desire to find out (Almaas; Epstein, Siegel and Silberman; Kabat-Zinn; Siegel, *Mindsight*). Art as a form of inquiry/research is introduced (McNiff, *Trust The Process*; McNiff, "Art-Based Research"; McNiff, "Artistic Expressions"). Art-based research is defined as "involving the researcher in some form of direct art-making as a primary mode of systematic inquiry.... Art based research ... is intended to include all artistic disciplines" (McNiff, "Artistic Expressions" (385-6). The perception of art as research is supported by Picasso who said, "I never made a painting as a work of art, it's all research" (Picasso qtd. in McNiff, "Art-Based Research" 29).

Artistic Exercises

A variety of artistic exercises are used within the classroom. Students engage in drawing with their non-dominant hand. They draw their journey, what has led them to be a midwifery student sitting in the classroom at the beginning of their first year of midwifery school. They are encouraged to take time to listen to themselves in terms of what wants to be expressed. It may emerge as a chronological tale or one or more particular experiences that were pivotal. Use of the non-dominant hand goes a long way in dispelling anxiety about final appearance and allowing right-mode activity.

Upside-down drawing is used to help students identify the state of accessing the right side of the brain. Rather than draw from preconceived notions of what they are looking at, they draw something unrecognizable (an upside-down drawing from a famous artist), paying attention to relationships of space and lines: "In drawing as in creative thinking—again paradoxically—it is sometimes valuable *not* to know what you are seeing, or what you are looking for. Preconceptions, whether they are visual or verbal, can blind one to innovative discoveries" (Edwards 26).

Drawing in this way calls for astute looking and being in present time. Students are often amazed at the accuracy of copying they can do when drawing with this approach. One of the main aims of the exercise is for students to notice when the right side of the brain becomes more dominant and the qualities that are present when the right side is dominant (Edwards 26).

Visual Thinking Strategies (Yenawine) are practiced in class by looking at slides of artwork. Students look at the artwork and are asked the following questions: What's going on in this picture? What do you see that makes you say that? What more can you find? (Yenawine 6-7). An attitude of not knowing, curiosity, and a willingness to look past initial impressions is encouraged: "When we describe rather than explain, we are bringing the experientially rich right side into collaboration with the word-smithing left hemisphere" (Siegel, *Mindsight* 114). Students also practice increasing their skills of observation through a variety of assignments based on work that is being done at Harvard Medical School using Visual Thinking Strategies (Naghshineh et al.). I think this area has great potential. Miller, who works as a consultant and educator, speaks to the value of aligning visual arts with medical school curriculum: "The experience of inquiring into the unknown through engagement can be difficult.... [I]t is tough work that is central to the practice of medicine. The experience of art-viewing helps to illuminate the qualities of this work, as well as capacities and habits that are essential to engaging fully with patients in the clinic." Miller identifies the following key connections between art observation and clinical practice:

> Make time for silent looking; know yourself as viewer; wonder; consider multiple right answers; state obvious details—and reach for elusive ones; prepare for those small

details to change everything; experience others' individual meaning-making processes. ... Experiences with art teach non-verbal, perceived, intuitive ways of knowing, and provide practice for building fluency between the domain of sensory perception and verbal language.

Schaff, Isken and Taylor describe an innovative program at the Kerk School of Medicine (University of Southern California) that is run in partnership with the Museum of Contemporary Art in Los Angeles. This program was initiated with the aim of "honing students' abilities to observe, describe, and interpret complex information" (1272). The value of students practicing skills of observation and interpretation in the safety of a non-clinical setting is recognized:

Each time we conduct the focus experience, a rich discussion occurs, leading to an inspired recognition that this collaborative, critical thinking process is parallel—and vital—to effective clinical practice. Individuals in both realms observe with intention, test hypotheses by integrating prior knowledge and comparing their evidence with that of other observers, imagine experiences beyond their own, and recognize that uncertainty is an inherent part of what they do. (1276)

Birth Art Project

In line with an approach of supporting the development of the whole person, for the past eleven years I have incorporated the birth art project into the course, with significant positive feedback from students. The assignment has three parts:

•Creating a piece or series of pieces in any art form to explore any aspect of what has been covered in the course.
•Writing a reflective piece discussing their process in approaching and working with this assignment.
•Presenting their piece to the class.

Though some of the students have some facility in the area of artistic pursuits, many do not. Regardless of previous experience, art making is always a journey into the unknown. I find this in itself is of great value as journeying into the unknown is also part of birth giving and engaging in this project can bring greater understanding of and empathy for this aspect of the birth journey. The project can be seen as a laboratory in which students can study and reflect on their approach in dealing with this kind of process. The importance of bringing curiosity and kindness to perceived barriers for both processes is emphasized. Nothing needs to be rejected. This correlates with the notion of flow in birth. Ina May Gaskin has beautifully highlighted the power of truth telling in labour, which can involve speaking/acknowledging barriers, with the resultant opening allowing for flow, the creative dynamism, to return to the birth process (*Spiritual Midwifery*; *Ina May's Guide* 134-5).

Part of the art of midwifery is to be able to sense when there is resistance to the flow and being skillful and creative in what will be of benefit to help restore flow to the situation. As we know, this may involve discussing fears, getting a woman moving, changing what is happening in the space, and looking holistically to see what is needed moment to moment. McNiff speaks to this skill from an artistic perspective: "The discipline of creation is a mix of surrender and initiative. We let go of inhibitions, which breed rigidity, and we cultivate responsiveness to what is taking shape in the immediate situation. The creative person, like the energy of creation, is always moving. There is an understanding that the process must keep changing" (*Trust the Process* 2). Nachmanovitch, a jazz musician, correlates this kind of process with improvisation: "We are all improvisers. The most common form of improvisation is ordinary speech.... Every conversation is a form of jazz. The activity of instantaneous creation is as ordinary to us as breathing. The ideal ... is moment to moment non-stop flow" (17, 19).

Students are encouraged to keep a journal about their process while working on this project, which assists them in writing their reflective paper. This aspect of the project has the potential to support lateral integration of the right and left hemispheres of the brain (Siegel, *Mindsight* 72). In their reflective papers, students speak of the personal impact the project has on them, including insights related to aspects of the art of midwifery:

> The lessons I learned during the creative process of conceiving the painting, including midwifery presence (Kennedy, Anderson and Leap) as well as the ability to surrender and to trust my inner self, are not only personally valuable, they are also important midwifery skills that I hope to use in my practice.... The lessons of surrendering and trusting despite the unknown are skills that I hope to share with my future clients as they approach aspects of their creative form: giving birth. (Bowman)

One student describes her initial reactions to the project, including dread, resentment, and fear, and her desire to avoid the project. She eventually found a way to navigate the situation and found it to be a rich learning experience:

> I learned about ... time and a re-definition of priorities ... I was convinced that art-time would be wasted school-time. Again, I was wrong. I learned about silence. The first time I worked on her, my doll, 5 hours passed without knowing it. And I didn't think "lost time." I thought what a peaceful break. I wonder if this is what they mean when they talk about presence? My mind was still, and yet I was whole. My mind was still, and yet it was concentrated. My mind was still, and yet I felt alert. I felt great. (Surm)

The resistance that this student initially felt correlates to how some women might experience the anticipation or experience of labour. A student's realization that initial reactions can be worked with and lead to uncharted territory and valuable new learning is useful in their future role of supporting women through challenging transitions.

Another student also spoke of her fear and initial resistance to the project. Consciously working through her barriers enabled her to explore what brought her to the profession and her intentions for future practice:

By giving myself permission to be curious about my intentions, I realized that my unique vision is about balance. Especially about the balance and protection of the mother-baby unit. ... Completing this project had incredible meaning for me. It gave me an opportunity to draw on my imagination and emotions around birth. Plus, helped me gain perspective on what my unique vision looks like. I will always cherish the work I did here, and plan to use it as a valuable starting point for my career. (Unrau)

One student created a dance incorporating a large egg, which she created, and the mythic stork feather. Her wish was to include the reproductive processes of all animal species. Her holistic approach to the project included paying attention to many "teachable influences," including lectures on fetal development, observing fetal movements by ultrasound, watching pregnant women move, listening to women's stories of their pregnancies, and incorporating the wide range of emotions expressed into her physical interpretation. Through a process of self-reflection and openness she gathered impressions, became clear on her mind's intentions, and trusted her body: "Through the process of developing this piece I reconnected with how important it is to trust in one's body. It is a magnificent tool.... It was amazing to observe how much the body, and not just my mind, had to contribute to the evolution of this birth conversation." (Emerson)

ARTISTIC CONCEPTS IN TEACHING THE ART OF MIDWIFERY

I believe that introducing artistic concepts can be an invaluable support in learning the art of midwifery. I see value in using different lenses that are more aligned with accessing the right side of the brain and its ability to see and operate holistically. We explore a few artistic concepts in class, though many more are possible. Examples of such concepts include: mark making, rhythm, vision/intention, perspective, space, balance, form, flow, harmony, design, working with the unknown, and presence. Flow has been touched on previously. I will expand on a few more concepts here.

Mark Making

When I engage with a piece of art often what strikes me the most is the quality of the line, brush stroke, or the artist imprint on whatever sculptural medium they are using, be it clay, wood, or stone. Presence and aliveness can be communicated directly through the mark. As midwives, we make our mark in a variety of ways as we work with expectant families, through speech, body language, and touch. Awareness of our impact in all of these areas is an invaluable skill for midwives. Kitzinger developed the following classifications of touch in childbirth: blessing touch, comfort touch, physically supportive touch, diagnostic touch, manipulative touch, restraining touch, and punitive touch (215-29). Gaskin emphasizes the importance for the midwife of what she calls "true touch" (*Spiritual Midwifery* 9-10). One way to support awareness in this area is to include touch as a strong thread (core competency) in our educational programs. This can be accomplished through ongoing reinforcement of its importance as a midwifery skill and through a variety of exercises.

Rhythm

Rhythm is a key component in the arts: dance, music, poetry, visual arts, etc. In birth, flow can manifest in particular rhythms. Tuning into rhythms can help connect one to flow. Looking through the lens of rhythm one hears the baby's heartbeat, the rhythm of contractions and vocalization, the rhythm of reassuring words, and observes rhythmic rocking and the rhythm the birth team finds in working together. Penny Simkin includes rhythm as a key component in teaching expectant parent about labour.

Vision/Intention

"To find our calling is to find the intersection between our own deep gladness and the world's deep hunger" (Buechner qtd. in Macy and Brown 169). I find that most students come into the midwifery program with a strong vision of serving childbearing families. In class, students are asked the following: How do you maintain and expand your vision? How do we support the unique vision of our clients? Students are encouraged to track how their vision develops and changes as they engage in the educational process.

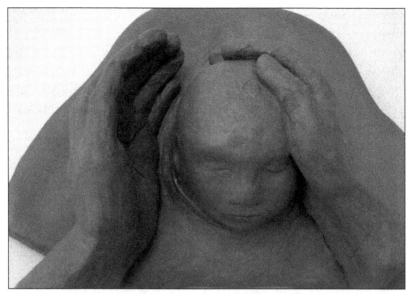

Jeanne Lyons, "The Welcoming," 2008, ceramic, 33 x 23 x 12 cm.
This sculpture reflects my vision of the importance of honouring and welcoming babies as they come into the world. In this sculpture the head has just emerged. The midwife's hands, being the first to touch the baby, are conveying information of what awaits in the outside world. The right hand conveys a grounded calm touch and lets the baby know that we are here, ready to meet him or her. The left hand conveys sheltering as well as openness. It speaks of holding space for the unknown possibilities of who this child is.

Listening is a key skill in the creative process. Though people approach their art in a variety of ways, I find listening is central to my approach. I listen for images. Sometimes they arise as complete images and sometimes as a glimpse of something that shows itself more as I work on a piece. It takes listening to oneself to discover one's vision in a similar way that it takes listening to women to hear what their vision/intention is for their birth. This kind of listening is connected to our intuition and sensing of our bodies to glean its wisdom. As we develop skill in this area we are more able to support our clients in listening to their bodies, which is key during birth. The wide range of possible visions is supported in the classroom.

Self-Awareness/Presence

Self-awareness is an important thread in teaching midwifery. While a strong knowledge base and excellent clinical skills are essential, our ability to be present greatly influences the course of care, affecting all our other competencies (Epstein, Siegel and Silberman; Kennedy, Anderson and Leap; Siegel, *The Mindful Therapist* 1-33). Skills for developing greater self-awareness and presence may include but not be limited to sensing, awareness of breath, self-observation, and reflection. I find introducing students to the conceptual framework and practice of "mindsight" to be of value:

> This seventh sense [mindsight] enables aspects of mind— thoughts, feelings, intentions, attitudes, concepts, images beliefs, hope, dreams—of oneself or others to be brought into the focus of attention. This capacity to perceive the mind ... enables us to gain deep insight and empathy. Mindful awareness contains the metacognitive processes that enable both awareness of awareness and the focus on the nature of the mind itself. (Siegel, *The Mindful Brain* 122-3)

With the new understandings in neuroscience of such states as presence, attunement, and resonance, (Siegel, *The Mindful Therapist*), I think we now have a tremendous opportunity to expand teaching in this area for midwives: "Some medical schools now include self-awareness as an explicit competency, with institutional investment in faculty and curricular time and foundation support" (Epstein, Siegel and Silberman 12). One of the profound opportunities of birth for all involved is to fully enter the present moment in ways that we are not usually called to do. Awareness of the newborn's state of presence is vital for midwives. How newborns are greeted and handled leave profound impressions on them as they enter this world (Klaus; Schore).

Not Knowing/ The Mystery

A journey into the unknown is a quality shared by art making and birth giving. In my experience, to sit in front of a blank canvas, a piece of clay, or a sheet of paper is a confrontation with the unknown. Most of our education is geared towards "knowing." How do we teach and support the skill of "not knowing"? According to Nachmanovitch, "Surrender means cultivating a comfortable attitude toward not knowing, being nurtured by moments that are dependably surprising, ever fresh" (21-22). I believe that the ability to embrace/tolerate the unknown is an important variable in the outcome of the birth process and that students' ability in this area will impact their ability to support clients as they traverse the profound and unknown rite of passage of birth. Even if a woman has birthed before, each birth is a unique journey. The ability to work with fear is an important skill to develop in this regard as fear of the unknown is a common human reaction. In my experience, one of the opportunities of birth is the realization that the present moment is the doorway for creative possibilities and change. It is the place where a woman in the throes of labour, having no idea how she will meet the challenge at hand, finds her resources to do so. I think honouring the challenge and value of not knowing, bringing awareness to this area that we work with on a daily basis, and highlighting its applicability to supporting women and their families in labour are important in our educational process. This can be incorporated with assignments and exercises that enable the student to experience working with the unknown so that they can reflect on their strengths and areas for further development in this area. I find the metaphor of "birth as an advisor" to be extremely useful when teaching midwifery students. I encourage students to be midwives in the space of the classroom to the best of their abilities. The metaphor of birth as a journey with an unknown outcome determined by everyone's participation is used.

Perspective

Flexibility in the use of perspective is a valuable skill in art as well as in supporting birth. Different information is available from different perspectives. While making art, sometimes my attention is focused on the details. At other times I need to step back and look at the piece from all angles, including upside down, to assess overall design, balance, etc. Midwifery encompasses a vast field of knowledge and skills. Using the lens of perspective, we can include microbiology to transcendence and everything in between. The art of midwifery requires knowing what perspective is useful at any given time. It includes the skill of entering into another's reality in an attuned way as well as the ability to step back and look at a situation with fresh eyes and see from a more distant vantage point what might be needed in any given situation. It includes the appreciation that different information is gleaned from different perspectives and the ability to move between perspectives is worth cultivating. This can also include the cultivation of empathy.

CONCLUSION

I encourage us to look with fresh eyes at what we cherish in birth and midwifery and see how we might best nurture and protect that which we cherish. Many midwives are exceptional practitioners of the art of midwifery. I think it is important to name what we do, value it as core competencies for midwifery, and make sure it is covered in what we teach student midwives.

What educational approaches will develop and nurture these future midwives? I believe there are many roads to this end. I have described some of my approach, with an awareness that there are many more possibilities for innovative scholarship. While there is great value in the left mode of thinking, if we have an imbalance in our methods of scholarship, I fear we will lose the heart of midwifery. We have a tremendous opportunity to incorporate a variety of modalities to develop ourselves and support our students in developing themselves to full potential, linking left and right modes for integrated and optimal functioning.

I have a vision that our work as midwives fosters a deep appreciation of the beauty of the birth process and supports childbirth as a transformational, empowering event that is realized for families and their communities; that babies come into the world healthy and welcomed and the natural power of bonding is supported; that the beauty and intelligence of the newborn is honoured; that the art of midwifery is central in our teaching, woven throughout the curriculum; and that as midwives we cherish the art of midwifery and find ways to maintain it in our practice and make sure that it is passed on to future generations of midwives.

WORKS CITED

Almaas, A. H. *The Unfolding Now: Realizing Your True Nature through the Practice of Presence*. Boston & London: Shambhala, 2008. Print.

Banaszek, Adrianna. "Medical Humanities Courses Becoming Prerequisites in Many Medical Schools." *Canadian Medical Association Journal* 183.8 (2011): E441-E442. Web. 15 July 2013.

Bowman, Jade. "Presence." *Birth Art Assignment*. University of British Columbia, 2012. Vancouver. Print.

College of Midwives of British Columbia. "Philosophy of Care." *College of Midwives of British Columbia*. N.d. Web. 1 June 2014.

Cooke, Molly, David M. Irby and Bridget C. O'Brien. *Educating Physicians: A Call for Reform of Medical School and Residency.* San Francisco: Jossey-Bass, 2010. Web. 15 Jan. 2015.

Davies, Lorna. *The Art and Soul of Midwifery: Creativity in Practice, Education and Research*. Philadelphia: Churchill Livingston Elsevier, 2007. Print.

Downe, Soo. "Debates About Knowledge and Intrapartum Care." *Essential Midwifery Practice: Intrapartum Care*. Eds. Denis Walsh and Soo Downe. Chinchester, UK: Wiley-Blackwell, 2010. 13-29. Print.

Downe, Soo, and Christine McCourt. "From Being to Becoming; Reconstructing Childbirth Knowledge." *Normal Childbirth: Evidence and Debate*. Ed. Soo Downe. London: Churchill Livingston, 2004. 3-24. Print.

Edwards, Betty. *Drawing on the Artist Within: An Inspirational and Practical Guide to Increasing Your Creative Powers*. New York: Fireside Book/Simon Schuster Inc., 1986. Print.

Eisenberg, Amy, Susan Rosenthal and Yvette R. Schlussel. "Medicine as a Performing Art: What We Can Learn About Empathic Communication From Theater Arts." *Academic Medicine* 90.3 (2015): 1-5. Web. 13 Jan 2015.

Elder, Nancy C., Barbara Toblas, Amber Lucero-Criswell and Linda Goldenhar. "The Art of Observation: Impact of a Family Medicine and Art Museum Partnership on Student Education." *Family Medicine* 38.6 (2006): 393-8. Print.

Emerson, Jenny. "Birth Art Assignment: Artist's Statement." *Birth Art Assignment*. University of British Columbia, 2012. Vancouver. Print.

Epstein, Ronald M., Daniel J. Siegel, Jordan Silberman. "Self-Monitoring in Clinical Practice: A Challenge for Medical Educators." *Journal of Continuing Education in the Health Professions* 28.1 (2008): 5–13. Web. 5 July 2011.

Gaskin, Ina May. *Ina May's Guide to Childbirth*. New York: Bantam Dell, 2003. Print.

Gaskin, Ina May. *Spiritual Midwifery*. Summertown Tennessee: The Book Publishing Company, 1977. Print.

Hall, Jennifer and Mary Mitchell. "Exploring Student Midwives Creative Expressions of the Meaning of Birth." *Thinking Skills and Creativity* 3 (2008): 1-14. Web. 14 June 2013.

Kabat-Zinn, Jon. *Full Catastrophe Living: Using the Wisdom of Your Body and Mind to Face Stress, Pain and Illness*. New York: Dell Publishing/Bantam Doubleday Dell Publishing Group Inc., 1990. Print.

Kennedy, Holly Powell. "A Model of Exemplary Midwifery Practice: Results of a Delphi Study." *Journal of Midwifery & Women's Health* 45.1 (2000): 4-19. Print.

Kennedy, Holly Powell, Tricia Anderson and Nicky Leap. "Midwifery Presence: Philosophy, Science and Art." *Essential Midwifery Practice: Intrapartum Care*. Eds. Denis Walsh and Soo Downe. Chinchester, UK: Wiley-Blackwell, 2010. 105-124. Print.

Kirkam, Mavis. "Sustained by Joy: The Potential of Flow Experience for Midwives and Mothers." *Sustainable Midwifery and Birth*. Eds. Lorna Davies, Rea Daellenbach and Mary Kensington. New York: Routledge, 2011. 87-100. Print.

Kitzinger, Sheila. "Authoritative Touch in Childbirth: A Cross-Cultural Approach. *Childbirth and Authoritative Knowledge: Cross-Cultural Perspectives*. Eds. Robbie E. Davis-Floyd and Carol F. Sargeant. Los Angeles: University of California Press, 1997. 209-232. Print.

Klaus, Marshall. "Mother and Infant: Early Emotional Ties." *Pediatrics* 102 (1998): e1244-6. Web. 9 June 2014.

Klugman, Craig M., Jennifer Peel and Diana Beckmann-Mendez. "Art Rounds: Teaching Interprofessional Students Visual Thinking Strategies at One School." *Academic Medicine* 86.10 (2011): 1266-1271. Web. 20 Jan 2105.

Kumangi, Arno K. "Perspective: Acts of Interpretation: A Philosophical Approach to Using Creative Arts in Medical Education."

Academic Medicine 87.8 (2012): 1138-1144. Web. 13 Jan 2015.

Lyons, Jeanne. *The Welcoming*. 2011. Saltspring Island, BC. Ceramic.

Macy, Joanna and Molly Young Brown. *Coming Back to Life: Practices to Reconnect Our Lives, Our World*. Gabriola Island: New Society Publishers, 1998. Print.

McLean, Cheryl. "Arts Alive and Thriving in Medical Education." *The International Journal of the Creative Arts in Interdisciplinary Practice* 8 (2009). Web. 3 July 2011.

McNiff, Scott. "Art-Based Research." *Handbook of the Arts in Qualitative Research Perspectives, Methodologies, Examples, and Issues*. Eds. J Gary Knowles and Ardra L. Cole. Los Angeles: Sage Publications, 2008. 29-40. Web. 19 July 2013.

McNiff, Scott. "Artistic Expressions as Primary Modes of Inquiry." *British Journal of Guidance and Counselling* 39.5 (2011): 385-396. Web. 15 July 2013.

McNiff, Scott. *Trust the Process: An Artist's Guide to Letting Go*. Boston: Shambhala, 1998. Print.

Miller, Alexa Rose. "Seven Habits to Improve Clinical Practice." *Arts Practica: Observation in Practice*. Arts Practica. 2012. Web. 15 July 2013.

Nachmanovitch, Stephen. *Free Play: Improvisation in Life and Art*. New York: J. P. Tarcher/Putman, 1990. Print.

Naghshineh Sheila, Janet P. Hafler, Alexa R. Miller, Maria A. Blanco, Stuart R. Lipsitz, Rachel P. Dubroff, Shahram Khoshbin and Joel T. Katz. "Formal Art Observation Training Improves Medical Students' Visual Diagnostic Skills." *Journal of General Internal Medicine* 23.7 (2008): 991-7. Web. 15 June 2013.

Odent, Michel. "Birth Territory: The Beseiged Territory of the Obstetrician." *Birth Territory and Midwifery Guardianship: Theory for Practice, Education and Research*. Eds. Kathleen Fahy, Marilyn Foureur and Carolyn Hastie. Toronto: Butterworth Heinemann Elsevier, 2008. 131-148. Print.

Reilly, Jo Marie, Jeffrey Ring and Linda Duke. "Visual Thinking Strategies: A New Role for Art in Medical Education." *Family Medicine* 37.4 (2005): 250-2. Print.

Schaff, Pamela B., Suzanne Isken and Robert M. Tager. "From Contemporary Art to Core Clinical Skills: Observation, Interpretation, and Meaning-Making in a Complex Environment." *Academic Medicine* 86.10 (2011): 1272–1276. Web. 13 Jan 2015.

Schore, Allan. "Attachment, Affect Regulation and the Developing Right Brain: Linking Developmental Neuroscience to Pediatrics." *Pediatrics in Reviews* 26.6 (2005): 204-217. Web. 15 June 2008.

Siegel, Daniel J. *The Mindful Brain: Reflection and Attunement in the Cultivation of Well-Being.* New York: W.W. Norton & Company, 2007. Print.

Siegel, Daniel J. *The Mindful Therapist: A Clinician's Guide to Mindsight and Neural Integration.* New York: W.W. Norton & Company, 2010. Print.

Siegel, Daniel J. *Mindsight: The New Science of Personal Transformation.* New York: Bantam Books Trade Paperbacks, 2010. Print.

Simkin, Penny. "The 3 Rs of Childbirth Preparation: Relation, Rhythm and Ritual." *Penny Simkin: Nurturing Positive Birth Memories Since 1968.* Penny Simkin, Inc. n.d. Web. 6 Jan. 2009.

Surm, Danika. "Circling Creativity: Reflections on the Process of Creating Birth Art as a Midwifery School Assignment." *Birth Art Assignment.* University of British Columbia, 2012. Vancouver. Print.

Unrau, Monique. "Birth Art Assignment." *Birth Art Assignment.* University of British Columbia, 2012. Vancouver. Print.

Yenawine, Philip. "Theory into Practice: The Visual Thinking Strategies." *Visual Thinking Strategies.* 1999. Web. 12 July 2013.

MARNI KOTAK

Birth is a Labour of Art

FOR ME, MY EXISTENCE AS AN ARTIST and a mother are deeply intertwined and reflect my belief that human life is the most profound work of art. Being a mother as an artist has the potential to unlock cultural institutions that have traditionally codified the maternal body as irrational, weak, and economically ineffectual (Liss 2). Giving birth and raising my child as a work of art challenges our capitalist society that glorifies products over people and the spectacle over authentic human experience.

I believe that the pressures upon women artists of the second wave to keep motherhood and art separate arose out of the dehumanizing, industrialized culture still dominant today, where children are viewed as mere diversions from real, more profitable work. In this paradigm, having children around, acting the way kids do, is often deemed "inappropriate" and ultimately considered a distraction from one's status as a self-determined, cultural producer. Children were not even allowed into the Woman's Building, a public outpost for women's art and culture that housed the influential CalArts Feminist Studio Workshop as well as galleries showcasing the work of female artists (Liss 2). This tendency continues today, as it still feels unconventional to bring my son into art galleries and radical to involve him in my performances; and I am turned away from applying for most residencies because I have a child.

However, of late, we see increasing voice given to the mother artist, both in academic and commercial venues, with a focus on representing the full spectrum of the maternal experience, especially non-idealized aspects. Natalie Loveless pioneered a series of

251

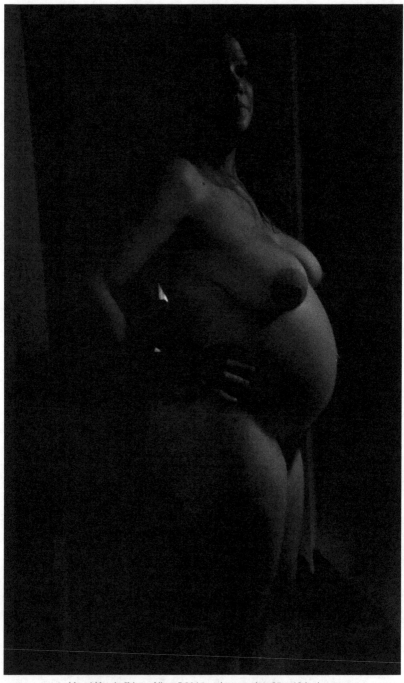

Marni Kotak, "Linea Nigra," 2011, colour c-print, 25 x 13 inches.
(Image courtesy of the artist and Microscope Gallery)

exhibitions with performances and talks centered around the inter-stices of motherhood and art with her *New Maternalisms,* which was first held at FADO art center in Toronto, Canada, in March of 2012 and reached as far as the Museum of Contemporary Art (MAC) in Santiago, Chile, in 2014. The 2014 Feminist Art Project Day of Panels organized by Myrel Chernick and Jennie Klein and entitled "The M Word" was entirely devoted to representations of the maternal in art and visual culture. And as Margaret Morgan writes, "The personal still is political but if feminism from the seventies was largely from the point of view of the daughter, ... it is high time for the voice of the mother—no, for lots of voices of lots of mothers, loud and strong, and talking back and talking over the discourse ... the urgently needed parrhesiastes" (232). So I will heed this call and add my voice in saying: giving birth and raising a child, creating a life, is a labour of art.

While there were not many women artists during the sixties and seventies that incorporated their children into their work within the spheres of high art, there were some pioneers from the second wave, such as Mary Kelly and Mierle Laderman Ukeles, whose work expressed the depth and intrinsic value of the complex experience of motherhood within broader social constructs.

Mary Kelly's seminal six-year work *Post-Partum Document* was revolutionary for its time in that it "established that the mother is anything but passive within the mother and infant/young child's relationship" (Liss 24), as well as postulated the inherent signif-icance and creative nature of maternal work. Kelly's production of the *Document* as a work of art in and of itself, as well as her narration of her own intersubjective participation in her child's development, solidify her role as an active force within the moth-er-child relationship; she creates its form, its documentation, its written interpretation. The mother isn't just a submissive, non-ex-pressive caregiver but an agent contributing to the development of a human being and of her own identity as a mother—and the *Document* is hard proof of this process. Andrea Liss writes of "Kelly's strategic use of autobiographical writing ... [which] allows the mother the truth of her experiences" (26). And through the materials she utilizes in the artwork and the diaristic style of her writings, Kelly's piece "rehabilitate[s] denigrated aspects of female experience, from needlework to maternity to female sexuality and language (Lippard xiii).

Mierle Laderman Ukeles's *Manifesto for Maintenance Art* and works with her own children also represented the voice of the parrhesiastes against the status-quo of their time. Ukeles struggled to be an artist in a world that told her she had to give up her career once she became a mother. Brilliantly, shortly after the birth of her first child, she penned her manifesto, proclaiming that the activities of traditional motherhood, including "cleaning, cooking, supporting, preserving" that were supposed to preclude her from being an artist, were in fact her "Art:"

> D.Art
> Everything I say is Art is Art. Everything I do is Art is Art. I am an artist. I am a woman. I am a mother. (Random order.) I do a hell of a lot of washing, cleaning, cooking, supporting, preserving, etc. Also (up to now separately) I do Art. Now I will simply do these everyday things and flush them up to consciousness, and exhibit them as Art. (Ukeles 2)

Ukeles subversively takes on the notion that there has to be a clear separation between the practices of art and mothering and that the activities traditionally understood as "women's work" are insignificant within the dominant cultural discourse. She is both a mother and an artist. And her motherhood is her "Art," is what is of greatest cultural value. Her manifesto actually opens with her delineating the difference between "The Death Instinct" of the male-dominated art world and "The Life Instinct" of her feminist maintenance art, which she defines as "unification, the eternal return, the perpetuation and maintenance of the species" (1). Ukeles is declaring her value for the transcendent potential of everyday human life, and her fight against the dehumanizing forces of society.

My exhibition/performance *The Birth of Baby X* presented the actual gestation, birth, and raising of my baby Ajax (aka Baby X) as a work of art. For the exhibit, held at Microscope Gallery in Brooklyn, New York, in October 2011, the entire gallery was

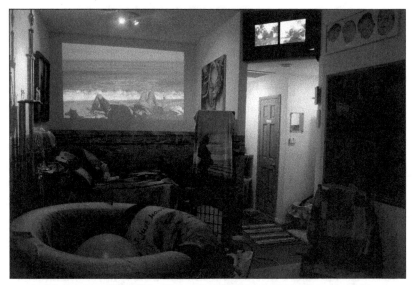

Installation view of "The Birth of Baby X" by Marni Kotak, 2011, Microscope Gallery.
(Installation View, image courtesy of the artist and Microscope Gallery)

installed to create my ideal homebirth center, and the show, culminating in the birth, entailed the weeks spent in the space preparing physically and mentally for labour and the days after, nursing and caring for the baby. The idea to give birth and raise my child as a work of art traced from a decade-long practice of creating work based upon my real life experiences, including re-enactments of my own birth, losing my virginity in a blue Plymouth, attending my grandfather's funeral, and practicing how to French kiss with my best friend in fifth grade, where we each covered our tongues with plastic baggies so as not to be "really" making out. The piece also drew inspiration from the pioneering work of Kelly and Ukeles in the spirit of representing the experiences of motherhood as the work of art itself.

The installation for *The Birth of Baby X* represented the kitschy style of my middle-class New England family appropriated and transformed to fashion an optimal sanctuary for performing the creation of a real life as art. The space incorporated an inflatable birthing pool, a video projection of myself with my husband on Marconi Beach in Cape Cod, the rocking chair my mother used to rock me to sleep, my grandmother's bed upon which Baby X was conceived, a kitchenette, a shower stall covered in photos from my *Baby Shower* performance series, and two ten-foot trophies dedicated to Baby X for being born and myself for giving birth. The exhibition also included works constructed from ephemera from my pregnancy and the birth, including an altar to Baby X's ultrasound, a trophy case containing my original positive pregnancy test, the bloody sheets from the birth sealed in clear plastic archival bags, a box of Texas soil to be the first earth for Ajax's feet to touch (a Texas tradition of my husband's family), and a print made from the baby's placenta with my husband, Ajax's father, Jason Robert Bell.

During the beginning of the exhibition, I spent time in the gallery preparing mentally and physically for the birth and talking to gallery visitors about my performance. The exhibition drew international media attention and critical response, opening discussions on issues of birth in our society. Birth, I discovered, is indeed a big business, which does not profit the women in labour. In the U.S., birth is largely expected to take place in hospitals with costly medical interventions, including a thirty-one percent chance of a C-section. Women are supposed to lie down, preferably with their feet in stirrups, which causes the pelvis to close by twenty-five to thirty percent, slowing down labour (Lake and Epstein xxix). Women are not informed by doctors that the methods used in hospitals that are supposed to help actually complicate the body's natural responses during labour and increase the risk of a "medically necessary" C-section (which is ultimately more convenient and lucrative for the medical establishment). And once a woman submits to medical interventions, to cover the hospital's potential liability, she must remain hooked up to a fetal monitor, so is not even free to move around.

Women routinely give their power over their own bodies and birth experience to doctors in hospitals; the result is that not many real representations of birth have been presented by woman artists, as it is next to impossible to create art in the context of hospital restrictions. In her introduction to *Women Writing Childbirth: Modern Discourses of Motherhood*, Tess Cosslett writes: "A central life-changing event for many women, childbirth needs to be made visible ... from a woman's perspective.... A 'medicalised'

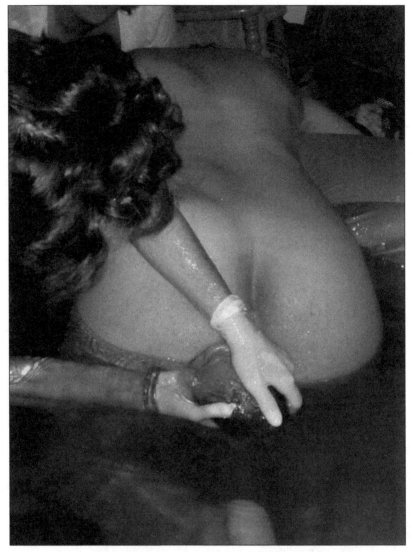

Marni Kotak, "The Crowing of Real Life," 2011, colour inkjet archival print, 18 x 24".
(Image courtesy of the artist and Microscope Gallery).

version of childbirth, in which women are objectified as machines for producing babies, has become increasingly dominant in the twentieth century. This medical discourse has taken institutional shape in the routines of hospitalized birth. Medical versions of childbirth reduce women to an object" (2).

In addition to the commercial benefits, the dehumanizing institution of hospital births appears to be another method for the patriarchy to control the powerful attributes of women that it fears. Tracing back to the Judeo-Christian tradition in the west, this anxiety has played out in various taboos that dictate that a woman is unclean from childbirth and needs to be purified afterwards. According to the Old Testament, she must "touch no hallowed thing, nor come into the sanctuary, until the days of her purifying be fulfilled" (Leviticus 12, 1-8). Julia Kristeva in *Powers of Horror: An Essay on Abjection* writes that the "evocation of the maternal body and childbirth induces the image of birth as a violent act of expulsion through which the nascent body tears itself away from the matter of maternal insides" (101). Birth pushes the body to its limits, out there on the border between life and death, and delivers the beauty of real life from the abject, from pain, blood, sweat and feces.

Deciding to give birth and raise my child as a work of art is taking the stand of the parrhesiastes, proclaiming that I and my child will live free from the reigns of the prevailing norms that do not serve my truth. Foucault describes this type of revolutionary expression in *Fearless Speech*:

> The parrhesiastes is someone who takes a risk. Of course, this risk is not always a risk of life.... If, in a political debate, an orator risks losing his popularity because his opinions are contrary to the majority's opinion, or his opinions may usher in a political scandal, he uses parrhesia. Parrhesia, then, is linked to courage in the face of danger: it demands the courage to speak the truth in spite of some danger. And in its extreme form, telling the truth takes place in the "game" of life or death. (Foucault 16)

By refusing to hide behind a white sheet and give birth in the socially prescribed institution of the hospital, to say that the act of giving birth and raising a child is itself a work of art and possesses inherent cultural value, is definitely contrary to popular opinion. Furthermore, birth and mothering is in fact a "'game' of life and death" (Foucault 16). *The Birth of Baby X* culminated in the live gallery birth of my son on October 25, 2011, at 10:17am.

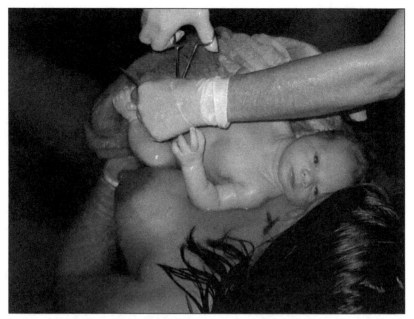

Marni Kotak, "The Birth of Baby X", 2011, colour inkjet archival print, 18 x 24".
(Image courtesy of the artist and Microscope Gallery).

People wanted to know why I chose to give birth in this way, and my response has been that for me, as an artist, the gallery is my temple where I honour what is most valuable to me, in this case, human life in general and the life of my baby specifically. But my choice to give birth outside of the normative confines of the hospital—where one is hidden away from the public, strapped to a bed for the convenience of doctors, even cut off from one's own body with numbing epidurals—was also driven by a feminist desire to represent the gestation, birth, and raising of a child as part of an ongoing artistic process, as well as to challenge the art world and society's taboo against the exposure of real birth and mothering practices. To those who would criticize me, I offer the following question: how are my life art practices with Ajax more threatening to my son's wellbeing than allowing him to be indoctrinated into various societal norms via the socially acceptable parenting practices of giving birth in a hospital, watching popular cartoons that are often disturbing or violent, playing with mass-marketed toys with high levels of safety recall, entrusting his schooling to

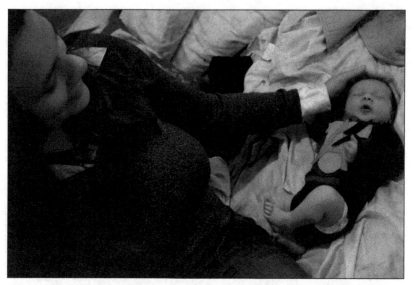

Marni Kotak and baby Ajax, from "The Birth of Baby X," 2011.
(Image courtesy of the artist and Microscope Gallery).

the state, and preparing him to find his niche in the prevailing consumer culture? Birth is a labour of art. After all, what other work of art could compare with the creation of an actual human being?

Over the past decade, there has been an emerging trend among a newer generation of feminist artists to represent specific aspects of their own maternal subjectivities. Natalie Loveless, in her catalogue for the 2012 exhibition that she curated called *New Maternalisms*, writes of "a recent upsurge in attention to the maternal ... all of which pay particular attention to the intersection between art and motherhood" (2). Artists such as Natalie Loveless and Lenka Clayton are demonstrating through their own embodied performances as mothers the inherent value in the everyday practice of real motherhood. These "artistic examinations of motherhood frequently pose inquiries into the mother-child relationship, from the close, yet volatile, connections ... to the changing collaborations and dependencies between mother and child" (Buller 8), even treating the interruptions and distractions inherent in parenting as valuable constraints from which to create art.

In her 2010 performance, *An Action a Day: Maternal Prescriptions,* Natalie Loveless asked five mothers with children under the age of two to perform with her in 84-day cycles, the length of time representing the duration of a trimester. On each day of the performance, Loveless outlined a specific action, derived from her own mothering practice with her son Orion, for them to perform with their children at home. Such playful and loving actions included: "Action 05: August 5, 2010, endure the nipple grab and the sharpness of little dagger-nails;" "Week 13:02, August 9, 2010, trace his ear with your finger, thinking of all the things he will hear in his life;" and "Week 23: 06, October 22, 2010, watch him eating his hand, mimic him with your own hand and see if he notices" (*Prescriptions*). The other artist mothers then in turn delegated a performance task back to Loveless, and Loveless documented it all through photography and writing on a blog. Loveless' ambitious performance demonstrates through its depth, specificity and tenderness, the complexity and beauty in everyday maternal work, as well as her commitment to hold it at the highest level of cultural value. What could be more important than the molding of a real life? As Loveless posits: What might we gain by taking seriously the *remaking* of selves and practices demanded by motherhood?" (*New Maternalisms* 10).

In her 2012-2014 *Artist Residency in Motherhood*, Lenka Clayton committed herself to completing an artist residency in her own home while caring for her two children, replete with the "fragmented mental focus, exhaustion, nap-length studio time and countless distractions of parenthood" (Clayton). Her radical decision to treat the disruptions and diversions that come with taking care of young children while doing one's own creative work as an essential part of her performance, rather than attempting to negate their existence, proves to open up a whole realm of possibilities in exploring the complex practice of mothering. Clayton states her *Residency* "subverts the art-world's romanticization of the unattached artist, and frames motherhood as a valuable site, rather than an invisible labour for exploration and artistic production"(Clayton). Loveless writes how Clayton's work "speaks both to the difficulties of producing work as a performance artist with a child as well as to the importance of working *with* maternal interruption in our social practices and not *against* it" (*New Maternalisms* 9).

In conclusion, I would like to assert that we have come a long way since the seventies where the common understanding among feminist artists was that women needed to keep their pregnancies, births and mothering practices out of their art. Yet, I also wish to acknowledge that we still have a long way to go before motherhood is recognized as the truly valuable artistic practice that it is. As Rachel Epp Buller states, "The complexities of mothering occupy the lives of many contemporary artists..., yet for both historical and present-day artists, motherhood has proven a problematic source of artistic inspiration" (1). Contemporary artist mothers demonstrate "through their work the range, complexity and contradictions of their conscious and unconscious desires, ... [and] contribute to the recognition of multiple maternal subjectivities" (Chernick and Klein 5). However, as Chernick and Klein acknowledge, "although feminism has made radical incursions into the male-dominated art world over the past thirty years, mothers and the representation of motherhood remain on the margins of art practice" (2).

However, if art created from the maternal experience is to take a more center stage in the art world, I believe more needs to be done by feminist artists to address "the elephant in the room" (as I heard it referred to at the recent Feminist Art Project day of panels) of money. Feminism has focused largely on issues with the patriarchy, and the consonant oppression of woman via relegation to lower status 'women's work.' However the lack of value ascribed to mothering runs deeper than the division of the sexes, and has to do with the entire capitalist underpinnings of our society. Caring for children just doesn't pay. So time spent with them is not considered as valuable as income-producing labour. Hence, time spent with them in art is also not considered as valuable as other more commercial art forms. And when it comes to birth, a woman's own experience of childbirth, of creating life, is not considered as valuable as how the hospital industry can profit from her labour.

When I was forced to return to work three months after having my son because my job did not have any paid maternity leave and we had run out of money, I realized very quickly how our culture did not value my role as a mother. The fact that Ajax needed me to nurture him, to feed him and make him feel safe was not important. What mattered was that I resumed my position in the dehumanizing industrial machine and earned a paycheck. And, as I don't have a trust fund, and am not supported financially by my husband, I have continued to struggle with this conflict throughout Ajax's early years, where I have had to juggle my income-producing work as a teacher, with my time spent with Ajax. If strides are going to made to elevate motherhood within art, then these larger underlying socioeconomic issues need to be addressed more in the work as well.

WORKS CITED

Bible. The Official King James Version. Leviticus, Chapter 12. Web. 31 May 2014

Buller, Rachel Epp. Introduction. *Reconciling Art and Mothering.* Farnham, UK: Ashgate Publishing Company, 2012. 1-12. Print.

Chernick, Myrel, and Jennie Klein. Introduction. *The M Word: Real Mothers in Contemporary Art.* Eds. Myrel Chernick and Jennie Klein. Bradford: Demeter Press, 2011. 1-17. Print.

Clayton, Lenka. n.d. Web. 31 May 2014.

Cosslett, Tess. Introduction. *Women Writing Childbirth: Modern Discourses on Motherhood.* New York: Manchester University Press, 1994. 1-8. Print.

Eisenstein, Zillah. *Capitalist Patriarchy and the Case for Socialist Feminism.* New York: Monthly Review Press, 1979. Print.

Foucault, Michael. *Fearless Speech.* Los Angeles: Semiotext(e), 2001. Print.

Kelly, Mary. *Postpartum Document.* Los Angeles: University of California Press, 1893. Print.

Kristeva, Julia. *Powers of Horror: An Essay on Abjection.* Trans. Leon S. Roudiez. European Perspectives: A Series of the Columbia University Press, New York. 1982. Print.

Lippard, Lucy. Foreword. *Postpartum Document.* Los Angeles: University of California Press, 1893. xi-xvi. Print.

Lake, Ricki, and Abby Epstein. Introduction. *Your Best Birth: Know all Your Options, Discover the Natural Choices, and Take Back The Birth Experience.* 1st Ed. Boston: Wellness Central, 2009. xxvii-xxxi. Print.

Liss, Andrea. *Feminist Art and the Maternal.* London: University of Minnesota, 2009. Print.

Loveless, Natalie. *An Action a Day: Maternal Prescriptions: Book Document.* Pdf.

Loveless, Natalie. *New Maternalisms.* Catalogue Essay. Toronto: Fado Performance, 2012. Print.

Morgan, Margaret. "Home Truths." *The M Word: Real Mothers in Contemporary Art.* Ed. Myrel Chernick and Jennie Klein. Bradford: Demeter Press, 2011. 213-233. Print.

Ukeles, Mierle Laderman. *Manifesto of Maintenance Art.* 1969. Web. 29 May 2014.

Split Open

THE VERY ACT OF BIRTHING FORCED ME to completely surrender to the throws of labour and natural delivery. There was no sidestepping the inevitable birthing.

Why had I not been told more about this initiation into being? Not my child's, but my own!

In this moment of birthing, I was *split open* at once. It was like a lightning bolt went in through the crown of my head right through the birth canal and split me open like a dry log under the axe. I had died and been reborn in that instant of my daughter's birth.

My child came through me—jettisoning me into the universe of space, time, and relations with all beings that are and would ever be. It was the only time in my life I can say I absolutely *knew* "G*d."

The mystery coursed through me. It was in me and of me. Every particle of my being became part of the matter of the universe. The world itself was changed, *split open*. From this place life emerged anew.

The very grit of being was the matter and communion of my universe. I was in the deepest vastest molecular spectacular oneness that opened me wider than vision can hold. It was particular and private and profoundly of something so much bigger than *everything* I had known.

And oh! What Child born of this push, this Bolt. This completely perfect immaculate energy was so much greater than the chemistry that wove the necessary ingredients together to bring her into being. Her Birth—through me—thrust me into that place of unnamed power and wisdom. In no time at all, life and death were one.

Is this divine divide visible only to those women who have had this experience?

Where were the philosopher mothers to guide me into the sacred nature of this psychologically critical rite of passage? (Were those best-qualified to write about it simply too exhausted, as I was, from middle-of-the-night feedings, diaper changes, mastitis, post-partum depression, worry about everything, and lack of sufficient child and personal support?) No amount of Babies R Us shopping trips could nourish the need to sanctify the depths of this experience. My motherhood was hungering for a feminist framework in which to honour this experience.

There was one wise elder woman I found, a psychiatrist and Jungian, who knew to wait and not medicate away the symptoms of post-partum depression that followed. She deeply knew how important it was to companion me and be present to my ravaging solitary journey into motherhood, and she understood that psyche needed time to honour and process the Split. I am forever grateful to Her. She acknowledged there was indeed a silence about this in our culture. She encouraged me to write about it all someday.

Now I wonder, and I ask you.... Have you been *Split Open*?

Flower of My Flesh

I. (2/8/60 for my daughter Elizabeth)

flower of my flesh i saw you bloom

tho
blossoms reach away
i will watch you grow
with hybrid style
with delicate
staminal
grace

tho blossoms reach away i saw you bloom

     a
     mere
     receptacle
     for birth
     was
     i
     stretched
     thin your bud
     was heaved was
     pushed full-
     blown
     the

pain all
trembling and un-
aided in the air re-
leased its shiny child
and pleasure
filled the
sharpened
depths

flower of my flesh i felt you bloom

and i
will follow you
through all the bendings
of your growing and
all the turnings of
you changing
until we shed
with scatter
on the wind

flower of my flesh i see you bloom

II. 3/22/94 for her son Levi (my heart)

flower of my flesh
i saw you bloom

      a seed writ large
      the first blossom of our love
      that special first

flower of my flesh
now grown, you bloomed again

      this life force
      of your own

was heaved was born
and made you new

flower of your flesh
i'll see him bloom

and be with him
at all the turnings
of each season
as he opens to his life

and watch the seeding
of his own, at each green time

THE STORY BEHIND THE POEM

When I was pregnant for the first time in 1959, I was working as a librarian at the Indiana State Library, with all the most recently published books at my disposal. Hot off the press, Marjorie Karmel's book *Thank You, Dr. Lamaze* was read in one sitting. Ms. Karmel described a new method of giving birth without drugs, a method that her French doctor modelled after his experiences in Russia at the time. It became known eventually as the Lamaze method of childbirth. The Mayo Clinic describes that the goal of this method is

> to increase confidence in your ability to give birth. Lamaze classes help you understand how to cope with pain in ways that both facilitate labor and promote comfort—including focused breathing, movement and massage. ("Pregnancy")

When we moved to New York, I was quite pregnant and immediately called Marjorie Karmel on the telephone for advice. She invited me to her home where I met Elizabeth Bing, who was called a Monitrice. Today she might be called a Doula or a labour coach or even a midwife. Now a pioneer in the field of natural childbirth, she then immediately began giving me and my husband breathing lessons for the early stages of labour at the rate of one a week. In 1990, she gave some historical perspective to her role in the field:

> Being considered a radical some years ago may sound strange to some of my younger colleagues today, some of whom now think of me as rather old-fashioned. Even though this may not be entirely true, it's a good healthy sign that our work is alive and moving forward in many new directions. ("About Lamaze")

Back in January of 1960, my husband and I never completed her course because my waters broke earlier than expected. We had to rush from our one-room apartment in Irvington, New York, to Mount Sinai hospital sometime after dawn. I remember arriving and beginning the breathing as Elizabeth had instructed. Meanwhile, a whole class of nurses came into my labour room to view the mother who wasn't screaming and marvel at my performance. Alan Guttmacher, an early president of Planned Parenthood and the famous doctor who founded the institute that bears his name today, even visited me. In the meantime, my husband had disappeared. He was on the phone with Elizabeth receiving instructions for the breathing technique during the final stages of labour. He returned just as I entered the transition stage. In the nick of time, as they said in those days.

They wheeled me into the delivery room, leaving my husband, Sandy, worrying in the hallway. He was not allowed to enter. I delivered my first child, Elizabeth, aptly named for that moment in history, on February 8, 1960, after quite a long labour. I wrote this poem shortly afterwards.

The poem that follows has another backstory. Elizabeth married in her late twenties, determined to have a child before she was thirty. She succeeded but the birthing was another story. Complications followed and she had a Cesarean delivery with her husband viewing the procedure. More complications followed in the marriage and soon afterwards they were divorced. She married again and delivered a boy avoiding another Cesarean. That's when I wrote the second poem. At this time, natural childbirth was much more mainstream. Someday I hope to write poem number three for my grandson, whose name is Levi, which means "my heart" in Hebrew.

WORKS CITED

"Pregnancy Week by Week." *Mayo Clinic.* 18 June 2014. Web.
"About Lamaze." *Lamaze International.* n.d. Web.

SUSAN HOGAN, CHARLOTTE BAKER,
SHELAGH CORNISH, PAULA MCCLOSKEY AND LISA WATTS

Birth Shock

Exploring Pregnancy, Birth, and the Transition to Motherhood Using Participatory Arts

THE BIRTH PROJECT IS FUNDED RESEARCH by the Arts and Humanities Research Council, UK. New mothers are being given the opportunity to explore their experiences of pregnancy, birth, and post-natal readjustments using different art forms: phototherapy, photo-diaries, and participatory arts. In The Birth Project, the arts are being used to interrogate this complex topic. We situate this endeavour in the context of an emerging practice of health humanities (Crawford et al.) art as social action (Levine and Levine) and visual research methodologies (Pink, *Advances, The Future*). This chapter will focus on the participatory arts work already undertaken to date with mothers. Our primary research interests are to explore how women experience birth, what factors contribute to a traumatic birth or post-natal distress, and furthermore what is distinctive and positive about an arts-based approach. This is a qualitative endeavour and we are addressing the research inquiries through the production of films, which have been edited to show footage that investigates these issues.

A GOOD ENOUGH BIRTH

Women may face challenges to obtain the kind of birth they want, whether at home or in hospital, whether they hope for a non-interventionist experience or an elective caesarean section. There are numerous factors that have an impact on any woman's experience. The decision to have a home birth carries its own set of challenges and involves making extra arrangements. This can require considerable strength of purpose—the prospective mother may encounter opposition or misinformation from doctors, midwives, or from family members who might need to be persuaded. Hospital protocols—which may be rigid and based on the "worst case" scenario—coupled with the unpredictability of birthing itself can override what women want and expect in terms of their birth experience; this leaves some women suspended on a spectrum from disappointed or let down through to traumatised, which can then have consequences for infant development and mental health (Knitzer, Theberge and Johnson).

The estimated costs of postnatal depression in England and Wales are at least £45 million per annum (Knapp et al.) and this was stated as a conservative estimate. Post-natal depression is a significant public health problem (Downey and Coyne; Almond; Oates et al.; World Health Organisation). The main cause of maternal death in the UK is suicide (Oates). Of course, *true* statistics on postnatal distress, depression, anxiety, and postnatal psychosis are impossible to gather as some women suffer in silence. Postnatal distress in all forms remains stigmatised and at odds with the idealisation of motherhood as a time of joy and wonder. It occurs at a time when women are regulated through the promotion of and enquiries about breastfeeding and through postnatal recovery check-ups (including the promotion of postnatal contraception as early as a few hours post-delivery), and are subject to potentially dismissive lines from family members and professionals, such as "It's just the baby blues—all women have them" or "Of course you're tired, its normal," or affront at reactions that fail to meet the broad expectation of happiness and joy at the creation of a new life. As well as risks to women themselves, which can be devastating, mother-baby interactions can be adversely affected. This in turn has consequences for the longer-term emotional, cognitive, and social development of the baby (Knitzer, Theberge and Johnson; NICE).

Although we have mentioned some of the ways that post-natal depression is commonly represented, this research is interested to develop a holistic picture of birth and the transition to motherhood. (Arguably, we need to explore the medical discourses which encapsulate many women's experience to be able to demonstrate the richness of experience outside of this discourse; we don't wish to label women). We are aware of critiques of the dichotomous dominant tropes of the radiant mother and those who can't cope—the hormonally unbalanced or unhinged. The transition to motherhood, as an important and highly contested rite of passage, is recognised. Discussion of the traumatised or depressed mother, if we are to adopt this language at all, needs to acknowledge a range of factors. These range from a disrupted sense of self-identity, compounded by sudden social isolation or discriminatory workplace practices, to societal reactions that may include restrictive expectations relating to behavioural change ("You're a mother now so..."), to idealised expectations of motherhood and mothering which are potentially oppressive in themselves, to an analysis of iatrogenic hospital practices (those practices which are illness-inducing, for instance, supine birthing postures in obstetrics; see Kitzinger). Rather than situating the new mother as inadequate, a feminist analysis is gentler in its judgement. Furthermore, feminist scholarship looks further still at the underlying discourses and critiques the inadequate models that underpin some dominant psychiatric theories about motherhood. The reductive application of theory is a structural issue insofar as it has an impact on services and on women's lives (Bordo; Hogan "Problems of Identity"). For instance, a generation of women have grown up worrying about leaving their infant in the care of another, believing that the baby could become traumatised or develop "attachment" problems; this has led to much unnecessary maternal misery and guilt (Hogan "A Discussion"). Sound anthropological research supports the idea that babies are resilient and will tolerate numerous regular caregivers and parenting styles; this is a finding that contradicts the reductive application of attachment theory ideology, that only mom will do, which is too prevalent in Western contexts (Blaffer Hrdy; Lancy). An edifice of practice has been built on faulty interpretation of theory resulting in much maternal anxiety and suffering (Hogan "A Discussion," "Post-modernist," "Dealing with Complexity"; "Maternal Ambivalence") and women circumscribing their activities unnecessarily. (Ironically, some of the women engaging in this project had difficulty using the crèche provision because the children were not used to using one.) Childbirth and the preparations for it are a contested site with regards to gender power relations and every aspect of its management is open to potentially highly inflammatory rival proscriptions (Hogan "The Beestings"). No wonder, then, that this is too a site of distress. Women's reactions must be seen as cultural, not merely biological and personal.

Confidential art-based support groups can offer a place in which maternal anxiety can be discussed, depicted, and explored (Hogan "A Discussion"). Women are invited to make art, which is then shared with others in the group. Formats vary but often include a period of sitting in a circle and taking turns to talk about the image produced and the experience of having made it, including articulation of their feelings. Socially unacceptable feelings of alienation from one's baby, for example, may be articulated. Because of the confidential nature of the art therapy support groups, women reported that they felt free to express feelings they are *unable to express elsewhere*. Self-identity is bound up with what we are capable of conceptualising and remembering, so it is not surprising that extreme fatigue, which disrupts these faculties, will prove challenging and destabilising. Hogan found that the effect of exhaustion was a recurrent theme throughout the art sessions ("A Discussion"; "Post-modernist"; *Revisiting Feminist Approaches*). Other key themes in the art therapy support groups run by Hogan were a sense of claustrophobia, disarticulation, shock, guilt, resentment, and loss of self, as well as a celebration of the new baby and joy. In the art elicitation group run as part of The Birth Project, not feeling cared for, not feeling heard, guilt, and shame predominated as themes.

Furthermore, often key relationships are re-examined in the light of pregnancy and birth (Swan-Foster). Hogan noted the challenge of pregnancy and childbirth to established notions of self-identity, suggesting that in the use of art materials, women are able to negotiate and articulate their new sense of self and mourn, if necessary, their lost self-identity. Hogan discusses a "ruptured sense of self-identity" that can be experienced by many new mothers:

> Ipseity, one's sense of individual identity, is arguably disrupted and dislocated by major trauma or abrupt change. In recent work on art therapy practice with new mothers

Hogan has explored this tremendous sense of loss. For some women it is immediate. For others, however, this is a feeling that creeps up on them more slowly, through a succession of little incidents: it is a slower realisation that their old self is irretrievably gone, a more incremental revelation. Here we are talking about psychic death and rebirth. (Hogan, "Post-modernist" 73)

New representations of self can be explored; though the seeming essentialism of "maternal subjectivity" might be brought into question, the challenges of a changed consciousness brought about by childbirth is acknowledged by some writers as potentially enriching. For example, Lisa Baraitser's *Maternal Encounters: The Ethics of Interruption* explores maternity as an encounter, or a series of encounters, which can be generative experiences, allowing maternal subjectivity to emerge in its own right. She describes this as

physical viscosity, heightened sentience, a renewed awareness of objects, of one's own emotional range and emotional points of weakness, an engagement with the built environment and street furniture, a renewed temporal awareness where the present is elongated and the past and the future no longer felt to be so tangible, and a renewed sense of oneself as a speaking subject. (4)

This sense of being in the moment and being jolted into the moment that Baraitser describes as potentially enriching is also reflected in parenting memoirs; here is an extract of a mother commenting on her son's enjoyment of a visit to a botanical garden:

Emile was in ecstasy fondling different plants, fingering dead leaves, running his hands over tree bark, chewing pampas grass, smiling. And I was sharing his moment of awe of being in the jungle of plants, excitedly watching squirrels. Surely his being there *enhanced my perception, helped me to sit longer, look more carefully, enjoy more fully…?* (Hogan, "Maternal Ambivalence" 8; italics added)

The 1970s in the U.S. saw a proliferation of art work that explored maternity, such as Mary Kelly's iconic *Post-Partum Document* (1973-1979), Susan Hiller's *10 Months* (1977-9), and Laura Mulvey and Peter Wollen's *Riddles of the Sphinx* (1977). (For a critical discussion of art that explores the maternal from the 1970s and since, see Betterton; Liss; and McCloskey). In the UK there has been a gradual emergence of birth being represented in visual culture in more complex ways than the ubiquitous supine, screaming, hospitalised depiction of women giving birth often seen on early television. (For an overview and analysis of birth in visual culture see Tyler and Baraitser). This new visual culture is starting to explore what has been described as "the taboo aesthetics of the birth scene" (Tyler and Clements 134). One of the threads taken up by The Birth Project is to explore the wider implications of the new visual culture of childbirth, thereby contributing to this relatively under-researched area.

Birth has become more visible in popular culture. Whether via television documentaries, such as *One Born Every Minute* (Channel 4, 2010 to present), or in dramas, such as *Call the Midwife* (BBC 2012 to present), there has been a veritable explosion in women capturing their birth experiences on camera and sharing these awe inspiring stories on social media. This relatively new development in visual representation of birth has resulted in a proliferation of representation of births on YouTube, in particular, where visual birth stories are shared with a global audience. The contemporary art world has also witnessed a growing number of artists grappling with birth as a topic, for example, the *Birth Rites Collection* and *MeWe*. *Birth Rites* is a growing collection of contemporary artwork that explores birth, with work such as Hermione Wiltshire's *Terese in Ecstatic Childbirth* (2008), Helen Knowles' *Heads of Women in Labour* (2011), *YouTube Series* (2012), and Jenny Lewis' and Liv Pennington's *Private View* (2002-2010). The *MeWe* project is an arts collective comprising visual artists, academics, writers, performers, poets, and film makers who share an interest in and create work about the maternal. A recent exhibition in the UK entitled *The Egg, The Womb, The Head and The Moon* (May 2014) featured original work exploring birth and transitions to motherhood created by members of the MeWe collective, artists such as Eti Wade, Helen Sargeant, Lena Simic, and Paula McCloskey. The photographer Jenny Lewis captures quiet, fragile, and miraculous moments in photographs such as *One Day Young* that challenge the increasingly "routine" perception of childbirth; whereas Eti Wade produces disquieting images, some of which render maternal anxiety as palpable.

ETHOS: A PARTICIPATORY ARTS APPROACH

Research techniques being used in The Birth Project include art elicitation and photography within a participatory arts framework. Using a participatory arts-based approach, our broad overarching questions are:

- •What role might arts and humanities engagement play in pre and antenatal care and provision, especially where post-birth trauma is being translated into bodily symptoms?
- •To what extent are iatrogenic clinically related birth practices implicated in post-natal distress?
- •Is *mutual* recovery between clinicians and the women and birth partners they care for possible through engagement through the arts? What form may this take?
- •What in particular does an arts-based approach offer?

PARTICIPATORY ARTS: MOTHERS MAKE ART

Two sets of workshops that have been run for The Birth Project will be discussed here. A participatory arts group, Mothers Make Art, has been facilitated by the artist Lisa Watts. Watts has a distinctive art practice called Live Art, described by Gorman as "an art practice that presents the living body to encourage a self-reflective exploration of subjectivity, art and knowledge production" (Gorman in Watts, *Significant Moments* 6). One facet of this mode of working is that is "engages with how the audience experiences the performing body's interaction with objects and materials" (Watts, *Art that Presents* 2).

Mothers Make Art asks questions in two main ways: What are the effects of participation in workshops for the makers of the art? And, then, what are the effects on others who experience as viewers the art that is produced? The Mothers Make Art group comprised eight women who live in a city in the north of England. They self-selected to participate in a series of twelve workshops. Some of the women were educated in the arts, some not, but all had an interest in visual arts and an openness to learn and to create. The brief was to use a participatory frame-work to enable the women to explore *any* topics they wished with respect to the birth experience and motherhood (Hogan, "Mothers Make Art").

Watts uses a number of self-devised experiential methods which involve, for example, members standing in a circle to explore "sameness" and "differentness." Each member is invited to step into the centre of the circle and to declare something about themselves that they believe may be shared by other members of the group. Watts describes the origins of these "declaratory" techniques as situated in consciousness raising:

> Consciousness-raising groups occurred throughout Europe and the United States and were organised by women with the intention of sharing women's "lived experiences" to "speak-out" common experiences of women that were not recognised politically. I have held on to some of the basic principles of these groups when working with the women's birth stories in my workshops. ... In my facilitation I used the legacy of the "consciousness-raising groups" that occurred from the 1970s onwards to provide an opportunity for the women to "speak-out" aspects of their birth stories. (Watts, "Contemporary Art" 2).

Further structured techniques were used to enable the partic-ipants to investigate the nature of meaning making and to con-struct and deconstruct works (physically and metaphorically). An important technique employed in the earlier workshops was the use of everyday objects: objects that were brought in by group participants (ornaments, clothing, mothering paraphernalia, toys) as well as the everyday objects that Watts brought (cling-film, tin-foil, kitchen paper).

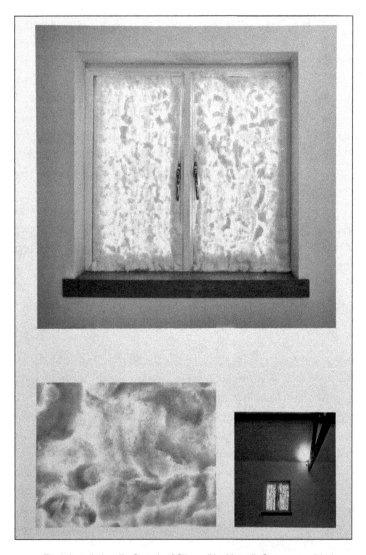

Fig 1: Installation. "In Search of Silence" by Hasmik Gasparyan, 2014.

During the second half of each session there was an opportunity to be "meditative" with objects supplied by Watts. Rather than making a representation or literal object referring to their birth or mothering, the women focused on the formal aesthetic qualities of the materials. This mode of working investigates materials with a focus on the materials capabilities, rather than starting with a predetermined vision of where the art making might go. Inven-

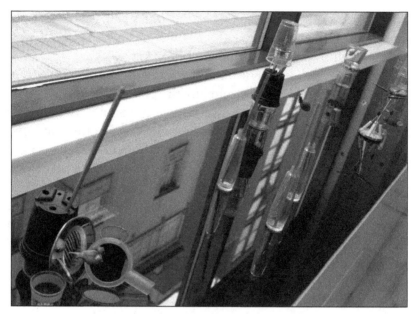

Fig 2 Installation. "Finding Equilibrium." Rachel Vedder, 2014.

tiveness and design may come to the fore. The use of materials to create installations was investigated. The actuality of the material was the focus and its capacity to generate meaning. This not only provided a self-reflective space and contrast to the structure of the first half, but functioned to give the women the skills and confidence to manipulate materials to be able to create their own original art piece at the end of the series (Hogan, "Mothers Make Art").

The art pieces were wide-ranging; one woman pegged up her boys clothes from the tiny newborn garments to the larger ones representing crazes and fads. With poems and a monologue, she acknowledged the preciousness and fleeting nature of each stage and an acute awareness of the transitory nature of experience. The work is emotive.

A further installation comprised a long row of cups containing all of the smells so familiar to mothers, from the bright pink sickly sweet smell of the Calpol (a ubiquitous liquid paracetamol) to lotions and baby food. One attendee reported that although her daughter was an adult, the smells immediately transported her back to her daughter's babyhood. Another remarked on the "chemical" quality of the smells, worrying what she was using on her baby! Another was repulsed by the food smell. Early parenting as a time of strong aromas and the power of smell as visceral were acknowledged (Hogan, "Mothers Make Art").

Hasmik's work used cotton wool to create a muffled peaceful space. She wrote this to accompany the piece: "I could not agree more with Professor Lesley Regan ... 'pregnancy is tightrope walking.' During these last nine months and even after, our mind is never silent. I want to look for silence. The one which is light positive and embracing." Audience members were invited to look at the installation photographs and then to put on headphones. The audio component, via the headphones, comprised a woman screaming in labour, which created a stark juxtaposition between that clamour and tranquil space depicted (Hogan "Mothers Make Art").

Rachel spoke of appreciating the time and space to make art work. She said that the work was about seeking equilibrium among the domestic, professional, and personal realms of her life, as well as exploring notions of what it is to be a good mother. She invited the group to say what her piece evoked: precariousness, balance, complexity, and giving the bulbs space to grow were a few of the reactions (see Hogan, "Mothers Make Art" for more detailed discussion and analysis of this workshop series).

THE ART ELICITATION GROUP:
ART THERAPY WORKSHOP SERIES

The second group of workshops was an art elicitation group explicitly for those who felt that they would like to work in a more intensive and therapeutic way with self-acknowledged, unresolved birth and mothering issues. If art-elicitation groups intend to delve deep into emotionally difficult subject matter, there is a strong case to be made that an art therapist is employed for this work, as artists may quickly find themselves out of their depth (Hogan and Pink). Trained art therapists also have a good understanding of ethical issues, which can be useful in working in multifaceted situations (Hogan, "Lost in Translation"). The facilitator for this project, Shelagh Cornish, was an HCPC-registered art psychotherapist with experience working with trauma, and consequently

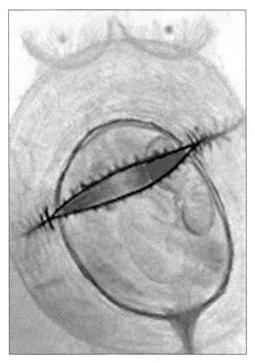

Fig. 3. Imagery from Art Elicitation Group. "Caesarean Section."

skilled in making a safe space and dealing with potentially emotive issues with sensitivity, should they arise.

The chosen overarching approach of the art elicitation workshops was included acknowledgment of "both the art and verbal disclosures in a supportive group with an emphasis on the individual in the group" in which participants have the opportunity of being truly understood and empathised with (Hogan, "Art Therapy" 33). Other aspects central to providing an effective, appropriate art elicitation frame and approach included gaining informed consent, clarifying the parameters of confidentiality and what is to become of images made, agreeing upon broad group aims (in addition to research aims), outlining the workshop process, negotiation of how and when the film crew would interact with participants, debrief, and supervision for the facilitator (Edwards; Hogan and Coulter). Normally, an art elicitation group would not be a therapeutic group per se, but would contain certain therapeutic features: it would be closed, supportive, and confidential and it might use directive or non-directive techniques from art therapy. However, because of the nature of the subject matter, the facilitator felt that an art therapy approach would be most appropriate in this instance and that the group would function as both a research vehicle and a therapeutic group.

The art elicitation workshop group comprises nine women who live in two cities, one in the East Midlands and the other in the north of England. The women's age ranges from mid-twenties to

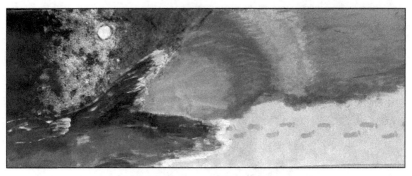

Fig. 4. Imagery from Art Elicitation Group.
"Journey with Tsunami."

mid-forties. The women were recruited primarily from local parent and toddler groups. They self-selected to participate in a series of twelve workshops to explore birth and related experiences. Only one woman was a professional artist, but all had an interest in expressing themselves through visual art.

A thematic art therapy approach was decided on by Shelagh Cornish as a means of offering metaphoric starting points that could be responded to as much or as little as each mother chose. This was with the intention of mediating depth of exploration. The sequence of themes chosen was designed carefully with the more challenging themes (and the potential for more depth of exploration) in the middle of the workshop series. The rationale for this design was that at the beginning participants would be developing relationships and "finding their feet" then, towards the end, they would need to focus on "completion and emotional closure" so they were ready to leave the group and, if necessary, be referred elsewhere.

Themes were offered as a starting point to stimulate imagination and were introduced through story-telling, poetry, guided imagery, and provision of artists' images. All themes came with the caveat that they could be interpreted and adapted as individuals chose; they were offered as a potential stimulus rather than an instruction (though sometimes themes can be hard to resist in group settings and there is a potential tension between a participant-led ethos and the use of themes, which we acknowledge). The structure of the group included consideration of women going back into their

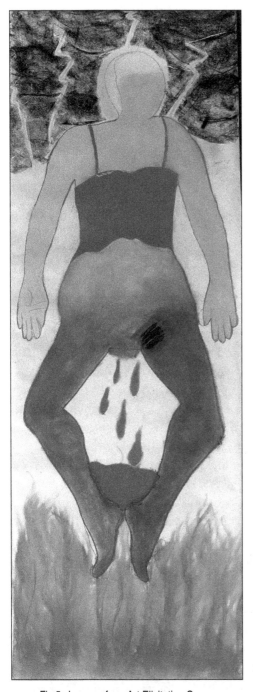

Fig 5 . Imagery from Art Elicitation Group.
"Image of Birth."

"everyday worlds" and resuming the care of their young charges and other responsibilities when debriefing at the end of each workshop was completed.

A number of common experiences emerged at the outset of the group. Topics included women saying their birth was not as expected, that many felt shame or inadequacy, distress, guilt, and anger at how the birth had gone. They all (bar one) felt the care they had received had been inadequate. During the initial sessions participants shared their experience of image making, talking in pairs and then together as a whole group. The women felt there had been a lack of preparation for birthing. They suggested that a lack of sharing of "real" birth stories had given them unrealistic expectations. They also shared their experience that communication with professionals prior to, during, and after the event had been limited.

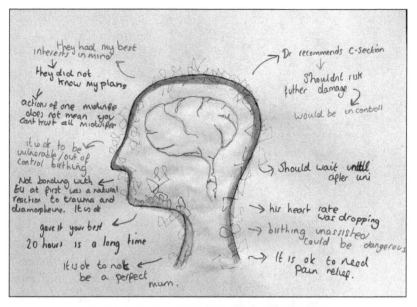

Fig 6. Imagery from Art Elicitation Group. "Mind Chatter."

Several mothers felt they had been left grappling with significant feelings relating to both psychological and physical aspects of their traumatic childbirth experience, with no network of professionals to share these with. They disclosed that when they tried to share feelings with friends and health professionals following discharge from hospital, they were not listened to. Rather, they were responded to with the message that they should now focus on having "a nice baby." They said this felt very shaming to them, and made them feel they could not share their distress with anyone. Real fear was also expressed that, should they pursue seeking psychological help, health staff may judge them as "failing" and feel they could not care for their baby, and therefore that the baby might be "taken away." The mothers felt that the focus of professionals seemed only on the physical health of the baby and whether breastfeeding was going well, and that the amount of post-childbirth support was wholly inadequate. The women expressed collective relief to hear other's experiences and feelings. That they had shared their own painful feelings and had not been judged made them feel "a bit better already." The role of image making was felt to be fun, relaxing, and anxiety-reducing, offering a chance to use art materials in a playful manner and to feel more comfortable with other mothers.

THEMES AND THE ROLE OF IMAGES

Recurring issues were fear, anger, anxiety, depression, shame, loss, and apparent symptoms of post-trauma response (such as invasive imagery). Women shared their experiences as to a sense of a lack of care by hospital staff and midwives alike, especially psychological and person-centred caring, being a parent and the losses and gains of that, as well as childhood memories of being a child and experience of being parented.

The theme of feeling let down by hospital staff through being "treated as a baby's deliverer not as a person," "having no control or say," "feeling scared, terrified, overwhelmed by the birthing experience," "feeling unprepared for the reality of childbirth," and "having no emotional or psychological support from staff" recurred throughout the workshop series. Through whole-body imaging, women created images that contained representations of how they experienced and felt now about their childbirth. Some of the images explicitly represented physical aspects of their experience. One picture was made of a caesarean section cut on one woman's pregnant belly revealing the baby contained within, and another a caesarean section operation with the woman lying terrified on the operation table surrounded by a large number of hospital staff. One woman represented the terror of the experience and the danger she had felt by creating a picture of herself lying down ready to give birth as she had imagined it would be, and then juxtaposing a second image of how it actually was having a forceps delivery. The painful delivery of a broken placenta was represented symbolically through red painted clay. Two images focused on the pros and cons of medical intervention, where one depicted a naked vulnerable self holding her baby.

Other images represented the journey through childbirth, from pre-pregnancy, pregnancy, dangerous childbirth, to the present and hopes for the future. Several picture sequences representing the journey, with a triptych-like feel, were created by three part 'narrative' sequences. One focused on a seascape that changes from a calm environment to a Tsunami threatening to overwhelm and destroy; this then moves to an image of "footsteps" in the sand with the woman apparently alive. Three sets of images seem similar in that they contain representation of women's lives before pregnancy and then depict the intensity of childbirth and the now of being a parent. Two others seemed more explicitly representational of the journey past and the journey future with descriptions of what had been experienced, achieved, lost and uncertainty about "what next" written on them.

Another important theme was that of the need for psychological and physical containment and safety. This was represented by an image of a clay foetus curled up in a nest, a self portrait in a foetal position, and a plasticine nest of eight eggs—perhaps representing the need for safety within the art elicitation group.

One woman's clay image is of a female warrior, resplendent with shield and sword, representing the view that for women to give birth, especially with little or no psychological support, "they have to be warriors."

Many images, however, were less representational and more metaphoric, symbolic, and multi-layered in nature where partial meanings were shared verbally or not at all. This is an advantage of an arts-based group, that material can be pictured and acknowledged, but not necessarily interrogated.

One woman's childbirth experience was described pictorially as well as in the following words: "I was feeling okay, and then suddenly nearly dead due to unwanted medical intervention that resulted in a huge loss of blood." The image is described as representing fear, "possibly terror," anger though "not quite rage," and feeling helpless and having no say in what was happening.

Later on, when the group as members got to know each other, some distressing fears began to emerge. During one session, the common fear that their baby might get hurt or might die was raised. One woman reported hallucinations and a dream of her baby drowning, and many shared fears that harm or death could befall their baby. These fears were pervasive for some. Women shared sadness for themselves and each other about how uncared for and uninformed they had felt, and relief that they could share and feel cared for in a supportive group: "That's what we're here for isn't it?"

SUMMARY AND CONCLUSION

All the women who undertook the art elicitation workshops said they had more awareness and understanding of what had happened to them as their feelings about events had been discovered and or expressed through the images made. Acceptance that feelings and experiences are valid through image making and reflection was agreed to be a powerful and transforming experience, in which accepting what I felt then, contrasted with an acknowledgment of 'this is how I feel now,' was shared by all participants. The group agreed that the sense of relief in sharing was very welcome and long awaited.

Women described the experience of image making as ranging from "initially anxiety-provoking in not knowing where to begin" to "a great way to engage with experiences when you don't even know what you feel yet" and "I never know what's going to come into my pictures which is exciting and I get to know myself."

One woman said that following the art elicitation workshops, she could now bear to consider another pregnancy and was feeling less fearful, saying, "My fear of childbirth is now in the past." Another shared that since coming to the group she could "stand up" for herself more often, both in terms of what she wanted as a mother and what she wanted for herself. Another said, "Something clicked last week through the image and I now feel able to say more openly how I feel with friends and family ... even to share 'ugly' feelings." Others said that the only treatments available to them were cognitive behavioural therapy and medication and that these were felt to be inadequate; one mother exalted, "I'm advocating for art therapy ... its *brilliant*." Another woman announced, "Coming here has helped me go through a door (transition) and take a place at university." She received much encouragement from others for this. Another reported that through image making she now knows more about who she is and what she wants and needs and that she has made changes in her relationships and employment. One woman described how she came to the group "feeling very angry, almost rage," but that the anger and feelings of shame are now largely resolved and that image making had a central role in this. Another shared that feelings of shame and feeling a failure were much less for her. Some noticed that feelings of loss had decreased since they had represented different losses visually. One woman shared that addressing childhood issues visually meant she could now parent how she wanted to and was generally feeling freer to express her emotions to herself and with others.

It has not been possible to summarise all the themes that arose in the workshops, the 'journey' though the experience was explored. As noted above, one participant was able to acknowledge distressing imagery regarding imagined harm to her baby. Being able to acknowledge such a thing is of value in mediating stress. Imagined images of babies being hurt are distressing for new mothers and liable to make some feel aberrant or deviant, or even potentially dangerous. Few baby books seem to acknowledge this phenomenon, the prevalence of which is unknown.

With a rather different tone from that of the art elicitation group, Watts' art practice is interested in encounter. This follows the work of Deleuze and Guattari (in O'Sullivan) who suggest that that the art encounter can challenge habitual ways of being and acting in the world, ways which are potentially destabilised and questioned. This is also the case for the art making process in art elicitation groups, which uses art therapy techniques. However, in the Mothers Make Art group there is a definite attempt towards exploring encounters with objects (and not in dialogue with oneself, as in much art therapy practice) but as a performance with the rest of the group acting as a witness. Watts' technique in particular would seem to draw on Deleuze and Guattari's sense of rupture and affirmation of the encounter. This lends a slightly different philosophical lens, a different attitude, to the Mothers Make Art group in that it represents a particular "way in" to questioning accepted assumptions about the birth experience and new motherhood (Hogan "Mothers Make Art").

Early findings from a preliminary analysis based on both groups would appear to corroborate research evidence that it is less the actual intervention itself in childbirth so much as *the quality of the engagement between health professionals and the birthing mother* which is of crucial importance—not to negate the reality of the pain of many procedures and complications in post-partum healing. So, for example, a woman might tolerate a caesarean section very well if it is negotiated in a way that does not feel disempowering. Women who feel neglected, negated, and "done to" are more likely to have unresolved feelings which may then translate into depression and other forms of distress. Lisa Watts reported distress in the Mothers Make Art group following from a perceived "lack of agency" in labour and in the early days following the birth: the inability to make informed decisions; not being treated with respect; and not being helped when "unable to help themselves" (Watts *Significant Moments*). In terms of iatrogenic practices, the difficulty of *resistance* was very powerfully articulated by one of the art elicitation group members who was also a medical doctor. She *understood* the possible consequences of induction, yet was overpowered by the pressure she was put under to accept an induction. Indeed, when she was told things weren't "progressing," she attempted to enter into a discussion and "they just said no—on the bed ... this is what we're doing." She had wanted a discussion with the doctor about the possible risks and benefits yet, despite her medical training, was unable to be sufficiently assertive to obtain this, and then felt she'd let herself down afterwards (Hogan "Mothers Make Art").

The cannula as a source of disempowerment and distress was another of the subjects articulated, as women didn't feel they could be removed once inserted, leading to discomfort and upset and, in one case, a ballooned "Hulk hand" that prevented the woman from removing an increasingly uncomfortable nightgown, which also later interfered with the skin to skin contact she wanted with her new-born (which in turn caused her worry about bonding).

As illustrated, supportive and therapeutic art groups can help mothers in the transition to new motherhood. In both groups, having time and space for personal and group exploration was valued. As of 2016, films will be available to elucidate groups' themes further (see www.healthhumanities.org).

The preparedness and courage of the participants, some of whom had never made art before, requires acknowledgement. Thanks to Dr. Lisa Watts for an elucidation of her innovative practice (a more detailed discussion of Watts' technique is available in

Hogan ("Mothers Make Art"). Thanks also to Sheffield Vision whose film work allowed the research team to get some insight into the ongoing group work. Particular thanks to Eve Wood. Thanks to Lynn Weddle for taking the photographs of the in- stallation work (copyright The Birth Project). Thanks too to our research assistant Kamaljit Kaur for helping with the MLA referencing and for her constructive remarks. Many thanks are due to Dr. Nadya Burton for her sensitive editorial suggestions. This research is being supported by the Arts & Humanities Research Council, UK via a Communities, Cultures, Health & Wellbeing Research Grant entitled Creative Practice as Mutual Recovery: Connecting Communities for Mental Health and Well- being. Ref. RGS. 117113. Award AH/K003364/1. Any comments about the conduct of this research can be directed to Professor Susan Hogan, who is also happy to discuss the project further: s.hogan@derby.ac.uk.

WORKS CITED

Almond, P. "Postnatal Depression: A Global Public Health Perspec- tive." Perspectives in Public Health 129 (2009): 221-227. Print.

Ayers, S. et al. "Posttraumatic Stress Disorder After Childbirth: Analysis of Symptom Presentation and Sampling." Journal of Affective Disorders 119.1-3 (2009): 200-204. Print.

Baraitser, L. Maternal Encounters: The Ethics of Interruption. London: Routledge (2009) Print.

Betterton, R., "Maternal Embarrassment: Feminist Art and Ma- ternal Affects." Studies in the Maternal 1 (2010):1-2. Print.

Blaffer Hrdy, S. Mother Nature: A History of Mothers and Natural Selection. New York: Pantheon Books, 1999. Print.

Bordo, S. "The Body and the Reproduction of Femininity." Writing on the Body: Female Embodiment and Feminist Theory. Eds. K. Conboy, N. Medina and S. Stanbury. New York: Columbia University Press. 1997. 90-112. Print.

Crawford, P., Brown, B., Baker, C., Tischler, V., and Abrams, B. Health Humanities. Hampshire: Palgrave, 2015. Print.

Downey, G, and J. C. Coyne. "Children of Depressed Parents:

An Integrative Review." *Psychological Bulletin* 108.1(1990): 50-76. Print.

Edwards, D. *Art Therapy.* 2nd edition. London: Sage, 2014 Print.

Hogan, Susan. "The Art Therapy Continuum: A Useful Tool for Envisaging the Diversity of Practice in British Art Therapy." *International Journal of Art Therapy* 14.1 (June 2009): 29-37. Print.

Hogan, S. "The Beestings: Rethinking Breast-Feeding Practices, Maternity Rituals, and Maternal Attachment in Britain and Ireland." *Journal of International Women's Studies* 10.2 (2008):141-160. Print.

Hogan, S. "A Discussion About the Use of Art Therapy with Women Who Are Pregnant or Have Recently Given Birth." *Gender Issues in Art Therapy.* Ed. S. Hogan. London: Jessica Kingsley, 2003. 148-173. Print.

Hogan, S. "Lost in Translation? Inter-Cultural Exchange in Art Therapy." *Creative Arts Across Cultures.* Eds. C. E. Myers and S. L. Brooke. Springfield, Il: Charles C. Thomas, 2014. Print.

Hogan, S. "Maternal Ambivalence and Motherhood Interrogated and Expressed Via Art Therapy." Conference paper delivered at the Feminist and Women's Studies Association Conference "Identity, Sexuality and Diversity," University of Bradford, UK, 13 July 2006. Print.

Hogan, S. "Mothers Make Art: Using Participatory Art to Explore the Transition to Motherhood." *Journal of Applied Arts & Health* 6.1 (2015): 23-32. Print.

Hogan, S. "Problems of Identity. Deconstructing Gender in Art Therapy." *Feminist Approaches to Art Therapy.* Ed. S. Hogan. London: Routledge, 1997. 21-48. Print.

Hogan, S. "Post-modernist but Not Post-feminist! A Feminist Post-modernist Approach to Working with New Mothers." *Creative Healing Through a Prism. Art Therapy and Postmodernism.* Ed. H. Burt. London: Jessica Kingsley, 2012. 70-82. Print.

Hogan, S., ed. *Revisiting Feminist Approaches to Art Therapy.* London: Berghahn, 2012. Print.

Hogan, S. and A. Coulter. *The Introductory Guide to Art Therapy: Experiential Teaching and Learning for Students and Practitioners.* Hove: Routledge, 2014. Print.

Hogan, S. and S. Pink. "Routes to Interiorities: Art Therapy, Anthropology and Knowing in Anthropology." *Visual Anthropology* 23.2 (2010): 1–16. Print.

Kitzinger, S. *Birth Your Way: Choosing Birth at Home or in a Birth Centre*. London: Dorling Kindersley, 2001. Print.

Knapp, M. et al., eds. "Mental Health Promotion and Prevention: The Economic Case." Personal Social Services Research Unit, London School of Economics and Political Science, January 2011. 1-43. Print.

Knitzer, J., S. Theberge and K. Johnson. *Reducing Maternal Depression and Its Impact on Young Children: Toward a Responsive Early Childhood Policy Framework*. Columbia: The National Centre for Children in Poverty, 2008. Print.

Lancy, D. F. *The Anthropology of Childhood. Cherubs, Chattel, Changings*. Cambridge: Cambridge University Press, 2014. Print.

Levine, Ellen G. and Stephen K. Levine. *Art in Action: Expressive Arts Therapy and Social Change*. London: Jessica Kingsley Publishers, 2011. Print.

Liss, A., 2009. *Feminist Art and the Maternal*. Minneapolis: University of Minnesota Press. Print.

McCloskey, P. *Art, Maternal and Matrixial Encounters*. Diss. University of Sheffield, 2013. Print.

National Institute for Clinical Excellence (NICE). "Antenatal and Postnatal Mental Health: Clinical Management and Service Guidance." NICE Guidelines (CG 45), February 2007. Web.

Oates, M. "Suicide: The Leading Cause of Maternal Death." *British Journal of Psychiatry* 183 (2013): 279-281. Print.

Oates, M. R. et al. "Postnatal Depression Across Countries and Cultures: A Qualitative Study." *British Journal of Psychiatry Supplement* 46 (2004): s10–16. Print.

O'Sullivan, S. *Art Encounters Deleuze and Guattari: Thought Beyond Representation*. New York: Palgrave Macmillan, 2006. Print.

Pink, S. *Advances in Visual Methodology*. Thousand Oaks, CA: Sage, 2012. Print.

Pink, S. *The Future of Visual Anthropology: Engaging the Senses*. London: Routledge, 2006. Print.

Swan-Foster, N. "Images of Pregnant Women: Art Therapy as a

Tool for Transformation." *The Arts in Psychotherapy* 16 (1989): 283–292. Print.

The Birth Trauma Association. *Post Natal Post Traumatic Stress Disorder*. Ipswich: The Birth Trauma Association, n.d. Accessed 12th May 2014. Web.

The Patient's Association. "Postnatal Depression Services: An Investigation into NHS Service Provision." 2011. Accessed 9 April 2014. Web.

Tyler, I. "Birth: An Introduction." *Feminist Review* 93 (2009): 1-7. Print.

Tyler, I, and Baraitser, L. "Private View, Public Birth: Making Feminist Sense of the New Visual Culture of Childbirth" *Studies in the Maternal* 5.2 (2013). Web. Accessed 26 August 2015.

Tyler, I. and J. Clements. "The Taboo Aesthetics of the Birth Scene." *Feminist Review* 93.1 (2009): 134-37. Print.

Watts, L. "Contemporary Art Making Methods for Interdisciplinary Research; Mothers Make Art." Unpublished paper. 2014.

Watts, L. *Art That Presents the Living Body*. Diss. Edinburgh College of Art, 2010. Print.

Watts, L. *32 Significant Moments. An Artists Practice as Research*. Sheffield: Arts Council of England, 2014. Print.

World Health Organisation (WHO). *Maternal Mental Health & Child Health and Development. Improving Maternal Mental Health Millennium Development Goal 5 – Improving Maternal Health*. Geneva: WHO, 2010. Print.

KORY MCGRATH AND LYNN FARRALES

Making Meaning of Stillbirth

S ENSITIVE LANGUAGE, REMEMBRANCE PHOTOGRAPHY, and
mementos have become integrated into stillbirth care practices
in North American health care institutions for parents and
families who have experienced the death of an infant. While representations reflect how families, caregivers, and society understand
stillbirth, they also help shape our relationship with birth, death,
and both as they occur together. From both subjective and objective points of view, this chapter will explore how words, images,
and artifacts come to represent multiple meanings of stillbirth in
a way that can both challenge and contribute to the silence, stigma, and emancipation of bereaved parents from ambiguity and
disenfranchisement, so that their experiences are recognized as
early deaths rather than pregnancy losses. Because language and
relics that make meaning of stillbirth imprint on a family's and
caregiver's understanding of this event and on future interactions,
current approaches to bereavement care and its implications will
be explored.

Making meaning is an expression of emotions wherein bereaved
parents and families create an "infrastructure" of their loss[1], using
words, tangible objects and images to symbolically and visually
narrate their individual experience (Cacciatore and Flint). Cacciatore describes meaning making as "a process that contributes
to bereavement adaptation" and includes an exploration of one's
personal understanding of the death, which may evolve over time
with new relevance (Blood and Cacciatore 78; Reagan; Kobler,
Limbo and Kavanaugh). Making meaning is, thus, an ongoing

296

process. It is not just making meaning when the body of the baby who has died is present, but it is also developing a language around the loss and making memories as the days, weeks, and years move onward. Some bereaved parents call this assembly of meaning the establishment of "parenthood" in the acute phase and "parenting" during the course of their own lifetime. Others also describe it as "healthy grieving," a term laden with its own social constructs of a medical framework as grief that does not fit within the prescriptive model of "health" is often pathologized (Howarth 128). Though stillbirth is often categorized as a "pregnancy loss," "to a mother and father, a stillbirth is no less a tragedy than the death of a newborn baby or child" (Mullan and Horton 1292). Thus, this chapter will describe meaning making from the perspective of child death. With regards to the ambiguous characteristic of grief after stillbirth, the construction and reconstruction of meaning making over time is that much more important (Caciattore and Flint). This ambiguity stems from the "lack of tangible evidence of the baby's existence" (Cacciattore and Bushfield 692). While language frames and contextualizes the descriptions of more concrete representations, items such as photographs and mementos come to represent the "only real, visual memory" making tangible and permanent an otherwise evanescent period of a very finite liminality (Caciattore and Flint 164; Layne, "He Was a Real Baby" 324; Van Guennep qtd. in Howarth 129; Linkman 86).

In this chapter, we aim to elucidate some of the cultural and standardized representations of stillbirth, how they reflect and reinforce silence around death, grief, and the intimacy of female reproduction, and how communities of bereaved parents adopt, resist, challenge, and reinvent the norms that exist surrounding stillbirth. Through an examination of language, imagery, and artifacts of stillbirth, we will consider origins, contemporary usages, opposition, and ingenuity. The vocabulary of stillbirth as it is used by individuals and communities will be considered, as language is but one manifestation of how meaning is made. An exploration of how stillbirth has come to be represented in photographs and mementos past and present will also be explored. We will conclude with a discussion on emergent practices of meaning making from the individual, private, collective, and public practice, wherein the "boundary between life and death is spatially and symbolically breached" (Gibson 146).

MAKING MEANING THROUGH LANGUAGE, PHOTOGRAPHS, AND MEMENTOS

Practices surrounding birth, death, and grief are informed by culture, faith, individuality, globalization, and technology, all of which are ever evolving. Therefore, there exists considerable variation and diversity in how bereaved parents, families, institutions, caregivers, and communities articulate the death of an infant at birth, and each word carries with it its own multiple meanings (Chalmers). A series on stillbirth in *The Lancet* highlights that "in many languages, the word stillborn suggests a meaningless venture" (Frøen et al. 1357). *The Canadian Oxford Dictionary* defines stillborn as: "1. (of a child) born dead. 2. (of an idea, plan, etc.) abortive; not able to succeed." The term stillborn is politically charged and contains multiple meanings and social consequences, leaving caregivers to struggle with a vocabulary that meets varied needs across cultural differences and individual preferences as a way to appropriately describe birth and death (Frøen et al.; Jutel). In addition, there is a paucity of language to describe the transformation of a parent-to-be that never comes to hold a living child. Bereaved parents do not relinquish their status of parent-identity, but rather "qualify simply by conceiving and giving birth" (Howarth 130-31; Mitchell et al. 414). Yet women and partners find themselves excluded from the parenthood category when they have no living children (Layne, "He Was a Real Baby" 323). In an autoethnographic essay about his experience of stillbirth, Weaver-Hightower describes himself as "a father and not-father" all at once (462). The quest to find language to articulate actual lived experience then becomes the catalyst for meaning making of stillbirth.

Cameron, Taylor and Greene analyzed fifty years of midwifery textbooks in Britain and considered how the language of ideology, rhetoric, and rituals (and their evolution) "shapes and reveals thought, knowledge and beliefs" (336). The language of perinatal death, written and edited by midwives, is traced from the late 1930s, where it is described as an event that is inevitable and a sign of the sacred, to the 1950s and '60s, where responsibility is placed on the mother as "being culpable." Cameron, Taylor and Greene then trace expressions of the fetus and baby as a person and an emphasis on need for support for the grieving in the 1970s and '80s as being informed by the feminist and reproductive rights movement. In the period from 1990 to 2004, content about how to make "good" memories following perinatal death were increasingly written by "user groups," such as bereaved parents. A critical analysis of the influence of class and religion on representations of perinatal death has come to be reflected in midwifery texts within the last decade (Cameron, Taylor and Greene 340). Likewise, Reagan's analysis of representations of miscarriage across time, seen as "hazard, to blessing, to tragedy"(359), mirrors how the language and texts of perinatal death inform authoritative language of care providers (Cameron, Taylor and Greene 340).

For statistical purposes, the terms miscarriage and stillbirth are separated in the literature and in medical documentation, yet academics, clinicians, and support organizations do not always disassociate miscarriage and stillbirth as uniquely distinguished from one another. The discourse thus often falls under the broad spectrum of "pregnancy loss," which itself includes early miscarriage, medical termination, and stillbirth (Robinson; MacConnell et al.; Forhan; Cacciatore "Position Statement"; Isle 34). Herein, we critique the term "pregnancy loss" and its incorrect proxy to bereaved parents and families of stillbirth as "losing" a pregnancy as opposed to more accurately describing the lived experience of infant death and birth.

The inclusion of stillbirth within the broad umbrella of "pregnancy loss" has been thought to perpetuate the ambiguity of parental grief (Cacciatore "Position Statement"). Likewise, the avoidance of the term stillbirth itself is thought to contribute to the minimization of the birth (Kelly and Trinidad). For some mothers, stillbirth as a term "captured a number of important realities: in stillbirth there is a birth, somebody was born, and someone did the birthing" (Kelly and Trinidad 13). In clinical practice, collapsing models of bereavement care into the broad category of "pregnancy loss" can also lead to difficulties. In her article "Pregnancy Loss," Robinson describes how the management of miscarriage has been influenced by stillbirth protocols with regards to viewing, naming, ritualizing, and memorializing the baby (171). Activities such as these may not be acceptable to all women who have experienced a miscarriage, suggesting that approaches to stillbirth may not be readily transferrable to miscarriage, although both may be categorized as a "pregnancy loss" (Reagan 366). It is only the shared experience of not having had a living baby that amalgamates groups across the spectrum and ultimately unites bereaved women, parents, and families (Layne, "Pregnancy" 610). Similarly, associating one's infant as an "is" versus "was" connects bereaved parents to one another and distinguishes them from "civilians," or parents of living children (Weaver-Hightower 462; Mitchell et al. 414).

Despite the common use of the term pregnancy loss to encompass a wide range of very unique situations, the language used to describe pregnancy is far more specialized. For example, women who are pregnant are often referred to in books and in the community as "with child" or "expecting." Thus, care providers need to be sensitive to "the values contained in words" when working with women whose pregnancies do not result in the live birth of an infant (Jutel 432). "Empty arms," a term sometimes used by parents, evokes strong metaphor (emptiness, empty cradle) that is both real and symbolic, perhaps in acquiescence to the dominant prescriptions of grief (Isle; Weaver-Hightower). Expressions of stillbirth as "silent" are also prevalent; "silent birth" and "born still" represent an antidote or resistance to the term stillbirth as medical terminology, while also playing into death-denial by using a soft qualifier to ultimately remove death. Could it be that stillness and silence are social constructs of a dominant patriarchal standpoint, one that has silenced and marginalized women throughout history and kept bereaved women out of "sight and sound" of new parents and their babies (Cameron, Taylor and Greene 338)? Or are these terms simply abstracts of the stillness and silence of death (though not generally of birth) (Ruderman 151), or more, the "unspeakable" infringement of the "natural" order of death (Mitchell et al. 414)? "Still a birth" unsettles, beseeching us to transgress death and see birth first, as bereaved parents often describe the event as having had a baby first, with a death that follows (Layne, "He Was a Real baby" 323).

In recognition of the importance of language and the cultural dissonance surrounding the origins of the term pregnancy loss, community groups who support and represent parents and families affected by stillbirth have become more deliberate about their messaging, thus exemplifying efforts at meaning making through purposeful choice of language. For example, the MISS Foundation, a U.S. non-profit serving bereaved families, has a position statement outlining why it has chosen to avoid the term pregnancy loss in its campaigns. The statement begins with a definition of stillbirth and miscarriage in order to contextualize its work (Cacciatore "Position Statement"). The resistance surrounding platitudes that promote the overcoming of stillbirth through a subsequent pregnancy and birth of a live infant implies that the "loss" is not solely that of a pregnancy but that of a child who is irreplaceable (MISS Foundation). Representations of stillbirth imprint on a family's and caregivers' understanding and future interactions with pregnancy, birth, and living children. Thus, one's choice of vocabulary has the power to either acknowledge or complicate a parent's experience. Conscientious and considerate use of language may even emancipate care providers and communities to recognize stillbirth as "early deaths rather than unproductive pregnancies," which is important to bereaved parents in their quest to have their babies and their grief recognized (Godel 266). For other bereaved parents, viability or gestation are not measures of personhood or existence (Jutel 430).

While it is important to consider the woman's experience as the point of departure for unpacking and reconceiving the language and culture of stillbirth, the experiences of fathers of stillborn infants are generally under-represented in the literature and ephemera surrounding stillbirth (Jutel; Cacciatore and Flint; de Montigny, Beaudet and Dumas "A Baby Has Died"; Weaver-Hightower). Could this be a consequence of gender standpoint hegemony over the realms of birth and parenthood (Smith)? It could be argued that as childbirth and parenting have traditionally been scripted as a woman's experience, men have been distanced out of and apart from these events, and have now come to feel underrepresented in the narratives of stillbirth, including support group newsletters, websites, poetry, and the like: "Gender does matter in material ways" (Weaver-Hightower 485). Nevertheless, father-specific blogs, social media portals, literature, and supports are slowly becoming more visible within a space historically dominated by motherhood (Davidson).

While the dominant narrative of stillbirth is sometimes gendered, it is not generally secular. "Angels" language and "angel-baby" imagery are prevalent in popular culture on parent blogs, social media posts, romanticized inscriptions on memorial stones, tattoos, t-shirts, materials of stillbirth support organizations and events, and even legislation in the American "Missing Angels Bills" (Godel; Layne, "He Was a Real Baby"; Keane; Mitchell et al.). "Angel" connotes a place; in the Christian construct maybe this place is Heaven where the baby is not actually *lost* but *somewhere*, if even an idealized place. Angel symbolism attributes the qualities of innocence and the sacred to the stillborn infant (Layne, "He Was a Real Baby"; Linkman). While the terms angels and angel-babies may resonate with some, it marginalizes others who do not iden-tify with these depictions. Individuals and groups are attempting to carve out spaces for grief and meaning making that are apart from angel-baby constructs and from the atheist, agnostic, and faith-neutral perspectives (Babyloss Support Group for Atheist and Agnostic Moms). Though meant to be sensitive to the diversity of experiences, bereaved parents who do not self-identify as being religious, nor make meaning through religious-based constructs such as angels, may feel compelled to make disclaimers prior to sharing their position for fear of harming others (as seen in Dudley). The inclusion of disclaimers in articles and social media content for the more widely held religious-based views and constructs is rare.

In the sixteenth and seventeenth centuries, stillborn babies in paintings, which provided a visual likeness before the advent of the photograph, were sometimes depicted as accompanied by angels, as if "being taken up to Heaven" (Mander and Marshall 237). For the grieving family who found comfort in faith, this may have offered some consolation. Presently, stillborn babies are sometimes adorned as guardian angels in photographs, clip art, or online graphics (Godel; Mitchell et al.). A recent movement in Canada is seeing women donating and repurposing wedding gowns to make infant-sized "angel dresses," which may soon be incorporated into hospital-issued memory boxes, along with other keepsakes such as the baby's footprints and photos (Allan). However, some might consider this as derogatory idol worship (Mander and Marshall 237). Standard practice in maternity care includes the assembly of immediate artifacts of stillbirth into memory boxes by caregivers as a gesture of comfort and sympathy for bereaved parents. Items often denote the place of birth and death, and include hospital wristbands, cot cards, the layette, and sometimes photos. Weaver-Hightower argue that "human institutions structure the experiences of stillbirth for those who suffer it" (477). It has also been documented that hospital-assembled mementos do not always reflect the parents' experience, culture, or parenting style, nor are they helpful for the healthcare provider (Noizet-Yverneau et al.). Because the traumatic nature of stillbirth places the bereaved under the guidance of the healthcare providers in the immediate loss context, Cacciatore ("Stillbirth") urges healthcare providers to use an evidence-based and patient-centered approach, while distinguishing their own beliefs and values from that of their patients.

Similarly, the promotion and practice of remembrance photography and memento making aims to facilitate attachment; however, it might also be utilized by bereaved parents to "resist disintegration and alienation," a way to emerge out of the silence of perinatal death (Godel 267). Collecting mementos such as a lock of hair is a simultaneous understanding of "that weight of flesh, that moment of death, preserved from its decay yet referring to it endlessly" (Lutz 135). Cot cards, baby hats, and wrist bands are also items collected from the births of living babies as keepsakes, just as items of significance, such as family photographs, letters, and funeral cards, might be collected from of a loved one following their death. These practices are simultaneously prescribed by norms, associations, traditions, and trends in birth and death, yet are not always appropriate or desired, culturally or otherwise.

Modern practices of stillbirth photography and collecting mementos, particularly locks of hair, are an evolution of *memento mori*, a Victorian-era practice (literally translated from the Latin as "remember you must die") where symbols or objects that remind us of death are utilized to illustrate one's experience with mortality (Linkman 83).

Relics speak of the truth of the loved body, which is a particularity that cannot be universalized, just as the relic can never be reproduced, copied, or multiplied. A kind of "dead commodity," they attest to the never before and the never again. (Lutz 135)

As much as Western society has become a death-denying and distancing culture in contrast to the customs of the nineteenth century, it could be argued that bereaved parents "unfettered on the Web" are in fact at the forefront of a "death integration into the world of the living" renaissance in their quest to make meaning of stillbirth through their similitude of Victorian-era practices, while they simultaneously risk having their grief "potentiate business opportunities" for the very outlets of their mourning (Lutz 127; Mitchell et al. 413). The commodification and commercialization of goods and services is not limited to grief, but is also prevalent in how parents prepare, encounter, and pay tribute to birth. Dominant imagery of pregnancy, birth, and parenting show glowing pregnant mothers and living, breathing, crying, breastfeeding pink babies. On the contrary, stillborn babies are erased from the "consumer face" of the birth space (Gibson 152). In a capitalist society/enterprise culture, does the death of a baby represent the death of a consumer (Howarth 130)? The link between the lack of recognition of stillbirth and loss of a consumer is illustrated in midwife Martha Roberts' 2013 poem "Silenced Families:"

Crying baby *silent*,
pulsing cord *still*,
signs of life *unseen*,
of families *invisible*,
to observing eyes,
to society that judges parenthood by:
nursery
stroller
carseat
crib
bottle
trappings of commercial motherhood.

Likewise, the baby that was to be born living is no longer recognized as a "patient" in the institutional birth space, but is segregated and classified as part the social dualism between the living and the dead, where the "scientific-rationale approach" and modern social norms distinguish between the end of medical care and the beginning of funeral professionals (Howarth; Ritchie). The disruption of the care trajectory between birth and death with stillbirth is a consequence of this dualism and important when considering stillbirth representations.

Photographs of stillborn infants are not only part of the culture of bereaved women and families, but an education aid about stillbirth's "visually, bodily aspects" (Weaver-Hightower 486). According to the website *Reconceiving Loss*, "Reading photographs links photography to literacy by establishing the idea that *photography is a language.*" In their study on representations of perinatal death in British midwifery textbooks, Cameron, Taylor and Greene highlight that an absence of information relating to the appearance of the infant has important implications for care, as midwives are not adequately prepared to provide accurate information to women and families (341). Even so, while stillbirth is more likely to affect under-represented groups of people, for example Inuit communities in the far North, these groups are not always portrayed in teaching resources, images, and texts (Jasen; Cameron, Taylor and Greene). The same exclusion is true for imagery of same-sex parents, fathers, grandparents, and older children affected by stillbirth. The omission of visible minority groups and family members in representations of stillbirth can be both stigmatizing and isolating for people who do not "see themselves" included as a part of the experience of stillbirth. Fathers, for example, need to be recognized as bereaved persons just as much as mothers are (deMontigny, Beaudet and Dumas, "Les Besoins"; Blood and Cacciatore). More research is also needed to understand the experience and depiction of stillbirth among same-sex parents (Blood and Cacciatore).

Artifacts of memorialization such as portraiture, headstones, and statues were at one time attributed to "identity politics," including lineage of the family, prominence in society, and personal wealth (Gibson 155). Now I Lay Me Down To Sleep

(NILM-DTS), a volunteer service, provides lasting photographic tributes to women and families who have experienced a stillbirth at no cost, and therefore transcends socio-economic status. The Little Spirits Garden in Victoria, BC, another example, makes available commemorative "Spirit Houses," stones, and flags to anyone who has lost a child "regardless of financial situation, location or time of loss" (*Saanich Legacy Foundation*). In the same fashion that memorialization becomes more accessible, so too does it transgress the private and the public realms of birth and death. Consider the representation of the butterfly on a door in the maternity ward, a symbol that notifies a death has occurred among the living. Or the Infant Memorial Garden at Mountain View Cemetery in Vancouver, BC, where "one stone for every infant" lies in a dry river bed to represent all of the babies that were buried anonymously, sometimes by the hospital or in an unmarked grave by a parent. These representations make the invisible visible. Consequently, it is interesting to consider what happens when the direct subjects and witnesses of the experiences of the stillbirth themselves begin to age and eventually die, and the photographs and mementos are transformed by the passage of time. Conversely, how might the passage of time transform the photo, as we are now seeing with age-progression photography (Carey)? Are the objects maintained as a living archive planned for "intergenerational transfer" as survivors look to engage successive generations in debate over their significance (Godal; Foote and Azaryahu; Linkman)?

Cacciatore and Flint describe non-traditional rituals to engage parents in the use of metaphors, symbols, stories, and ceremonies beyond the immediate collection of mementos and photographs following an acute loss. For example, "scrapbooks, memorial web-sites, commemorative jewelry, auto window stickers, personalized Christmas cards and ornaments, balloon releases, volunteering and participating in random acts of kindness, and tattoos" were found to be non-traditional rituals and symbols in Cacciatore and Flint's study of bereaved parents whose children's ages at time of death ranged from stillbirth to fifteen years old (166). Could it be that online memorials, as counterculture to traditional newspaper obituaries, help the baby to have an ongoing presence in the virtual forum, which opens opportunities for parents and others to visit, communicate, and establish a type of relationship with their child in death? Here, infants remain in the charge of the parent, as opposed to being limited to the "constraints of the hospital or the funeral home" (Mitchell et al. 415-16). As a transient form of meaning making, some bereaved mothers who find comfort in the "ability to mother after their baby is gone" are also adopting breast milk donation (Lourgos). One's journey through grief can be facilitated meaningfully in any number of individualized ways (Kobler, Limbo and Kavanaugh).

Not surprisingly, since a language around grief after stillbirth is not readily available, creative expression through poetry and visual arts has been offered as an option to bereaved parents (Jones). In 2014, the Vancouver-based organization Still Life Canada: Stillbirth and Neonatal Death Education, Research and Support Society hosted an art workshop for bereaved parents. Not only were tangible objects produced to symbolize the collective experience for use in future awareness and educational campaigns to combat ambiguity and stigma, but also through this silent process, the participants experienced a state of oneness that countered the aloneness and disenfranchisement of stillbirth. This creative strategy can also be used for young children. An Early-Childhood Educator in Toronto developed a felt board so that young children could make their own meaning of the death of a sibling using felt cut-outs rather than being prescribed meanings by parent(s), caregivers, and/or prefabricated resources (Oliveira).

LIMITATIONS AND IMPLICATIONS FOR PRACTICE

This chapter has focused specifically on the unique facets of representations of stillbirth. Making meaning for women and families who have experienced a miscarriage or medical termination has similar but separate challenges. To elucidate the particularities in the lived experiences of those who have had the experiences of miscarriage and medical termination is also of importance. As seen with the exploration of stillbirth, to prematurely generalize among categories ignores the diversity and can be potentially marginalizing.

Though beyond the scope of this chapter, an exploration of the limited number and prominence of public memorials regarding stillbirth as an "officially sanctioned category of death" is an area of important future discussion (Gibson 152,156). Though it is an event so prevalent, the absence of such public memorials removes bereaved families from public recognition of the experience and trauma of stillbirth and the sadness of lives that will never be lived (Weaver-Hightower 477; Gibson 156). Moreover, "the lives and deaths of women and other publicly marginalized identity groups are generally under-represented in public memorial-culture" (Gibson 155).

For some bereaved women and families, rituals (prescribed or customary) surrounding stillbirth may not provide comfort to their grief, especially if what is put in front of them does not speak to them or approximate the profundity of their grief (Romanoff and Terenzio). While the narrative herein was written by two women with very different experiences and interpretations of stillbirth, we recognize our point of privilege as educated, middle-class, working professionals. The commentary is limited at best to our experiences of North American culture, and may not translate to how stillbirth is represented to individuals and organizations elsewhere. What is universal as being important to bereaved parents is the concept of consent in the creation of bereavement mementos (Warland et al.). According to Blood and Cacciatore, "Promoting postmortem photography in a manner that will help parents surpass an inhibitory context of stigma requires sensitivity, awareness, and clinical wisdom" (231). On challenging normative representations, Cacciatore states:

> Less emphasis should be placed on ... standardatization.... [F]ocus should be on relational caregiving that underscores the uniqueness of each patient and their family, recognizes culture, and encourages affirmative, rather than traumatizing, provider reactions ... based on authentic, mutual relationships. (Cacciatore and Bushfield 694)

This can be accomplished by "guided participation," wherein, as a jumping-off point, caregivers ask women and families what is important to help guide and engage them in meaningful represen-tation-making, especially in this context of traumatic grief (Kobler, Limbo and Kavanaugh). Furthermore, restoring the centrality of parents through the standpoint of language is an important task in care, as this empowers women and families (Jutel 433). For example, utilizing the term "parental bereavement" as opposed to "perinatal bereavement" acknowledges parenthood and thus the grief of child death (Mitchell et al. 413).

For the woman, her pregnant and postpartum body may be-come "lost' in the discourse and rituals of making meaning of stillbirth as the focus shifts to her baby who has died (Jutel 428). At the same time, the pregnant body may epitomize where the infant's survival ended and the very image may be problematic for parents and families who have experienced stillbirth. Images of the pregnant body, typically absent from websites and leaflets of stillbirth support organizations, underscore how symbols of the pregnant body might be imagined by the viewer as a trigger or as continuing forward as life-giving. Care providers should be sensitive that for families who have experienced stillbirth, future interactions with facets of pregnancy, birth, and parenting may carry associations of risk or fear. Though the majority of births (and deaths) in Canada take place in the hospital setting, a place associated with life-saving technologies, one's understanding of pregnancy and birth is disrupted by the event of stillbirth. As technological advances are increasingly able to maintain the lifespan of humans, thus challenging how and when we define death, we must consider how the technology of maintaining the lives of earlier gestational ages may eventually disrupt the very definition of stillbirth (Jutel 430).

CONCLUSION

In death and bereavement, we often look to the things that are left behind as a way to make meaning of someone's life and what they meant to us (and us to them). When very little is left behind, as with stillbirth, making meaning of the death is that much more challenging. Given the trends in biomedical prescriptions around grief, it may be that caregivers will be challenged to dismantle the boundary between life and death and to engage in the intangibles as bereaved parents continue to make meaning with the ever-growing presence of material legacies (Howarth 134). With ninety-eight percent of the annual 2.6 million stillbirths worldwide occurring in low- and middle-income countries, stillbirth is now carving out a space in global agendas where it has been historically absent in discussions of maternal and child health (Lawn et al.). This discussion is filtering into mainstream and social media and beginning to infuse the culture of stillbirth with new political meaning. Local community initiatives are being buoyed by this global attention as their work is now given context on a larger scale. Solidarity between individuals and groups around the issue is also facilitated by the global attempt to bring "stillbirth out of the shadows" (Mullan and Horton).

This discussion on meaning making, from language to relics, from the individual, private, collective, and public practice, across time and space, has aimed to illustrate how parents, families, and communities make sense of stillbirth. Through an examination of the social and cultural norms, innovations, and counter-culture of stillbirth representation, we have demonstrated how and why people may ascribe, challenge, and resist social prescriptions of birth, death, and grief.

As bereaved parents and families amplify their voice, they are infusing silence with new meaning. Stillbirth is silence = Silence is stillness. Bereaved parents are conceiving a kind of counterculture of death and grief by giving meaning to "being with death" when there is stillbirth. A quiet revolution is challenging caregivers to learn how to "be with" the silence and the stillness of birth and death. This will require self-awareness, an understanding of supporting difference, and great reverence in being guided by what innately unfolds, rather than directing a parent's experience.

[1]We acknowledge the death-denying quality of the word "loss," but recognize its usage in the mainstream to describe all types of deaths. In her scholarly paper "What's in a Name," Jutel critiques the language surrounding perinatal death but fails to be critical of her own use of the word "loss" (431).

WORKS CITED

Allan, Bonnie. "Sask. Women Giving 'Angel Dresses' to Grieving Families." *CBC News*. May 2014. Web. Accessed June 4, 2014.

Babyloss Support for Agnostic and Atheist Moms. Facebook Group. Web. Accessed May 25, 2014.

Blood, Cybele, and Joanne Cacciatore. "Parental Grief and Memento Mori Photography: Narrative, Meaning, Culture and Context." *Death Studies* 38.1-5 (2014): 224-33. Print.

Cacciatore, Joanne. "Position Statement of the MISS Foundation." MISS Foundation. 2010. Pdf.

Cacciatore, Joanne. "Stillbirth: Patient-Centered Psychosocial Care." *Clinical Obstetrics and Gynecology* 53.3 (2010): 691-699. Print.

Blood, Cybele and Joanne Cacciatore. "Psychological Effects of Stillbirth." *Seminars in Fetal and Neonatal Medicine*. 18.2 (2013): 72-82. Print.

Cacciatore, J. and S. Bushfield. "Stillbirth: The Mother's Experience and Implications for Improving Care." *J Soc Work End Life Palliat Care* 3.3 (2007): 59-79. Print.

Cacciatore, Joanne and Melissa Flint. "Mediating Grief: Postmortem Ritualization after Child Death." *Journal of Loss and Trauma* 17.2 (2012): 158-172. Print.

Cameron J., J. Taylor, and A. Greene. "Representations of Rituals and Care in Perinatal Death in British Midwifery Textbooks 1937-2004." *Midwifery* 24.3 (2008): 335–343. Print.

Carey, Tanith. "Can an Age-Progressed Picture of a Dead Child Really Help Bereaved Parents?" *The Guardian*. 16 May 2014. Web. Accessed June 4, 2014.

Chalmers, Beverley. "Cultural Issues in Perinatal Care." *Birth* 40.4. (2013): 217-219. Print.

Davidson, Deborah. "A Technology of Care: Caregiver Responses to Perinatal Loss." *Women's Studies International Forum* 31.4 (2008): 278-284. Print.

de Montigny, Francine, Line Beaudet, Louise Dumas. "A Baby Has Died: The Impact of Perinatal Loss on Family's Social Networks." *Journal of Obstetric and Gynecological and Neonatal Nursing* 28.2 (1999): 151-6. Print.

de Montigny, Francine, Line Beaudet, Louise Dumas. "Les besoins des mères et des pères en deuil d'un enfant." *Perspectives Soignantes* 17 (2003): 89-108. Print.

Dudley, Carly Marie. "Voices and Differences." *Still Standing Magazine*. 11 Dec 2013. Web. Accessed May 25, 2014.

Foote K. E. and M. Azaryahu. "Toward Geography of Memory: Geographical Dimensions of Public Memory and Commemoration." *Journal of Political and Military Sociology* 35.1 (2007): 125-144. Print.

Forhan, Mary. "Doing, Being, and Becoming: A Family's Journey Through Perinatal Loss." *American Journal of Occupational Therapy* 64.1 (2010): 142-51. Print.

Frøen, J. Frederik, Joanne Cacciatore, Elizabeth M. McClure, Oluwafemi Kuti, Abdul Hakim Jokhio, Monir Islam, Jeremy Shiffman. "Stillbirths: Why They Matter." *The Lancet* 377.9774 (2011): 1353-66. Print.

Gibson, Margaret. "Death and Grief in the Landscape: Private Memorials in Public Spaces." *Cultural Studies Review* 17.1 (2011): 146-61. Print.

Godel, Margaret. "Images of Stillbirth: Memory, Mourning and Memorial." *Visual Studies* 22.3 (2007): 253-269. Print.

Howarth, Glennys. "Dismantling the Boundaries between Life and Death." *Mortality* 5.2 (2000): 127-138. Print.

Ilse, Sherokee. *Empty Arms: Coping After Miscarriage, Stillbirth and Infant Death*. Minnesota: Wintergreen Press, 1982. Print.

Jasen, Patricia. "Race, Culture, and the Colonization of Childbirth in Northern Canada." *Social History of Medicine* 10.3 (1997): 383-400. Print.

Jones, Kara L.C. "Creative Expressions of Grief." *They Were Still Born Personal Stories About Stillbirth*. Ed. Janel C. Atlas. Plymouth, UK: Rowman & Littlefield. 2010. 184-184. Print.

Jutel, Annemarie. "What's in a Name? Death before Birth." *Perspectives in Biology and Medicine* 49.3 (2006): 425-434. Print.

Keane H. "Foetal Personhood and Representations of the Absent Child in Pregnancy Loss Memorialization." *Feminist Theory* 10.2 (2009): 153–171. Print.

Kelley, Maureen C. and Susan B. Trinidad. "Silent Loss and the Clinical Encounter: Parents' and Physicians' Experiences of

Stillbirth: A Qualitative Analysis." *BioMed Central Pregnancy and Childbirth* 12.1 (2012): 1-15. Print.

Kobler K., R. Limbo, K. Kavanaugh. "Meaningful Moments: The Use of Ritual in Perinatal and Pediatric Death." *The American Journal of Maternal/Child Nursing* 32.5 (2007): 288-295. Print.

Lawn, Joy E. et al. "Stillbirths: Where? When? Why? How to Make the Data Count?" *The Lancet* 377.9775 (2011): 1448–1463.

Layne, Linda. "He Was a Real Baby With Baby Things: A Material Culture Analysis of Personhood, Parenthood and Pregnancy Loss." *Journal of Material Culture* 5.3 (2000): 321–345. Print.

Layne, Linda. "Pregnancy and Infant Loss Support: A New, Feminist, American, Patient Movement?" *Social Science & Medicine* 62.3 (2006): 602-13. Print.

Linkman, Audrey. *Photography and Death*. England: Reaktion Books, 2012. E-book. 28 Dec 2013.

Lourgos, Angie Leventis. "Donating Breast Milk After Her Son's Death, Mother Helps Another Baby Survive." *Chicago Tribune*. 15 Feb 2014. Web. Accessed June 4, 2014.

Lutz, Deborah. "The Dead Still among Us: Victorian Secular Relics, Hair, Jewelry, and Death Culture." *Victorian Literature and Culture* 39.1 (2010): 127-142. Print.

MacConnell, Grace, Megan Aston, Pat Randal, Nick Zwaagstra. "Nurses' Experiences of Providing Bereavement Follow-Up: An Exploratory Study Using Feminist Poststructuralism." *Journal of Clinical Nursing* 22.7-8 (2013): 1094-102. Print.

Mander, Rosemary and Rosalind K. Marshall. "An Historical Analysis of the Role of Paintings and Photographs in Comforting Bereaved Parents." *Midwifery* 19.3 (2003): 230-242. Print.

MISS Foundation. "Being Effectively Present: An Invitation to Caregivers." MISS Foundation. n.d. Web. Accessed June 22, 2014.

Mitchell, Lisa M., Peter H. Stephenson, Susan Cadell, Mary Ellen Macdonald. "Death and Grief On-line: Virtual Memorialization and Changing Concepts of Childhood Death and Parental Bereavement on the Internet." *Health Sociology Review* 21.4 (2012): 413-431. Print.

Mullan, Zoë, and Richard Horton. "Bringing Stillbirths Out of the Shadows." *The Lancet* 377.9774 (2011): 1291-1292. Print.

Noizet-Yverneau O., C. Deschamps, F. Lempp, I. Daligaut, G. Delebarre, A. David, C. Barbie, P. Morville, N. Bednarek-Weirauch. "Memory Boxes in the Neonatal Period: Caregivers' Opinions After 1 Year of Practice." *Archives de pédiatrie:organe officiel de la Sociéte française de pédiatrie* 20.9 (2013): 921-927. Print.

Oliveira, Suzanne. Presentation in "Birth and Its Meanings" class. Ryerson University, Toronto. Fall 2013.

Reagan, Leslie J. "From Hazard to Blessing to Tragedy: Representation of Miscarriage in Twentieth-Century America." *Fem Stud.* 29.2 (2003): 356-78. Print.

Reconceiving Loss. "Core Concepts of Photography." n.d. Web. Accessed May 14, 2014.

Ritchie, David. "Loss, Grief and Representation: 'Getting on With It.'" *Double Dialogues: Art and Pain* 4 (2003). Web. 28 Dec 2013.

Roberts, Martha. Personal communication, May 31, 2014

Robinson, Gail Erlick. "Pregnancy Loss." *Best Practice & Research Clinical Obstetrics and Gynaecology* 28.1 (2014): 169–178. Print.

Romanoff, Bronna D., and Marion Terenzion. "Rituals and the Grieving Process." *Death Studies* 22.8 (1998): 697-711. Print.

Ruderman, D. B. "The Breathing Space of Ballad: Tennyson's Stillborn Poetics." *Victorian Poetry* 47.1 (2009): 151-171. Print.

Saanich Legacy Foundation. 2013. Web.

Smith, Dorothy E. "The Relations of Ruling: A Feminist Inquiry." *Studies in Cultures, Organizations and Societies* 2.2 (1996): 171–190. Print.

"Stillborn." *Canadian Oxford Dictionary.* 2nd ed. 2004. Print.

Warland, Jane, et al. "Caring for Families Experiencing Stillbirth: A Unified Position Statement on Contact With the Baby." An International Collaboration. *MISS Foundation.* 2011. Pdf.

Weaver-Hightower, Marcus. "Waltzing Matilda: An Autoethnography of a Father's Stillbirth." *Journal of Contemporary Ethnography* 41.4 (2012): 462–491. Print.

3.
LOOKING AT PARENTING

Kids Aren't Cute

L ET'S GET A FEW MORE THINGS STRAIGHT about kids. Kids aren't cute. Kids aren't cute, but they are little and little is cute, but it's only the little that's cute, not the kid. Think about it, a six-foot newborn would not be cute. Not only are kids not cute, they don't like cute things. They don't even like primary colours. Given the chance, they always go for the black remote control. They don't want fuzzy stuffed animals; they want to turn the oven on. They want to drive the car. They want to work that new table saw. They only play with toys because that's all they can reach. In the last nine years, I've spent quite a bit of time around kids and I, for one, have seen their true colours, and they're not cute.

This is my theory: we adults just try to make our experience of children cute to lessen the intensity of existing with them. Children are a complex labyrinth of life at its rawest, a penetrating mirror into ourselves. That's why it rubs me the wrong way to hear kids passed off as being "cute." All right, in my own selfish way, I want to argue for kids to make my job title as mother appreciated as more than quaint and sweet. I want the grit and glory of motherhood revealed through the splendor of our charges, just as lion-tamers are revered because of the ferocity of lions. Therefore, I wish to systematically argue for adjectives other than cute when describing kids. Okay? Here we go.

Kids are deep. They thwack you up-side the head with insights when your guard is completely down. Accompanying Stella in the bathroom at a Mexican restaurant, she's sitting on the toilet pushing and she announces to me quite off the cuff, "I have in-

317

finity love. Once until I give a love another love comes back to me." Which reminds me of another point concerning the deepness of kids. Kids love infinity. Once they hear about it, that's all they talk about for the next month. Month? Year. Year? Years. I hear them arguing, "I have infinity smart." "Oh yeah? Well, I have two infinity smart." "If you have two infinity smart then that means you don't even know what infinity is." "I do too." The word after infinity that they love is googolplex. And they are very pleased if they can memorize and casually drop in conversation the word antidisestablishmentarianism.

Kids are racist. On the playground a mother walked by and gushed over my cute little Josephine in the carriage. Her five-year-old son was walking behind her and stopped at our carriage after his mother had passed. Looking me straight in the eye he said, "That baby is black." I said, "Yes, I know, she was adopted from Africa." Not dissuaded from his purpose, he continued, "And she's going to stay black."

Also kids are selfish. Driving in the car, Leo's in his car seat, i.e. philosopher's stone, and he asks, sounding a little worried, "Is grandma going to die?" I reply, "Someday she will, yeah, but she's had a good full life and we'll be sad for ourselves when she dies, but we won't need to be sad for her." Going a little deeper he asks, sounding a little more worried, "Are you going to die, Mommy?" "Someday I'll die, but I take really good care of my body and I try to be safe so I will probably have a lot of good life left in me." He seems mildly reassured but is still thinking. "And will Daddy die?" "Someday, but he's probably got a lot of good life left in him too." Then it hits him and he freaks, "AM *I* GOING TO DIE?" Kids are fundamentally rooting for ol' number one, themselves. Case in point, Leo asked me if he could get a tarantula. I explained that I have an irrational fear of spiders and could never, really never, live in the same house with a spider. He thinks a moment and then, not giving up hope of living with a spider, asks, "Do you think you'd move out if you and dad got a divorce?"

Kids are linguistic. They're daily putting our language in a salt shaker and turning it upside down, doing to our language just what we revere Shakespeare for having done. Stella, weeping that Leo hurt her says, "He stepped on my toe [weeps more] and it was my youngest." They're masters of hyperbole. In declaring her love, she stated earnestly, "I love you so much I could pull my brains out." They're ever-surprising with the unexpected turn of phrase. When walking into the room where my sister and I were sitting on the bed talking, Stella proudly announces herself: "My name is Stella, I have blue eyes and a teeny crotch."

And kids can render you speechless with statements and retorts to which there really is no reply. For instance, one day Leo came running up to me breathless, checking over his shoulder, and said, "Stella's going to tell on me." Another time I was giving one of my impassioned lectures to our teenage foster-daughter who lived with us for two years: "It's not like there is any one thing I want you to be. You don't need to be a teacher or a doctor. I just want you to be happy." To which she said, "Yeah, but what about what I want?"

In addition, kids are spiritual. Waiting at the bank drive-through one day Leo at four years of age said, "God is a good story ... so is Spiderman. Are we just stories too?"

Also, kids are savvy. One time I got a cheap flight back to Wisconsin with a three-hour layover in O'Hare. I said to Leo after two hours waiting at the airport, "We get to take two planes to Grandma's, aren't we lucky?" He replied, unimpressed, "I don't want to be that lucky."

Kids are surrealistic. One evening walking on the Pearl Street mall, we happened upon some teenagers swing dancing for tips. I said to Leo, "Wouldn't that be a fun thing for you to do when you're a teenager?" He surmised the scene and responded, "I only want to dance with Chinese girls wearing red dresses."

Don't forget, kids are imaginative. Furthermore, their understanding between reality and fantasy is still reluctantly developing. One day, Leo and I were under the covers, we were going down for our nap and I was making up a story for him like I did every afternoon. In this story, Leo was floating upwards into the clouds. He moved his arms and legs as though swimming and found he could propel himself through the air. He tucked his head quickly between his legs and somersaulted. Then he made his way over to a cloud. It was unthinkably soft. He felt very tired and yawned an enormous yawn. Then he lay down on the soft cloud and nestled in for a nap. Feeling a slight chill, he pulled a downy blanket from the cloud. Then I whispered to an almost-asleep Leo, "Let's not finish the story. Let's fall asleep together inside the story." Leo's eyes tripled in size, "But what would happen then?" His mind was on fire. I soothingly replied, "Let's wait and see. Close your eyes and fall asleep." Leo closed his eyes but his thoughts raced and collided into all the imaginable possibilities. The task proved too great. The very possibility of a nap had vanished. This kind of imagining is more Einsteinian than cute.

My final point of contention as to why people think kids are cute is that it's because there is a widespread misnomer that kids are funny. Kids aren't funny. Have you ever heard a kid try to tell a joke? It goes on and on and it's always one you've already heard. Kids can be silly but that is a very non-inclusive variety of low humour based on the same fart noise made over and over again. It's generally not funny at all to adults but, rather, annoying. Okay, kids can be funny when they unknowingly juxtapose bizarre combinations in an earnest effort to make sense of a situation. For instance, one day Leo walked up to me with a snotty nose that was suffering from some severe leakage and asked with scientific curiosity, "What's inside my head besides the stuff that comes out of my nose?" And, lastly, they can create the unintentional pun, made all the funnier by their complete ignorance of what they are really saying. My good friend and her daughter were cuddling in bed and my friend said to her girl, "This is what Mommy and Daddy do in bed sometimes, it's called spooning." The little girl thought about that for a few moments and then asked, "Do you and Daddy ever fork?"

I rest my case.

Paternal Loss and Anticipation

An Artist's Perspective

MATERNITY IS BECOMING A VISIBLE PRESENCE on the contemporary art scene. Around the world, artists like Rineke Dijkstra, Katharina Bosse, Maru Ituarte, Mariángeles Soto-Díaz, Zorka Project, Kate Kretz, Gail Rebhan, and Jess Dobkin address pregnancy, lactation, the postpartum body, the mother-child relationship, and societal expectations of mothers. Some creative practitioners use their maternal position as a point of activist departure, turning to social and political engagement to effect cultural change for parents and children.[1]

While many artist-mothers have confronted cultural taboos to speak more fully to their own lived experiences and to challenge heteronormative, raced, and classed expectations of motherhood, the counterpart depictions and voices of fatherhood are much fewer and farther between. This essay will introduce one such artist-father who engages with complex issues of paternity as a means to consider not only his personal situation but also cultural expectations of child development.

LOSS

Raw. Blunt. Misshapen. Unembellished clay, iron, and steel twist together in irregular ways, starkly contrasting the perfect geometry of the circle and square in which they are inscribed. Wires and rods seek to bisect the circle but they become tangled, lost in the unruly form of contorted clay. Nails protrude, strongly individual yet tenuously connected to each other.

321

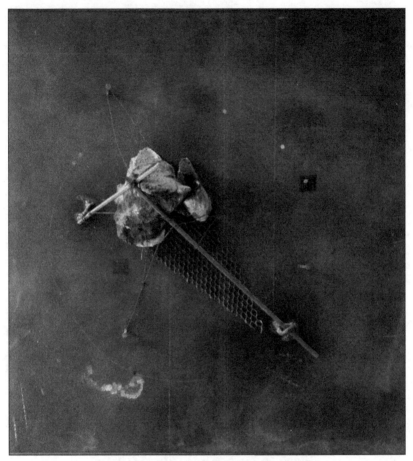

Figure 1: Merrill Krabill, Untitled, 1994. Mixed media.
Collection of Bethel College Math Department.

After he and his wife experienced miscarriage, American artist Merrill Krabill embarked on a series of mixed media sculptures exploring the difficult and often conflicting emotions that accompany the journey toward parenthood. While the forms are non-representational, they contain a host of possible emotions—grief, anger, pain, despair. Krabill treats the medium with an aesthetic that seems wholly appropriate to conveying the loss of life. Crumpled pieces of clay, fired but unglazed, appear to be discarded remnants, perhaps the leftovers of some more finished piece. Krabill pierces his ceramic forms with large nails and iron rods, imparting a sense of physical pain and destruction. And yet, the mass of clay refuses to be subordinated, suggesting a tension where life clings tenaciously under threat of submersion. For Krabill, sorrow and fear live alongside awareness of the miracle of birth. As he reflects, "It isn't so much shocking that pregnancies end early as it is that they sometimes result in new life" (Krabill, "Re: postpartum show"). One can imagine the artist's process of grief borne out through the sculptures as existing structures and forms are poetically reduced to fragments.

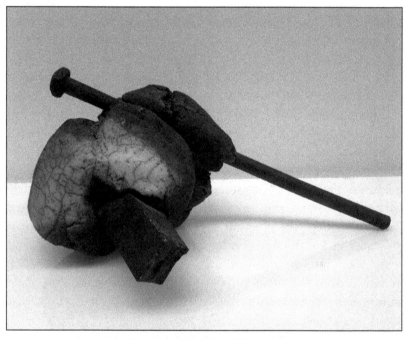

Figure 2: Merrill Krabill, Untitled, 1990. Mixed media.
Collection of Bethel College, Gift of Bob Regier.

Krabill's treatment of clay in an intentionally unaesthetic manner speaks to his schooling in an era immediately after the Process Art movement of the 1960s, a period during which artists focused on the practice of making rather than on the eventual end product. U.S. and European artists explored widely varied three-dimensional media such as felt, rubber, and latex. Ceramic artist Peter Voulkos and his colleagues in California revolutionized the medium of clay by stripping it of functionality and moving it from the realm of craft to that of art (MacNaughton). Voulkos emphasized the process of facture through his treatment of the medium: by hitting and cutting at the clay, Voulkos conveyed energy and emotion in the resulting forms. Krabill's manipulation of ceramic chunks speared with metal rods vividly communicates the strong, even violent, emotions present during the making. Like artists of the Process movement, Krabill frequently works with abstraction and asserts that specific perspectives on the work come only later, after he has wrestled in the studio with the material forms. While he began the miscarriage series with identifiable content, he acknowledges that for him it felt "a bit clumsy to work in that way, with subject matter that connects with a more specific narrative" (Krabill, "article").

Miscarriage and infant loss are still relatively taboo topics in the visual arts, but Krabill's sculptures do not exist in isolation. Rebecca Baillie used her own blood to draw a portrait of her miscarried son as a way "to understand the somewhat unreal and fleeting experience of miscarriage" (Baillie). Similarly, Tabitha Moses transformed miscarried blood into a chart of island forms linked to phases of the moon: "Constructing this map was a way to salvage grace and meaning from an incomprehensible occurrence" (Moses). For both artists, the physical and emotional bodily experience of miscarriage became the conduit for the art.

A father's interpretation of such loss necessarily differs, markedly separate from the pregnant / not pregnant body, and so Krabill comments at times from the margins. Through his sculptures, Krabill offers a voice from the outside looking in, not experiencing the physical trauma but wholly invested in the emotional experience. Nick Johnstone laments pregnancy, birth, and breastfeeding as "the paternal trilogy of being condemned to the role of observer" (96). An observer need not be passive, however, nor uninvolved. German photographer Fred Hüning turned his lens on his wife, and later his child, to capture the rollercoaster of emotions on their shared journey into parenthood. Hüning's trilogy of photo books, *Einer, Zwei,* and *Drei,* portrays the trauma of their loss of a child to stillbirth, as well as the trepidation and joy that accompany a second pregnancy and birth. The photographs become a cathartic tool for dealing with grief and reveal the intensity of birth and death within family cycles (Bright 72). Hüning himself is never pictured in the photographs but we know that the father exists behind the camera, implying family structure and paternal attachment. Both Hüning and Krabill offer profoundly nuanced experiences of fatherhood and visibly mark that which is often unseen.

ANTICIPATION

Science interprets the vagaries of nature and anticipation becomes laced with uncertainty. What gifts will this child bring? Who will recognize her gifts?

In a conceptual series of photographs, Krabill reflected on his family's experience of awaiting the birth of Emily, who they knew

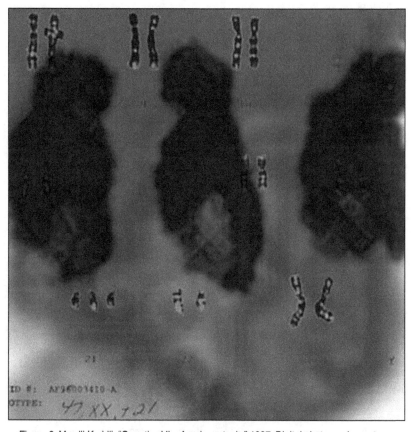

Figure 3: Merrill Krabill, "Genetics VI—Amniocentesis," 1997. Digital photograph montage.

would be born with Down syndrome. *Inquiry into Gifts* layers together markers of nature and human measurement, which at times compete with each other. Through the photographs, Krabill touches on parental and societal expectations, considerations of "normalcy," fear and pain, and the possibility of spiritual revelation.

The series of digitally layered photographs charts elements of the family's experience from initial diagnosis to several years into Emily's growth. *Genetics VI—Amniocentesis* (figure 3) enlarges

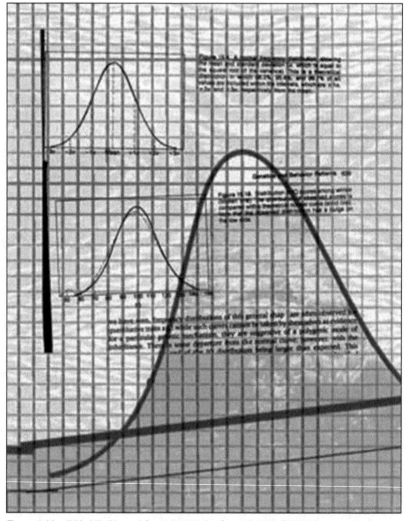

Figure 4: Merrill Krabill, "Normal Curve I—with the Ocean," 1997. Digital photograph montage.

the triplet (rather than paired) chromosomes in the twenty-first set, combining the image with the amniocentesis report, all that they knew of the baby girl at that point. *Normal Curve I—with the Ocean* layers natural and human-defined curves—ocean waves superimposed by multiple forms of bell-shaped curves that illustrate standard distributions of normalcy. Knowing that Emily will hit growth and development milestones at different times than is considered "normal" in our society, it at all, Krabill encourages us to reconsider our expectations: "Comparing similar information and experiences in a general way and specific physiological data statistically are valuable tools, but that information is often used as some kind of measure of a child's success" (Krabill, *Inquiry*). Many of his photographs include images of nature, implicitly questioning human categorization of children like Emily as non-natural. *Wheat I* (figure 5) juxtaposes a bell curve with a field of yellow wheat.

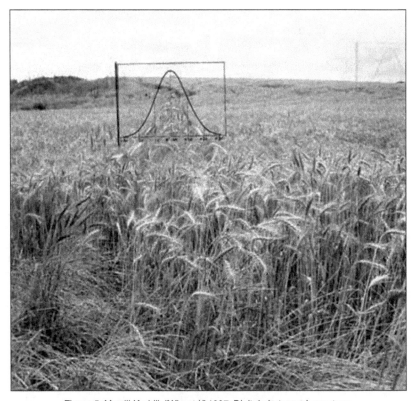

Figure 5: Merrill Krabill, "Wheat I," 1997. Digital photograph montage.

In one section, the wheat has grown far taller than the rest of the field, mimicking the curve Krabill layers on top. Embracing the diversity to be found in nature, Krabill positions it as a teachable moment, suggesting that "the natural world is changing to fit the model of what normal should be like" (*Inquiry*).

Krabill's use of bell curves speaks to the parental and societal tendency to want to document, to quantify, child growth and development. Among artists, Mary Kelly's *Postpartum Document* is the classic example of this tendency: a 135-part pseudo-scientific record of the mother-child relationship in the extended postpartum period. Significantly, though, Kelly never photographically pictured mother or child, who were instead represented by journal entries, records of early attempts at language, and physical remnants such as onesies and soiled diapers. Kelly avoided representing the mother's body because of her particular context within 1970s feminism, in part to avoid the male gaze and also to open up the mother-child conversation beyond just autobiography (Kelly 23). For Krabill, though, the photographs of the *Inquiry* series seem almost wholly removed from the mother's body. Perhaps because of the father's remove from the physical experience of pregnancy, Krabill's focus instead becomes the growing child and his own anticipation, not only of parenthood but also of how she will be received in this world.

At the same time, though perhaps unintentionally, Krabill enters into a photographic tradition of making visible marginalized populations. Diane Arbus famously pictured the pariahs of society, giving her attentions to circus sideshow performers, conjoined twins, and mentally and physically disabled children. Scholars debate whether Arbus' intentions were more voyeuristic than sympathetic, since she referred to her subjects as "idiots" and "freaks" (Gross 170). Although the language represents common parlance of the time, the words still establish a substantial emotional distance between photographer and photographed. A significantly different feel— still unsentimental but less objectifying—comes through when the photographer is invested in the communities depicted. Catherine Opie first came to attention for her large-scale colour portraits that sought to give visibility, and thereby grant social legitimacy, to her queer and transgendered communities in Los Angeles. Photographer Debbie Rasiel's recent body of work makes visible the faces of autistic children and their caregivers around the world. Beginning from a personal position as mother to an autistic child, Rasiel captures the "tense moments, dysregulated facial expressions, and misshapen hands" that are common across social and cultural divides, yet grants her subjects individuality as well. In *Inquiry into Gifts,* Krabill makes no claims about picturing the world of Down syndrome as Rasiel does with autism, but by making visible his experience with Emily, he raises larger societal questions about expectations for both parents and children.

Running through both of Krabill's series is a considered relationship with the divine, a topic addressed nearly as infrequently in contemporary art as fatherhood. Perhaps as a way to make sense of the unexpected and the traumatic, Krabill draws on religious narratives and the natural world, seeking to understand his experience of fatherhood as something much larger than himself. The mixed media sculptures, whose piercings and perpendicular juxtapositions make oblique references to crucifix forms, play with a push and pull between suffering and healing. They are at once damaged and patched together. Krabill asserts, "There is a richer understanding gained through being broken and healing, than there is in an unblemished posture" ("Re: article"). The photographs, too, address not only his individual experiences of fathering a child with Down syndrome but also his broader worldview and conception of the sacred, positioned as an inversion of who is last and who is first:

> It can be those who are the least influential who have the most to teach, who understand some important things better. That Upside Down Kingdom thinking seems to pervade my work. Real joy and peace come out of being broken and healed instead of avoiding ever feeling pain. The sacred is messy and earthy and nearby instead of unblemished, perfect, and distant. ("Re: article")

FURTHER CONTEXTS

The rarity of fatherhood as a theme for contemporary artists stems partly from the stratified cultural perceptions of mother-hood versus fatherhood. For women to both have children and hold down a job is still seen as trying to "have it all," while for men, doing both is socially expected and culturally rewarded. As James Levine and Todd Pittinsky argue in *Working Fathers: New Strategies for Balancing Work and Family,* "When a wom-an works outside the home, our society assumes she must feel a constant tug-of-war between her 'job self' and her 'parent self.' But *working father* is seen as a redundancy.... The prevailing assumption is that men do not feel that tug-of-war between their 'job selves' and their 'parent selves'" (17). Stated another way, a man's juggling of work and family is generally ignored in the United States. In *Redefining Fatherhood,* Nancy Dowd argues that even though more fathers engage more consistently with raising children than ever before, "father care remains rooted in the assumption that the mother will be the primary caregiver" (86). Thus, while it may seem logical, even obvious, for women to engage with and critique the institution of motherhood in art and scholarship, the same has not always held true for men.

Negotiating parenthood within a creative life may be no less momentous for men than for women, yet there are fewer visible examples. In a recent anthology of male authors writing about fatherhood, Lev Grossman candidly reflects, "Even as a child I could see that appealing depictions of fatherhood in popular cul-ture were, at least in the 1970s and 1980s, thin on the ground.... Fathers were most often seen taking out the trash in sitcoms. They were almost never seen composing works of genius" (16). Gross-man, and many other contributors to the anthology, feared that fatherhood would be incompatible with the creative life. Indeed, as Grossman writes, fatherhood "kick[s] the shit out of your life plan" (18). But Grossman and others also discovered along the way that their new roles as fathers significantly informed their writing. Not all turned to writing about the father-child relationship—in fact, most did not—but many acknowledged the shift as deep and profound, affecting all parts of their lives and often changing their writing dramatically.

A similar anthology could, and perhaps should, be written by artist-fathers, but up to this point, very little has been published about their experiences. Historically at least, male artists could celebrate their progeny in ways that female artists could not. When American artist Leon Golub's wife, artist Nancy Spero, gave birth to their first child in 1954, Golub produced a large lithograph entitled *Birth I*. Stylistically similar to Golub's other totemic and mythological work from the time, *Birth I* in fact marks his entry into parenthood, a visual proclamation of his achievement of father-hood status in a public manner that would have been unthinkable for Spero and her female peers at the time. For Myrel Chernick, her maternal status meant that a New York curator dismissed her work out of hand, declaring babies to be "boring" (256). Parisian curators repeatedly rejected Diana Quinby's drawings of the pregnant maternal body as "too intimate," "taboo," and "unshowable" (153). Renee Cox's now-famous *Yo Mama* series emerged from the hostility she encountered while pregnant during graduate school. For male artists, however, as for men in general, children have long been regarded culturally as accessories, signs of stability and maturity. Alison Bain suggests, "Elevated above everyday reproductive tasks, the figure of the male artist is idealized and romanticized for his ability to reveal the creative, imaginative, and aesthetic value in the ordinary. Part of the sacrifice that seems to be almost socially expected of the male artist is the eschewing of family life" (252). For heroicized artists of the twentieth century such as Pablo Picasso, wives, mistresses, and children functioned as tangential accoutrements—objects of interest but not of particular emotional and physical investment.

Fathers of the last twenty years, however, many of whom in-vest more in parenting than previous generations, have begun to realize the negotiations necessary to combine active parenting with active art-making. Krabill has acknowledged the cyclical nature of work and family, where parenting sometimes precludes a focus on professional priorities ("Re: article"). In her study of contemporary artist-fathers, Bain argues that "dominant discours-es of masculinity in the visual arts do not sit comfortably with fathering practices" and have left some feeling illegitimate in both realms (249). Rather than believing they can "have it all," in the language of popular culture for contemporary women, many of the men Bain interviewed "reject the possibility of success at both artistic labour and domestic labour" (256). They choose one over the other instead of trying to do both at once. While few other studies address artist-fathers in particular, broader sociological studies point to the need to redefine U.S. cultural understanding of fathers' roles and change institutional frameworks in order to account for fathers' greater involvement with children (e.g., Marsiglio and Roy).

Through his photographic and sculptural investigations, Merrill Krabill navigated a rocky path that was significantly informed, though not defined, by his journey of fatherhood. More than simply personal explorations, both of Krabill's series became for him greater meditations on humanity and the natural world—moving past private pain to question cultural definitions of normalcy and realize the miraculous nature of life beyond our understanding. As Krabill notes, "There is a sadness, I suppose, but the overwhelming sense is of how beautiful the connection is sometimes between people who care about each other" ("Re: article"). In a time when a critical mass of artists addressing themes of fatherhood seems overdue, Krabill's work offers a nuanced model for artists who might seek entry into the theme in a manner larger than autobiography.

[1]Presenters at two recent conferences emphasized varied maternal and political intersections among contemporary artists. Martina Mullaney, founder of *Enemies of Good Art,* Andrea Francke, of the project *Invisible Spaces of Parenthood,* and many other maternal artist-activists spoke at *Motherhood and Creative Practice,* a two-day conference at London South Bank University in June 2015, and at *The Mothernists,* a three-day conference put on by *m/other voices* in Rotterdam, the Netherlands, also in June 2015.

WORKS CITED

Baillie, Rebecca. "My Son 22.10.11" *Studies in the Maternal* 5.1 (2013). n.pag. Web. 5 May 2014.

Bain, Alison L. "Claiming and Controlling Space: Combining Heterosexual Fatherhood with Artistic Practice." *Gender, Place, and Culture: A Journal of Feminist Geography* 14.3 (2007): 249-65. Print.

Bright, Susan. *Home / Truths: Photography and Motherhood.* London: Art Books Publishing, 2013. Print.

Chernick, Myrel. "Reflections on Art, Motherhood, and Maternal Ambivalence." *Reconciling Art and Mothering.* Ed. Rachel Epp Buller. Surrey, UK: Ashgate, 2012. 255-65. Print.

Dowd, Nancy E. *Redefining Fatherhood.* New York: New York University Press, 2000. Print.

Gross, Frederick. *Diane Arbus's 1960s: Auguries of Experience.* Minneapolis: University of Minnesota Press, 2012. Print.

Grossman, Lev. "Daughter Pressure." *When I First Held You.* Ed. Brian Gresko. New York: Berkley Books, 2014. 15-22. Print.

Johnstone, Nick. "Mothering Fathers." *Home / Truths: Photography and Motherhood.* Ed. Susan Bright. London: Art Books Publishing, 2013. 94-99. Print.

Kelly, Mary. "Notes on Reading the *Postpartum Document.*" *Imaging Desire.* Cambridge, Mass.: The MIT Press, 1996. 20-25. Print.

Krabill, Merill. *Inquiry into Gifts. Merrill Krabill.* 2003. Web. 15 March 2014.

Krabill, Merill. "Re: article." Message to the author. 29 April 2014. Email.

Krabill, Merill. "Re: postpartum show." Message to the author. 10 February 2013. Email.

Levine, James A. and Todd L. Pittinsky. *Working Fathers: New Strategies for Balancing Work and Family.* San Diego: Harcourt Brace and Company, 1997. Print.

MacNaughton, Mary Davis. *Clay's Tectonic Shift: John Mason, Ken Price, and Peter Voulkos, 1956-1968.* Los Angeles: J. Paul Getty Museum, 2012. Print.

Marsiglio, William and Kevin Roy. *Nurturing Dads: Social Initiatives for Contemporary Fatherhood.* New York: Russell Sage Foundation, 2012. Print.

Moses, Tabitha. "Islands of Blood and Longing." *The Egg, the Womb, the Head and the Moon.* 11 November 2013. Web. 30 May 2014.

Quinby, Diana. "Art About Motherhood—The Last Taboo? Reflections of an American Artist in Paris." *Reconciling Art and Mothering*. Ed. Rachel Epp Buller. Surrey, UK: Ashgate, 2012. 151-64. Print.

Raisel, Debbie. *Picturing Autism*. Soho20gallery. May 27-June 21, 2014. Web. 14 June 2014.

Two Mums and Some Babies

Queering Motherhood

G AY AND LESBIAN PARENTS ARE A NEW FRONT in parenting
research. Coining the term *lesbian baby boom*, Morris,
Balsam and Rothblum indicate the numbers of lesbian
mothers has increased rapidly over the last two decades. Following
that paper, there has been a good deal of research that explores
the experience of lesbians as parents. Much of this research (see
Lubbe; Tasker and Patterson) has focused primarily on family
identity. In one study, Lubbe found that the children of lesbian
parents were aware of their non-standard familial identity and its
impact on society. These children were aware that the reactions
from strangers ranged from acceptance and apathy to outright
hostility. Taking this idea further, Tasker and Patterson argue
that disclosure is an important consideration of lesbian parents.
In deciding when and to whom they will disclose, lesbian parents
also needed to consider how this disclosure will impact their children. In line with Fukuyama and Ferguson, Tasker and Patterson
suggest that "different aspects of identity are salient in different
contexts for instance, at home, with extended family, in relation
to the child's school, or parental work" (11).

However, research has not really addressed how individuals position themselves through different discourses of parenthood and
sexual identity or how these positions challenge heteronormative
familial patterns. We acknowledge that the routes to parenthood
have been widely explored (see Erich, Leung and Kindle; Lev "Gay
Dads") and other factors affecting a family's cultural and social
circumstances have also been explored, in particular, issues affecting

a family's status, such as disability (D'Aoust) and race (Bowen).

The families of gay and lesbian parents take many forms (Tasker and Patterson; Patterson and Riskind). This paper offers an analysis of one account by one family. Using a journal entry as its basis, the paper offers an opportunity to see into the lives and home of one family parented by a lesbian couple. This couple has been together for six years and has four children. The family has a mix of foster-to-adopt and birth children between the ages of one and six. One of the women is an academic; the other is a stay-at-home mother. The family is located in one of Australia's capital cities and lives in a suburban area, close to schools, parks, and shopping centres. The analysis elaborates how this lesbian family challenges heteronormative modes of performing family in ways that outdo discourses of family on their own terms, with a particular focus on how the speaker in the data positions herself and is positioned in terms of queering discourses of motherhood.

QUEERING MOTHERHOOD: A THEORETICAL FRAMEWORK

As this paper examines queering motherhood, it draws extensively on several theoretical domains. The paper is broadly informed by a body of knowledge known as queer theory and in particular the term queer (Ault) and Berlant and Warner's understanding of heteronormativity. These theoretical ideas are married up, for the purpose of this study, with Butler's concept of performativity (*Gender Trouble*) and Bernstein's thinking the unthinkable. We recognize these theoretical ideas work across and sometimes between structuralist and poststructuralist ways of understanding social phenomena, but they are drawn together in tension in this paper to make it possible to think through the data by elaborating competing tensions.

As a body of knowledge, queer theory is disparate and uneven (Jagose). There is no definitive and precise way to write about what queer theory is because queer itself disrupts this notion. To queer is to disrupt heteronormativity, "to make strange, to frustrate, to counteract, to delegitimized, to camp up—heteronormative knowledges and institutions" (Sullivan 1). Berlant and Warner define heteronormativity as "the institutions, structures of understanding, and practical orientations that make heterosexuality seem not only coherent ... but also privileged" (548). Heteronormativity makes it possible to think about heterosexuality as normal and unquestionable and makes other ways of doing sexuality unthinkable. Most importantly, heterosexuality is so normalized as to be unmentionable, hence the imperative to "come out" (i.e. disclose) as lesbian, for instance. This normalization is produced by the unspoken, unquestioned normalcy of heterosexuality: there is no imperative to "come out" as heterosexual because heterosexuality is imbued with an implicit "sense of rightness" (Berlant and Warner 548); it is so normal that it needs no mention. Thus, to queer in this paper denotes "proclivities, practices, or sympathies [that] defy the strictures of the dominant [heteronormative] sex/gender/ sexual identity system" (Ault 322).

Butler's (*Gender Trouble*) account of gender queers heternormativity because it is grounded in notions of performativity. Butler suggests the gendered self is fabricated, something which is "manufactured and sustained through corporeal signs and other discursive means" (*Gender Trouble* 136). For Butler, gender is "*a corporeal style*, an 'act' as it were, which is both intentional and performative, where '*performative*' suggests a dramatic and contingent construction of meaning" (139, original italics). The performance of gender occurs within what Butler calls the heterosexual matrix. It is not possible to stand outside performing gender; "it is the *effect* of a regulatory regime of gender differences in which genders are divided and hierarchized *under constraint*" (Butler, "Critically Queer" 22, original italics). Within a heterosexual matrix, people are compelled to perform gender in ways that align with heterosexuality. Gender becomes a repetitive, reiterative performance of what it means to be heterosexual, as a hierarchized, privileged position in western culture. It is expected that femininity is performed by women in accordance with heterosexual norms (and therefore in relation to having relationships with males). This "cannot be thrown off at will" ("Critically Queen" 23), hence the marginalization of those who perform gender in ways that transgress expectations of heterosexuality.

We have linked the work of Butler (*Gender Trouble*) on gender as a performance with the work of Bernstein. Bernstein argues that there are two classes of knowledge, the thinkable and the unthinkable or the mundane and the esoteric. His work draws extensively on Durkheim (Moore and Muller) in that all societies distinguish between sacred or esoteric knowledge on the one hand and the mundane or profane knowledge on the other. Esoteric knowledge is sacred because it was traditionally associated with the church; it is concerned with theoretical or abstracted knowledge and the ability to make new knowables. The other, profane knowledge, was defined by Bernstein as "knowledge of the other ... of how it is (the knowledge of the possible)" (157). Religion was previously associated with the knowledge types we now associate with academic or theoretical learning because, as Wheelahan argues, this knowledge allows individuals to project beyond the present into an as yet unknown future or alternative world. Thus, it is proposed that the ability to promote a new familial structure, and live within that, is associated with esoteric knowledge.

Bernstein states that "the line between these two classes of knowledge/practices is relative to any given period, and that the principles generating both classes are also relative" (181). He also argues that "in small-scale, non-literate societies ... the division between the 'thinkable' and the 'unthinkable' ... was affected by the religious system, its agents and their practices" (181). However, in industrialised societies such as modern Australia/US/UK, the division is governed rather differently, although, Bernstein argues, it is similar in the sense that it establishes an order. He argues that power is distributed with the ability to think the unthinkable and that those who have access to the ability to think the unthinkable have differentiated access to power, to knowledge, and to control over themselves and their societies. They are the powerful in our society.

While this thinking the unthinkable referred, in Bernstein's work, to industrialized, "school" knowledge, this paper argues that the problems many lesbian and gay couples with families face is that they disrupt the established order and force a delegitimation of heteronormative familial structures. In effect, these families upset the traditional mum + dad + children structure associated with the nuclear family. While much of the research into lesbian and gay families has already troubled this assumption, it does so through a lens of white privilege. In addition, as Lev argues, "for LGBT parents there is the added pressure to raise heterosexual and gender-conforming children, or risk familial and societal condemnation that their 'lifestyle' created or encouraged these behaviors" ("A Review" 285-6). Thus, heteronormativity can be seen to invade many areas of their lives. It is this emphasis on the normative discourse of family that suggests that lesbian mothers think the unthinkable in a sense that they are working within a space that regulates "the realization of that potential, in the interests of the social ordering it creates, maintains and legitimates" (Bernstein 182). For Bernstein, it is this potential that is concerned with the production of discourse, rather than the reproduction of discourse.

DATA ANALYSIS

The text will be analysed using Critical Discourse Analysis (CDA). CDA is a method that examines the role of discourse in social practice (Diriker). It attempts to make visible power relationships that are frequently hidden and is useful to analyse how normative discourses are challenged. CDA does not have a specific direction of research nor a single theoretical framework. As a result, it can be useful as an interpretive framework (see van Dijk; Fairclough and Wodak), which, in the case of this paper, is applied to analyse the narrative in a journal entry.

The approach to CDA that has been taken by this paper is the Discourse Historical Approach (DHA). The approach examines discourses that construct inclusion and exclusion, difference and sameness for different groups (Wodak, "Critical"). Because of its emphasis on difference and sameness and inclusion and exclusion, it is useful for this narrative text to explore how difference and inclusion operate in queer families. It applies multiple theories and methods to practical problems by examining the "relation-ships between various 'symptoms'" (Wodak, "Friend of Foe" 64). Symptoms are defined as the evidence of discourse in social practice and are seen in the context of the discursive event, usually a linguistic utterance (Reisigl and Wodak). In the DHA, symptoms are the first stage of analysis.

The Wodak ("Critical") model of the Discourse Historical Approach has been adapted by this paper and an emphasis on argumentation strategies and we-you discourses have been added. There are four tools traditionally associated with linguistic analysis using the Wodak model: perspectivisation, or the speaker's perspective; self-representation strategies, which position the speaker positively; argumentation; and intensification and mitigation strategies. The latter refers to the strategies the speaker uses to mitigate the other or intensify their status. In addition to the four linguistic analysis tools proposed in Wodak's model of the DHA, Reisigl and Wodak have proposed that the argumentation strategy tool could be used to further examine the argumentation strategies speakers use. Argumentation strategies make it possible to analyse: (a) the degree of association a speaker has with their argument; (b) the complexity of the argument that the speaker uses; and (c) the speaker's ability to demonstrate their point of view using argumentation (Titscher et al.; Wodak, "Critical"; Reisigl and Wodak).

The *three dimension analytic apparatus* was an earlier tool of the Discourse Historical Approach (Titscher et al.). This study has used the three dimension analytic apparatus because the apparatus explores strategies that construct we-you discourses. Matouschek, Wodak and Januschek developed the three dimension analytic apparatus to examine the strategies that speakers use to define those who belong and those who do not through an analysis of the construction of a *we-you discourse* (Matouschek, Wodak and Januschek; Titscher et al.).

In this study, we traced the we-you discourse through the linguistic analysis of the argumentation strategies. A representation of the model we used can be seen in Figure 1, below. In this model, we have adapted Wodak's model in her 2006 work, "The Discourse Historical Approach."

DATA

A journal reflection was chosen by one lesbian parent for analysis in this chapter. This reflection centres on her life as a parent, particularly that of a busy working parent:

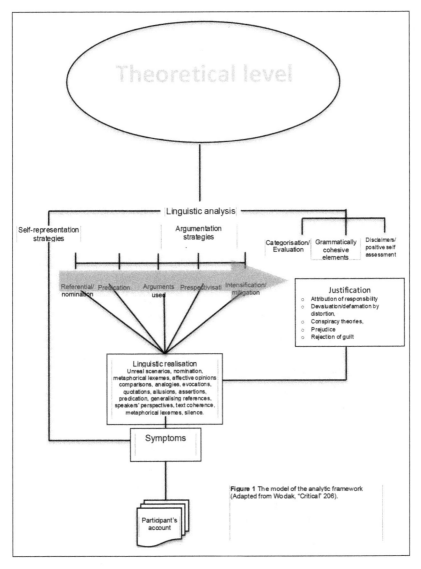

Figure 1 The model of the analytic framework (Adapted from Wodak, "Critical" 206).

I started to reflect on [my experience of motherhood] while I was away from my family, on an international business trip. My four children were home with their other mother, the stay-at-home parent, while I worked away from them for two weeks. It wasn't the first time I left them, and it certainly won't be the last, either.

"I don't know how you do it," women say. "I couldn't leave my children." I often wonder if they say this to fathers.

The struggle with them understanding it is because I am female. Our situation confuses them more because I was the mother that got pregnant and gave birth. (We have a mixture of birth and adopted children).

When we planned our family, we agreed that I would be the one to do the fertility treatment, to get pregnant, but she was present beside me the whole time. She held my hand during the process; she was holding my hand during the birth. I had some romantic notion about the big belly (it was simply awful, actually!) and she was keen to be mum, but not get pregnant herself. I never wanted to be a stay-at-home mum, and it worked well for us, with a large family, that she did. It was the ideal situation—win, win!

The challenge for many is how to position us. People want to put us into heteronormative titles, probably because of our SAHM/ Working parent dichotomy. If we both worked part-time and parented, or both worked full-time, perhaps people would be less eager to try to categorise us. We acknowledge that we've taken on traditional roles of the stay-at-home parent and the provider and this automatically results in a female/male comparison. Had I not given birth, and if I was not feminine presenting, people would say, "She's like a dad." Had my partner given birth and if she was more feminine presenting, people would say, "She's clearly the mum." As it is, they're confused. Like stay-at-home fathers, we don't fit the common mold of parenting. Parenting is being redefined, but it's not for any political reason. It's just what works for families: our circumstances and our preferences.

For us, labels are unnecessary. We are both mothers, though I find I tend to call myself "parent" rather than "mother." The children call me Mama. My partner, on the other hand, identifies strongly with the term Mum.

I'm busy, but I'm involved—I drive my children to school, I volunteer on the School Committee, I teach them to read, I go to meetings with their teachers, I bake for their lunches, I know their friends' parents. Perhaps if I was a father, people would say, "What a great dad—to be so busy

and still so involved." As a mother, however, people pity
me for travelling away. They shake their heads and they
say, "I don't know how you do it," not with admiration,
but with confusion. Labels shouldn't matter, but they do.

To begin the analysis, the symptoms of discourse were first identified. It is proposed that there are five symptoms in this account.
The first deals with the work/life balance question. Examples
include the statement "I worked away for two weeks." The second symptom is the concern the speaker has for the ways people,
especially women, discuss her situation. For example, the speaker
states, "Women say, 'I couldn't leave my children.' I often wonder
if they say this to fathers." The third symptom is familial solidarity
and includes the statement, "We planned our family, we agreed."
The fourth symptom deals with family roles, for example, "Like
stay-at-home fathers, we don't fit the common mold of parenting."
Finally, the fifth symptom deals with what the speaker does in the
family, such as "drive my children to school, I volunteer on the
School Committee, I teach them to read, I go to meetings with their
teachers, I bake for their lunches, I know their friends' parents."
These all suggest that the speaker is concerned about both the
ways that she is perceived in the wider community as well as what
it means to be a mother who gave birth but does not stay at home.
She is also aware of how her situation challenges the traditional
heteronormative roles of mother and father and family. These
represent self-representation strategies in that they allow her to
represent herself as a mother/primary breadwinner. It involves her
positioning herself through the discourse of both mother and worker.
In addition, she justifies the positive self-assessment using a rejection of guilt. The symptoms here that can be seen to demonstrate
this are those associated with the roles she plays in the family.
In addition, the symptom that deals with the way others see her
was significant. She identifies how they say things to her but she
wonders whether they say the same to fathers.
The argumentation strategies are concerned with arguments
used. Arguments are built on several linguistic devices including
affective opinions, such as the symptom that deals with the ways
others see her; she justifies her situation by questioning the different

expectations of mothers and fathers. Another linguistic device is analogy; the narrative is composed of several analogies. These two devices, arguments and analogy, build the speaker's perspective on her situation and also allow her to form an argument about her role in the family. Clearly, she is a loving mother who cares deeply for her children but, just like an increasing number of heterosexual women whose partners stay home, she is able to earn more money and enjoys her career, so she goes to work.

Interestingly, she notes the way she is involved: "I drive my children to school, I volunteer on the School Committee, I teach them to read, I go to meetings with their teachers, I bake for their lunches, I know their friends' parents." Although there is no doubt there are other ways she is involved, this list emphasizes her involvement in school and education. Perhaps this makes sense, given she is an academic. However, it is interesting that she is creating a culture around her children's school identity, more so than the at-home activities. It could be because her partner is taking care of most of the at-home activities, so the school side allows her a role. Similarly, she prefers to call herself "parent" rather than "mother," another aspect of identity revealed within the quote. She does not explain why. Perhaps this name is chosen because her partner clearly identifies as "mum" and despite her children having two mums, she can clearly separate her role from that of her partner. Alternatively it may be an aspect of identity, based on gender perceptions. Despite presenting herself as feminine, the term "mother" may have gender-based implications.

DISCUSSION

The linguistic devices suggest a we-you discourse has been constructed. The speaker clearly feels that she is positioned through a you-discourse to the majority of parents' we-discourse. While there might be multiple you or we discourses, there is only one we-you discourse. Thus, while there may be multiple constructions of family, this account constructs her family as separate but equal. The linguistic devices suggest that she understands she is not like the majority of parents, and that her family is not like the majority of her children's friends' families. However, they are comfortable and have organized their roles and this is the familial structure that suits them. There is a power in the you-discourse position because it allows the speaker to not only justify her different familial structure but also be comfortable in a situation and an environment that is the best for her family.

The we-you discourse speaks to specific aspects of the theory. The narrative suggests the speaker queers heteronormativity because she does not perform gender in ways that align with heterosexual expectations. She is, as Butler argues, performing her gender in a way that is different to the other mothers. While the speaker was the mother who gave birth to the birth children, she is not the stay-at-home parent. This element of her parenting suggests that the "corporeal signs and other discursive means" (Butler, *Gender Trouble* 136) this family uses to create and construct its family is occurring within the heterosexual matrix. The effect of the regulatory regime of gender differences is troubling for the observers, as the participant says in her account: "The challenge for many is how to position us." These troubling moments highlight the heterosexual matrix at work where instances of dissonance occur in gendered expectations and performances. Dissonance is signalled in almost undetectable behaviours and gestures such as using the word "parent" rather than "mother."

Challenging normative discourses of parenting, working outside a traditional parental discourse, is a further aspect of the construction of the we-you discourse. She appears to construct a we-you discourse because, as the participant says, "they're confused. Like stay-at-home fathers, we don't fit the common mold of parenting." It may be that she is performing a you- to a we-discourse of heteronormativity. It is clear there is no outside of being heterosexual or performing femininity as woman who wants to be at home with her children ("I don't know how you do it. ... I couldn't leave my children"). The speaker is being positioned in relation to a majority of parents' we-discourse—we are the heterosexual norm and you queer that norm in how you "defy the strictures" (Ault 322) of dominant sexed and gendered discourses about what makes a proper mother.

In addition, the speaker's account suggests a thinking of the unthinkable. The account suggests that, in some of the interactions with which the speaker is involved, hers is the first non-heterosexual family that others have encountered. While there are an increasing number of lesbian families (Breshears), the account suggests that this is the first time many commenters have encountered this structure. There are several anecdotes in the account, for example, "'I don't know how you do it,' women say. 'I couldn't leave my children.' I often wonder if they say this to fathers. The struggle with them understanding it is because I am female."

Thus, this family presents an unthinkable, a sacred, to these women. The family is a new knowable to these women, while, at the same time, a new order. This new order challenges the traditional nuclear family order and suggests, in line with Bernstein, that this is a powerful family precisely because it provides an identity position for this family that sits comfortably with their identity.

Further, it is this power that challenges the normative, heterosexual family structure. It also realizes a potential "in the interests of the social ordering it creates, maintains and legitimates" (Bernstein 182). It challenges the women who observe this family to consider, in many ways, the normative discourses they have adopted and, in some cases, through which they are encouraged to position themselves. However, it is this challenge that allows lesbian mothers to produce, rather than reproduce, non-normative discourses of family—discourses of family that queer heteronormativity. It appears from this account, and the theoretical discussion that follows it, that this family has an enormous freedom from the oppressive expectations of heteronormative parenting. Further to this, they perform family in ways that outdo heteronormativity on its own terms. They represent a visible, spectacular example of how to do parenting in ways that defy the boundaries of heterosexual, gendered motherhood and make malleable the boundaries between thinkable and unthinkable families. They are a powerful example to which other mothers, and potential mothers, who queer the performance of family might observe and be inspired by.

CONCLUSIONS

Although a growing body of research has examined lesbian and gay family forms and the diversity therein, researchers have tended to overlook how the parents themselves are positioned by, or are positioned within, discourses of family and parenting. This paper has analysed an account of one family from the perspective of a lesbian parent's journal narrative. The analysis demonstrates the tensions that come with performing parenthood, and specifically motherhood, in certain ways that transgress heteronormative expectations. Performing feminine gender as a lesbian mother who has a career not only disrupts the boundaries of heterosexuality but also queers how we expect mothers to do gender in the heterosexual matrix. This lesbian mother is always already unthinkable within and between these heteronormative discourses.

With the ever-growing interest in amassing stories and statistics about lesbian and gay family forms and lives, researchers can sometimes neglect what can be learned from the minutiae in texts written by these parents. This paper has sought to address this gap grounded in the notion that if we are ever to outdo heteronormativity on its own terms, we need to further examine how lesbian and gay parents position themselves within these sometimes oppressive discourses of family. Queer has the disruptive potential to make thinkable and possible the fracturing of heteronormative expectations because "queer marks a suspension of identity as something fixed, coherent and natural" (Jagose 98). The account of a lesbian family in this paper suspends motherhood, feminine gender, and parenthood as fixed, coherent, natural "things." Embracing the power of queering these discourses, to make them bend and stretch, may in fact make them thinkable in terms of how they might yield and fall away.

WORKS CITED

Ault, Amber. "The Dilemma of Identity: Bi Women's Negotiations." *Queer Theory/Sociology*. Ed. Steven Seidman. Cambridge: Blackwell Publishers, 1996. 311-329. Print.

Berlant, Lauren and Michael Warner. "Sex in Public." *Critical Inquiry* 24.2 (1998): 547-566. Print.

Bernstein, Basil. *Class, Codes and Control*. Volume 4. London: RKP, 1990. Print.

Bowen, A. "Another View of Lesbians Choosing Children." *Lesbian Parenting: Living with Pride and Prejudice*. Ed. Katherine Arnot. Charlottetown, PEI: Gynergy Books, 1995. 253-264. Print.

Breshears, Diana. "Understanding Communication between Lesbian Parents and their Children Regarding Outsider Discourse about Family Identity." *Journal of GLBT Family Studies* 7.3 (2011): 264-284. Print.

Butler, Judith. "Critically Queer." *The Routledge Queer Studies Reader*. Eds. Donald E. Hall and Annamarie Jagose. London: Routledge, 2013. 18-31. Print.

Butler, Judith. *Gender Trouble: Feminism and the Subversion of Identity*. New York: Routledge, 1990. Print.

D'Aoust, Vicky. "Non-Existent & Struggling For Identity." *Disabled Mothers: Stories and Scholarship by and about Mothers with Disabilities*. Eds. Gloria Flax and Dena Taylor. Toronto, Canada: Demeter Press, 1995. 276-296. Print.

Diriker, Ebru. *De-/re-contextualizing Conference Interpreting: Interpreters in the Ivory Tower?* Amsterdam: John Benjamins Publishing Company, 2004. Print.

Erich, Stephen, Patrick Leung, Peter Kindle. "A Comparative Analysis of Adoptive Family Functioning with Gay, Lesbian and Heterosexual Parents and their Children." *Journal of GLBT Family Studies* 1 (2005): 43-60. Print.

Fairclough, Norman and Ruth Wodak. "Critical Discourse Analysis." *Discourse As Social Interaction*. Ed. Teun van Dijk. Thousand Oaks, CA: Sage, 1997. 258-284. Print.

Fukuyama, Mary and Angela D. Ferguson. "Lesbian, Gay, and Bisexual People of Color: Understanding Cultural Complexity and Multiple Oppressions." *Handbook of Counseling and Psychotherapy with Lesbian, Gay, and Bisexual Clients*. Eds. R.M. Perez, K.A. DeBord, K.J. Bieschke. Washington, DC: American Psychological Association, 2000. 107-131. Print.

Jagose, Annamarie. *Queer Theory: An Introduction*. New York: New York University Press, 1996. Print.

Lev, Arlene Istar. "Gay Dads: Choosing Surrogacy." *The British Psychological Society Lesbian and Gay Review* 7(2006): 72-76. Print.

Lev, Arlene Istar. "A Review of 'Gay and Lesbian Parents and

Their Children: Research on the Family Life Cycle; Who's Your Daddy? And Other Writings on Queer Parenting; Becoming Parent: Lesbians, Gay Men, and Family.'" *Journal of GLBT Family Studies* 6.3 (2010): 341-348. Print.

Lubbe, Carien. "The Experiences of Children Growing Up in Lesbian-Headed Families in South Africa." *Journal of GLBT Family Studies* 4 (2008): 325–359. Print.

Matouschek, Bernd, Ruth Wodak, Franz Januschek. *"Notwendige Maßnahmen gegen Fremde?": Genese und Formen von rassistischen Diskursen der Differenz*. Wien, Austria: Passagen, 1995. Print.

Moore, Rob and Johan Muller. "The Growth of Knowledge and the Discursive Gap." *British Journal of Sociology of Education* 23.4 (2002): 627-637. Print.

Morris, Jessica, F., Kimberley F. Balsam, Esther D. Rothblum. "Lesbian and Bisexual Mothers and Nonmothers: Demographics and the Coming-Out Process." *Journal of Family Psychology* 16 (2002): 144–156. Print.

Patterson, Charlotte J. and Rachel G Riskind. "To Be a Parent: Issues in Family Formation among Gay and Lesbian Adults." *Journal of GLBT Family Studies* 6.3 (2010): 326-340. Web. 16 March 2013.

Reisigl, Martin and Ruth Wodak. "The Discourse-Historical Approach (DHA)." *Methods of Critical Discourse Analysis*. 2nd ed. Eds. Ruth Wodak and Michael Meyer. Thousand Oaks, CA: Sage, 2009. 87-121. Print.

Sullivan, Nikki. *A Critical Introduction to Queer Theory*. Armadale, Vic: Circa Books, 2003. Print.

Tasker, Fiona, and Charlotte J. Patterson. "Research on Gay and Lesbian Parenting: Retrospect and Prospect." *Journal of GLBT Family Studies* 3.2 (2007): 9-34. Print.

Titscher, Stephan, Michael Meyer, Ruth Wodak, Eva Vetter. *Methods of Text and Discourse Analysis*. Thousand Oaks, CA: Sage, 2000. Print.

van Dijk, Teun. "Multidisciplinary CDA: A Plea for Diversity." *Methods of Critical Discourse Analysis*. Eds. Ruth Wodak and Michael Meyer. London: Sage, 2001. 95-120. Print.

Wheelahan, Leesa. "Competency-Based Training, Powerful Knowledge and the Working Class." *Social Realism, Knowledge and the Sociology of Education: Coalitions of the Mind.* Eds. Karl Maton and Rob Moore. London: Continuum International Publishing Group, 2010. 93-109. Print.

Wodak, Ruth. "Critical Discourse Analysis." *Qualitative Research Practice.* Eds. Clive Searle, Giampietro Gobo, Jaber Gubrium, David Silverman. London, UK: Sage, 2004. 197-213. Print.

Wodak, Ruth. "The Discourse Historical Approach." *Methods of Critical Discourse Analysis.* Eds. Ruth Wodak and Michael Meyer. Thousand Oaks, CA: Sage, 2001. 63-94. Print.

Wodak, Ruth. "Friend or Foe: The Defamation or Legitimate and Necessary Criticism? Reflections on Recent Political Discourse in Austria." *Language and Communication* 22.4 (2002): 495-517. Print.

BETTY ANN MARTIN

Go the Fuck to Sleep Prince George?

Juxtaposing Cultural Representations of Motherhood and Exploring the Politics of Authenticity

NOTED ANTHROPOLOGIST CLIFFORD GEERTZ defines culture as "the ensemble of stories we tell ourselves about ourselves" (448). In keeping with this theory, Fred Inglis suggests that identity is formed through a process whereby we observe and "inhabit the narratives of how to live" available within a given culture ("Culture and Sentiment" 2). Such narratives generally reflect the dominant discourse and accepted range of meanings in relation to socially defined roles. In terms of the negotiated meaning of motherhood, however, there is a growing tension between competing narratives and representations that highlight the juxtaposition between culturally constructed fantasies of maternal perfection and the lived experience of mothering.

The idealization of motherhood and the supposedly "natural" and intuitive quality of maternal instinct are perpetuated and commodified by the conflation of celebrity, maternity, and brand cultures, which together capitalize on a seductive combination of "knowability with distance" (Inglis, *History of Celebrity* 11) to sell popularized images of maternal eminence. A litany of celebrities, such as Beyoncé, Jessica Alba, and Angelina Jolie, have translated their motherhood into a profitable brand consistent with the ideology of the "new momism," (Douglas & Michaels 20) which celebrates empowerment through maternity while simultaneously reinforcing an idealized and unattainable image of "mother." More than these celebrities, however, Kate Middleton's foray into motherhood has prompted a following by women who believe that by investing in her "royal" brand of maternal identity they position themselves as "a little more attractive and glamorous" (de Botton). It is estimated that the commodification of Kate's maternity garnered £247 million for the UK economy after George's birth, and it is projected that it will yield £150 million in the weeks following the birth of Princess Charlotte ("It's a Girl!"). Everything from commemorative biscuits to royal totes, as well as the host of consumables that Kate deems worthy of her royal progeny, are fodder for the mommy-making capitalist machine. However, in spite of women's attempts to reproduce and, thereby, claim Kate's particular brand of mothering as their own, the dominant cultural narrative of maternal flawlessness embodied by Kate is founded on spurious claims to "knowability" and authenticity that obscure evidence of the artifice and inaccessibility of such representations. In this manner, fantasy and cultural misdirection become powerful influences in the formation of maternal identity while simultaneously engendering feelings of inadequacy as women come to know a parenting reality that is drastically different from the dominant fiction perpetuated by popular culture.

In stark juxtaposition to Kate's royal brand of maternity, there are emergent countercultural representations that document the reality of birth and motherhood and seek to deconstruct the myth of the "natural" mother, her complete fulfillment, and infallibility. So, in spite of the fact that culture's contemporary fascination with celebrity motherhood has found a locus in the image of Kate Middleton, as evidenced by "the Kate effect" ("Kate Middleton Causes"), I would argue that the trend in maternal representation is toward the proliferation of a growing countercultural voice that resonates with the authenticity of women's lived experience. While the dominant culture and its available discourses are a conduit for identification and the production of meaning in a mother's interpretation of the narrative of her own maternal performance, cultural inscriptions and expectations are meaningfully challenged by alternative representations of maternity that liberate women to freely negotiate the meaning of mothering and inhabit the narrative embodied by their own experience.

After the birth of a child, women re-story themselves in relation to their maternal role and inevitably look to culture for messages that will inform the transformation of their identity. For Giroux, "struggles over popular culture ... represent a different but no less important site of politics. For it is precisely on the terrain of culture that identities are produced, values learned, histories legitimated, and knowledge appropriated" (187). Giroux goes on to explain that culture is the medium through which the process of assuming collective and individual identities is initiated and through which we come to "understand and narrate the self in relation to others" (188). Similarly, Stuart Hall suggests that we decode cultural messages toward an understanding of identity ("Encoding/ Decoding" 130). These messages generally reflect the dominant hegemonic discourse; however, a negotiation of their meaning is often initiated by the realization that our experience, or story, is somehow different from the prevailing cultural narrative. According to Judith Butler, identity (especially as it pertains to gender) is not "natural" or fixed, but perpetually re-presented and performed and in accordance with cultural imperatives (140). The subversion of prescribed boundaries occurs when alternative experience finds expression, and expression finds power through replication in discourse. The performance of maternal identity, therefore, is liberated from the oppressiveness of cultural inscriptions through the emergence of authentic representations of parenting within popular culture. By generating discourse around previous sites of silence and taboo, diverse experiences and realities are explored which find resonance with women seeking a frame of reference for the meaning of their own experience. This process enables a re-signification of motherhood beyond the idolization encouraged by constructed images of celebrity mothers like Kate Middleton. By embracing stories of imperfection and alterity, women transgress the cultural myths of motherhood and find community with other women through acts of re-signification whereby the socially constructed maternal pedestal, and its accompanying quest for perfection, may potentially be abandoned.

At stake in the tension between competing representations of motherhood is women's sense of competence and feelings of adequacy in relation to their maternal role. Jennifer Senior alludes to the complexity of negotiated meanings of parenting in the introduction to *All Joy and No Fun: The Paradox of Modern Parenting* (2014): "There's the parenting life of our fantasies, and there's the parenting life of our banal, on-the-ground realities" (1). Alternative discourse around parenting challenges culturally informed fantasies and normalizes common parental struggles. Though identity, as Butler argues, is performed in response to available meanings and cultural dictates, performance resonates with truth when grounded in narratives of personal experience that represent the reality of motherhood. Through recourse to a politics of truth in storytelling, Erma Bombeck's *Motherhood: The Second Oldest Profession* (1984), Nancy White's album *Momnipotent* (1991), and more recently Adam Mansbach's book *Go the Fuck to Sleep* (2011) as well as the website www.theshapeofamother.com (2007) have become sites of resistance to the prevailing cultural supposition that parents are perfect beings, engaged in an endlessly gratifying task. Ultimately, culturally fuelled maternal fantasies that incite a drive to perfectionism and engender a "disembodied" knowledge (Shields 184) of motherhood are challenged by the growing prevalence of authentic representations of parenting that validate personal experience as an "expert text" (Shields 180) and credible narrative worth inhabiting in the quest for the meaning of motherhood.

Before the advent of Kate Middleton and the current fascination with consumable representations of celebrity motherhood, writers like Erma Bombeck were already sensing a need for an alternative discourse around the lived experience of mothers. In *Motherhood: The Second Oldest Profession*, Bombeck's challenge to the prevailing cultural narrative of maternity resonated with women whose experiences, like hers, had been vastly different from the images of maternal perfection that dominated the popular culture mainstream. The text's open-hearted honesty about the less glamorous aspects of motherhood found such a large and embracing audience that it spent an entire year in the number one spot on the *New York Times* best-selling non-fiction list in 1984 (McDowell). In *Motherhood*, Bombeck satirizes the sitcom mothers of the 1950s and '60s as angels of the house who never seemed to lose their patience or their figure:

> They never lost their temper [or] gained weight. ... Their collective virtue was patience. There was no situation

too traumatic for them to cure with milk and cookies, no
problem that could not be resolved in twenty-four minutes,
plus four minutes for commercials and two minutes for
theme and credits. (9)

Bombeck's humour is rooted in the disjunction between cultural
representations of maternal flawlessness and the imperfect truth
of her own experience. She concedes that real work of birth and
motherhood had been such a well-kept cultural secret that for a long
time she was "afraid to laugh at the contrast, for fear no one else
would" (4). Overall, the text is a humorous treatise on the humanness
of the maternal experience that features multiple representations
of motherhood through individualized narratives that offer a wide
range of possibilities for identification and meaning. The form is
consistent with Bombeck's assertion that "motherhood is not a
one-size fits-all, a mold that is all-encompassing and means the
same thing to all people" (4). Though we may presume motherhood
to be synonymous with the ideals of devotion, personal sacrifice,
and perfection, she cautions that not all mothers "give standing
ovations to bowel movements" (4). By satirizing the dominant
cultural standard, Bombeck breaks the silence concerning the often
banal existence of mothers, applauds and normalizes imperfection,
and paves the way for a growing number of contemporary popular
culture representations that liberate the parental identity from its
limitations through recourse to an alternative discourse around
parenting grounded in authentic experience.

Bombeck's work highlights popular culture's influential role in
the social construction of motherhood and women's on-going negotiation of maternal identity and, therefore, prefigures women's
contemporary vulnerability to commodified representations of maternity generated by the "celebrity-industrial complex" (Podnieks
88). The myth of perfection, embodied by the June Cleavers and
Carol Bradys of the '50s and '60s, generated an intense admiration
and idolization that has been replicated in relation to celebrity
moms of the current generation. For example, the meaning of Kate
Middleton's pregnancy, birth, and early experience of motherhood
have been heavily constructed by the media and carefully decoded
by women seeking identification with a maternal image that is

relatable, yet exclusive. *Hello!* magazine reports that "no birth in history has been as anticipated as baby Prince George's" ("It's a Boy!" 3) and, by implication, no mother's actions scrutinized more closely than those of the Duchess of Cambridge. During pregnancy, Kate was celebrated as "brilliant, beautiful, and blooming" ("Kate's Pregnancy Parade" 71) at the center of a "picture-perfect parade of maternity fashions" ("KPP" 68). This alliterative testament to Kate's flawless prenatal appearance manufactures an alluring fantasy, a narrative women are tempted to inhabit; yet, this representation operates in sharp contrast to women's lived experience of the less than blissful aspects of pregnancy.

In reality, pregnancy is a strenuous time for many women, both physically and emotionally. The musical compilation *Momnipotent* by Nancy White features alternative representations that expose and validate the often unspoken facets of the maternal experience. Her song "It's So Chic to be Pregnant at Christmas" openly and humorously explores the litany of physical complaints that often accompanies late pregnancy:

> No, I enjoy being pregnant at Christmas/ Though my identity is draining away.... / And I may suffer from gravid senilis-/ (and heartburn and nausea and charleyhorses/ and overwhelming fatigue and frequent/ micturition and vari-cose veins and swollen/ankles and shortness ... of breath and That Tired/ Achy Feeling in the Groin)-/ But I won't be alone on New Year's Eve! (White, "It's So Chic")

While the humour is self-deprecating, the message is comforting in its honest proclamation: pregnancy can be very uncomfortable and not altogether glamorous. White's account of the prenatal body in disrepair offers hope to women whose own experience of pregnancy falls short of the cultural fantasy of blissful elegance, exemplified by celebrities like Kate Middleton. Kate's combined style and independence, demonstrated by her rejection of the "frumpy frocks and tent-like smocks beloved of maternity brands of the past" ("KPP" 71), generate a vicarious empowerment for countless women who perform their maternal role through identi-fication with her image; however, it is ultimately the realization of the degree to which royalty renders her distant that women begin to feel apprehensive about their ability to close the gap between the reality of their own experience and the iconic quality of Kate's maternal brand.

Commodified representations of stylized maternity, endorsed by celebrity culture, allow women to indulge fantasies of empowerment through vicarious status. In truth, we look to celebrities to "perform our significant actions for us" (Inglis *History of Celebrity* 231) in much the same way that theatre functions to mirror and cathect emotional energy. The cult of celebrity invites a kind of maternal mentorship whereby new mothers perform their identity as a reproduction of the character and beliefs particular to a given celebrity and confirm this process of identification through conspicuous consumption. As Allison Clarke argues, "the process of 'becoming a mother' involves simultaneity of materiality and social conceptualization" (56) and it is ultimately through consumption that women "make their babies and themselves as mothers" (59). However, by watching Kate's maternal performance unfold "perfectly" on the world stage, women become invested in misleading assumptions about the meaning of their own maternal performance and identity.

Kate's flawlessness has been marketed in popular culture, to the point of saturation, with reference to everything from her relationship to her style, to the supposed predestination of her maternal success. Kate and William are referred to as the "perfect match" ("Fairytale" 36) and hers as the "picture-perfect pregnancy" ("KPP" 72). Kate is also described as an exemplary child, owing to her mother's superlative parenting: "If Catherine was the perfect baby, it's because Carole was an ideal mom" ("Kate's Baby Days" 63). In other words, Kate's success as a mother is constructed as prefigured in the image of Carole, who is said to be the "perfect maternal blueprint" (Wade and Robey 93). The image of Kate's maternal perfection has been reified and marketed as an ideal to which women are invited to aspire through brand loyalty. According to Angela McRobbie, celebrity culture advances the notion that the only avenue to "respectable" motherhood involves a project of self-actualization that denies subjectivity in favour of "self-perfectability" through consumption. However, the implied failure of such an enterprise engenders feelings of inadequacy and anxiety that ultimately serve the capitalist agenda to sabotage authenticity by persuading women to indulge fantasies of maternal renown through a futile struggle to reproduce unattainable representations of maternity.

Within the realm of popular culture, the dominant narrative of idealized maternal perfection is often aligned with the essentialist presumption of an innate maternal instinct. Indeed, it is noted that Carole "took to motherhood like a duck to water" ("KBD" 64) and that "her children were always the neatest, cleanest students at their school with well-brushed hair and shiny shoes" (Wade 79). Such anecdotal evidence supports the cultural construct that Kate's "natural" predisposition to mother is the product of a matrilineal endowment. The narrative of Kate's maternal aptitude is further reinforced by the comment that "Kate has taken to motherhood much as she did to royal life, with ease and a smile" (Cupido 49). The attempt to market Kate's supposedly predetermined, intuitive ability to mother supports the essentialist fallacy that women have an innate maternal competence and that maternal proficiency is evidence of a perfected femininity. This fallacy is challenged by feminist theorists, including Simone de Beauvoir who argues in *The Second Sex* that "one is not born, but rather becomes [a] woman" (283). In the same way, one is not born, or naturally inclined, to mother, but becomes a mother through a complex social process of participant observation, imitation, and consumption, which reflects careful attention to the stories our culture tells us about the meaning of motherhood. However, the danger of the narrative of Kate's perfection and "natural" affinity for motherhood is that women's acceptance of this fabrication precludes a recognition of the value of individual experience as a credible, "expert text" (Shields 180) and liberatory source of meaning in a woman's personal quest to understand what it means to be a mother.

The narrative manufactured to sell Kate's maternal brand is a pseudo-heroic epic in which she is portrayed as a glamorous, yet down-to-earth, royal heroine whose "happily ever after" is a function of cutting-edge individualism, informed by the power of maternal intuition. In popular cultural, this image is reinforced in the celebration of Kate for "pioneering a whole new approach to 'bump chic'" ("KPP" 71). She is said to have "thrown away the rule book and revolutionized pregnancy fashion" ("KPP" 71). Kate's revolutionary status extends beyond style to her tendency to break with royal tradition, as suggested by the fact that she intends to be "a hands-on mom with help from minimal staff" ("Royal Nursery" 51). Similarly, in Kate's pursuit of a "normal" upbringing for Prince George, she is said to be determined "to break new ground" by "combining her respect for royal tradition with the influence of her own upbringing" ("Royal Nursery" 51). The media's construction of Kate as a deferential yet fashionable rebel with a trailblazing spirit has captured the imagination of both women and mothers worldwide who long to identify with an accessible yet radical brand of motherhood. In Kate, women glimpse the constructed image of a maternal pioneer, and it is through identification with Kate as the embodiment of the "new momism" that women seek to define their own pioneering experience of motherhood.

While Kate's role as revolutionary is attractive, equally saleable is her conventional beauty and her status as "princess mom" ("Inside Kate's Life"). It is not difficult to imagine that this dual signification is at the heart of the "Kate effect," as it speaks to a generation raised on Disney who fetishize the familiar story of the commoner turned princess, but who long for a locus of self-identity and site of imagined happiness beyond this childhood fantasy. Therefore, motherhood, embodied by Kate in the figure of a royal trend-setting heroine with a penchant for both style and grace, is presented as a natural extension of an empowered princess' love story, a narrative easily inhabited by women seeking a continuation of this fantasy in their own lives. The evolution of this fantasy is best illustrated by the recent birth of Charlotte Elizabeth Diana, whereby the "Kate effect" is reproduced and the legacy of royal femininity is renewed; the familiar narrative of the princess begins anew and Kate's branding as "flawless mom" is reinscribed. Kate's image of maternal resilience is reinforced by her appearance on the hospital steps, in full makeup and carefully coiffed, just hours after Charlotte's birth; however, her portrait-ready perfection has the power to immortalize the cultural myth of idealized motherhood.

Media coverage of Kate's transition to motherhood furthers the fantasy of an idyllic maternal experience by drawing attention to and expanding upon the pre-existing narrative arch of the "fairy-tale" storyline. *Hello!* magazine reports that "in the latest chapter of their joyous love story, the Duke and Duchess of Cambridge take on parenthood" ("Fairytale" 47). This chapter continues with the celebration of Kate's maternal prowess as confirmed in reports that "she balances royal duty with diaper duty—and makes time for her marriage" ("Inside Kate's Life"). Predictably, the media indulges reader expectation of a "happily ever after" in its account that "parenting has brought [Kate and William] more joy than they ever could have imagined" ("Fairytale" 47). Missing from this tale, however, is the truth of maternal fatigue and the many frustrations that necessarily accompany life with a newborn. This narrative has no sub-plots of disillusionment or struggle but rather reproduces a discourse of bliss and fulfillment in which Kate is said to be "enjoying every minute" ("Fairytale" 50) of motherhood. Ultimately, Kate's royal brand of ecstatic parenting reifies maternal identity through a narrative fantasy of perfection and predestined satisfaction that has the potential, through its inaccessibility, to heighten maternal insecurity regarding the disjuncture between authentic experience and culturally fabricated fairytales of motherhood.

This constructed image of Kate does not represent maternal experience grounded in reality but rather a cultivated fantasy, a kind of disembodied knowledge far removed from more authentic ways of knowing. Indeed, the perceived fissure between popular culture's idealized image of parental omnipotence and the lived experience of early motherhood has given rise to a counter-hegemonic discourse, which openly negotiates the meaning of motherhood through representations that unabashedly confront the realities of parenting. These representations document and bear witness to the truth of maternal struggle and imperfection and, subsequently, liberate mothers from cultural fantasies of parental bliss. The implications for identity are manifold. While cultural messages overwhelmingly reflect the dominant discourse, as embodied by Kate, negotiated meanings are formed in accordance with the realization that experience in the particular is removed from the dominant narrative constructed in relation to that experience (Hall, "Encoding/Decoding" 137). Hall touches on the instability of identity and meaning in general when he writes, "We should think ... of identity as a 'production,' which is never complete, always in process, and always constituted within, not outside, representation" ("Cultural Identity" 222). It follows, therefore, that representations of maternal identity inform women's negotiation of the meaning of that identity at the site of popular culture. While Judith Butler maintains that gendered identity is not innate, but performed in response to culturally imposed mandates, I would argue that the expression of identity approaches authenticity when it is meaningfully negotiated in response to the tension between social expectation and personal experience. Through this process of negotiation, then, women have the power to resist the dominant narrative of infallibility as a source of definitive meaning in the formation of maternal Selfhood. In this way, alternative representations and discourse, which celebrate diversity and validate both the reality of motherhood and the authenticity of personal experience, liberate women to embrace the less than perfect elements of their own parenting journey.

In terms of authenticity of maternal experience as explored through alternative and counter-hegemonic discourse, one need look no further than Nancy White's *Momnipotent* (subtitled "Songs for Weary Parents") for representations of personal experience that normalize the imperfections of motherhood while simultaneously inviting women to identify with a more human understanding of what it means to be a parent. In the title track "Momnipotent," White challenges the basic supposition that there is some inherent claim to absolute power or knowledge that can be made through maternal identity:

Sometimes I feel like the other mothers/ Are the real mothers,/ And me, I'm just playing a role,/ And I don't know my lines,/ And the writing is SO bad./ Sometimes I feel like the other others/ Are so organized,/ And their kids eat tofu and sleep through the night,/ While at our house the chaos is driving me mad. (1-9)

By honestly engaging the insecurity that accompanies the maternal role, White confronts the illusion that the meaning of "mom" has any relationship, in real or discursive terms, with omnipotence. Ironically, women do not feel the power of the pedestal that society has erected for mothers, but rather the insecurity generated by daunting cultural expectations. In alluding to motherhood as a "role" for which women often do not "know [their] lines," White highlights the performative aspect of maternal identity, as well as the degree to which women actively attempt to negotiate the meaning of their "role" in relation to perceived social pressure. In keeping with Butler's theory, the performance of motherhood is revealed in White's lyrics to be a process of continual renegotiation that is highly sensitive to cultural cues. In truth, women often rely on the dominant cultural discourse around mothering to inform the performance of their maternal script due to the profound insecurity generated by the excessive demands of motherhood. Media coverage of celebrity mothers, such as Kate Middleton, contributes to the social construction of the meaning of maternity by advancing a script that perpetuates the illusion of bliss and perfection. However, counter narratives, such as those highlighted in the music of Nancy White, ground the image of motherhood through the humorous admission of the unspoken insecurities and frustrations of the parenting experience.

Fundamental to any reclamation of the authenticity of maternal experience is the emergence of true stories, which acknowledge that the joy of parenting is often mitigated by moments of deep disillusionment. By breaking the silence on the reality of parental frustration and insecurity, White (like Bombeck before her) paves the way for other "on the ground" parenting narratives such as *Go the Fuck to Sleep* by Adam Mansbach, which has been celebrated as a "refreshingly honest" take on the "familiar and unspoken tribulations about putting your child down for the night" (Neill). It is this element of the unspoken, yet universally shared, lore of parenting that becomes a site of both familiarity and solidarity in Mansbach's treatment of the bedtime routine. The text has the lilting lullaby quality of a child's traditional storybook yet highlights the exasperation of the weary parent through recourse to repetition of the profane: "The cats nestle close to their kittens,/ The lambs have laid down with the sheep./ You're cozy and warm in your bed, my dear./ Please go the fuck to sleep (1-4)."

Throughout the text, profanity becomes the common thread of refrain as the parent endeavours, using all manner of persuasion, to lull the sleep-resistant child: "The eagles who soar through the sky are at rest/ Like the creatures who crawl, run, and creep./ I know you're not thirsty. That's bullshit. Stop lying./ Lie the fuck down, my darling, and sleep (9-12)."

The language in Mansbach's book provokes an intense negotiation of the meaning of parenthood through the tension highlighted between the tale's soothing rhyme, rhythm, and pastoral imagery, and the expletives used to represent the absolute despair of a parent beyond patience—a less celebrated but universally understood manifestation of parental identity.

The success of Mansbach's text is that parents recognize their own image in this confessional portrait of parenting life in the trenches. By marring fantasy with profanity, Mansbach exclaims society's shared, secret knowledge of the experience of parental disillusionment. In response to this breach of taboo, Mansbach says, "A lot of these frustrations are not permissible to talk about. We're not completely honest because we don't want to be bad parents" (Hetter). However, through recourse to both humour and transparency, Mansbach, like White, opens a discursive space that exposes the reality of parenting and works to deconstruct the dominant myth of perfection and create a more grounded site of identification for parents struggling to situate the meaning of their own experience. The spectre of imperfection is empowering in that it expands the range of signified meanings of parenthood and, thereby, promotes the relevance of experiential knowledge as a source of authentic expression. Popular cultural representations that engage the less glamorous truths of parenting, rather than advancing a single narrative of bliss and infallibility, validate the diversity of personal ways of knowing by recognizing the breadth of meanings born of experience and, thereby, generate sites of connection and resonance for both fathers and mothers.

The necessary validation of the truth of lived experience in the quest for an embodied knowledge of the meaning of motherhood is demonstrated most clearly at the site of the maternal body. This quest involves challenging many of the taboos associated with the unspoken experiences of motherhood. For example, exposure and acceptance of the postpartum body are essential to a grounding of women's conception of maternal reality. Kate Middleton's first appearance with Prince George was perfectly manufactured, and equally well received, except for the controversy incited by the visibility of her postpartum belly. For some, it was as if tangible evidence of the reality of birth had marred the carefully constructed image of Kate's perfection. The debate raged about whether the unhidden presence of her postpartum bulge signified a distasteful reality or women's liberation. One fashion blogger wrote, "In all honesty, the dress was not pleasing to the eye, neither was the stomach. I hope she gets her post-maternity bod soon" (Free Britney). However, the majority of commentary seemed to celebrate Kate's "bravery" for displaying the post-pregnancy bump. British motherhood guru Siobhan Freegard commented:

> In a couple of minutes on the steps of the Lindo Wing, Kate has done more for new mums' self-esteem than any other role model. Sadly too many celebrities often have ultra fast tummy tucks or strap themselves down to emerge in tiny size 6 jeans, leaving everyone else feeling inadequate. Kate shows what a real mum looks like—and natural is beautiful.... [O]n her first appearance as a new mum she's proved herself a healthy role model for real mums around the world. ("Royal Mummy Tummy")

Discussion generates a space for meaning to actualize and, in spite of these diverse impressions, the scrutiny of Kate's maternal body unearthed cultural taboos relating to the postpartum period. As one columnist writes, "Criticism of the Duchess of Cambridge's post-baby bump is sparking a global discussion about the need for greater understanding of what happens to women's bodies during pregnancy" (K.Clarke). In other words, contemporary society's understanding of maternity has been so mediated by popular cultural that the truth of pregnancy and its physical legacy must be re-presented and reclaimed as part of the natural process of reproduction.

The cultural misconceptions and expectations that shape the meaning of the maternal body, and mothering, are challenged by the website www.theshapeofamother.com, where women post unaltered images and share personal narratives exploring the manner in which motherhood has shaped/reshaped both their body and identity in light of the physical changes of birth. Stacy, a mother of seven, blogs:

> I love this site because it is the only place I have ever found that speaks of the profound changes that women go through and the unique challenge that we face to experience it in the 21st century. Some days it surprises me that women can muster any confidence at all, given the images and verbiage we are forced to ingest every day; all around us. I like to be reminded of the normalcy of these changes.

In response to her photos and post, another mother comments: I am "learning to enjoy the reality of the female body after birth. I wish that real pictures like the ones you've posted were shown more frequently instead of the airbrushed myth that we get sold!" (KT). The site fosters a sense of communal identity and solidarity around the post-pregnancy material reality of the body. The site's creator comments on the politics of generating a space for women to both celebrate and lament changes entailed by the transition to motherhood:

> The post-pregnancy body is one of this society's greatest secrets; all we see of the female body is that which is airbrushed and perfect, and if we look any different, we hide it from the light of day in fear of being seen.... Sure we all talk about the sagging boobs and other parts, but no one ever sees them. Or if they do, it's in comical form, mocking the beauty that created and nourished our children. (Bonnie)

So, while Kate's postpartum belly initiated a popular cultural awakening to the truth of the maternal body after birth, theshapeofamother.com normalizes the postpartum body in a manner that enables women to re-figure and reclaim the meaning of motherhood through connection with other women in the context of a social-networking community. By celebrating the diversity of maternal representation, women develop a shared understanding that there is no single "shape of a mother." Through a virtual mosaic of pictorial and alternative narrative explorations of identity, this website generates multiple sites of resonance for moms seeking affirmation of their own experience. The diversity of voices and imagery invites inclusion by documenting and validating the changes experienced by real maternal bodies as physical signs of a deeper transformational narrative shared by all mothers.

Culture is the site of negotiated meaning in relation to identity; representations, and their accompanying discourses, form the mediating lens through which these negotiations are undertaken. Indeed, Hall argues that "meaning is never finished or completed, but keeps on moving to encompass other, additional or supplementary meanings" ("Cultural Identity" 229). With regards to the meaning of motherhood, celebrity culture invites "imitation founded on admiration," (de Botton) where admiration is based on notoriety rather than evidence of maternal wisdom. In this way, traditional knowledge and rites of passage have been replaced by pop culture icons to which communities of followers look to perform the role formerly reserved for wise women or elders (Giddens 204). In lieu of authentic guidance, dominant cultural representations encourage women to consume manufactured images of motherhood that promise to satisfy fantasies of empowerment but alienate women from the wisdom potentially acquired by dwelling in the story of their own experience (Shields 183). The narrative construction of Kate's brand sells the story of a people's princess, like Diana before her, with a pioneering approach to motherhood characterized by a flawless grace. This narrative is at once familiar and appealing in terms of its possibilities for identification and imitation; however, acceptance of Kate's story as the defining narrative in the quest for the meaning of motherhood engenders feelings of inadequacy in women whose experience does not conform to a "fairytale" of maternal bliss.

When myths mediate maternal experience and form the basis of an identity actualized through consumption of a particular brand (celebrity personality or product), rather than through wisdom gained from personal understanding, reality becomes a site of secrecy, especially concerning the maternal body and the truth of parental frustration. As a result, alternative representations of parenting, such as those offered by Erma Bombeck, Nancy White, and Adam Mansbach, as well as those featured on www.shapeofamother.com, create a much needed space for maternal re-signification that subverts normative assumptions by rejecting essentialist fallacies and by challenging the discourse of maternal fulfillment and infallibility, such as that advanced by the image of maternal royalty embodied by Kate Middleton. Narratives highlighting the authenticity of personal experience engender a sense of inclusion by re-figuring oppressive and inaccessible representations of maternity. Alternative discourse around motherhood legitimates personal experience as a source of embodied knowledge and encourages women to resist parenting fantasies constructed for cultural consumption with an investment in conformity. So, while signification of maternal identity is constantly shifting, performed and re-presented in relation to competing discourses, women's increasing validation of their own experience in the ongoing negotiation of Selfhood signals a cultural shift toward a more grounded appreciation of what it means to be a parent. Ultimately, representations that expose taboos, celebrate diversity, and validate authentic ways of knowing liberate women to inhabit the narrative of their own experience and, thereby, reclaim a more personal knowledge of motherhood.

WORKS CITED

Bombeck, Erma. *Motherhood: the Second Oldest Profession.* New York: McGraw-Hill, 1983. Print.

Bonnie. "Welcome." *The Shape of a Mother.* BlogHer: Life Well Said, 2007. Web. 25 April 2014.

Butler, Judith. *Gender Trouble: Feminism and the Subversion of Identity.* New York: Routledge, 1999. Print.

Clarke, Alison. "Maternity and Materiality: Becoming a Mother in Consumer Culture." *Consuming Motherhood.* Eds. Janelle S. Taylor, Linda L. Layne, & Danielle F. Wozniak. New Brunswick,

NJ: Rutgers University Press, 2004. 55-71. Print.

Clarke, Katrina. "Kate Middleton's Post-Baby Bump Sparks Debate over What 'Normal' Women Look Like after Giving Birth." *National Post* 25 July 2013. Web. 12 May 2014.

Cupido, Erica. "Mommy Moments." *Hello!: Kate's World* 2014: 49-53. Print.

de Beauvoir, Simone. *The Second Sex*. New York: Knopf Inc., 1952. Print.

de Botton, Alain. "Don't Despise Celebrity Culture—The Impulse to Admire Can Be Precious." *The Guardian* 31 January 2014. Web. 24 May 2014.

Douglas, Susan J. and Meredith W. Michaels. *The Mommy Myth: The Idealization of Motherhood and How It Has Undermined Women*. New York: Free Press, 2004. Print.

"A Fairytale Love Story." *Hello!: Kate's World* 2014: 36-47. Print.

Free Britney. "Kate Middleton's Post-Baby Body Media Coverage: Disrespectful to Women? *The Hollywood Gossip* 28 July 2013. Web. 25 April 2014.

Geertz, Clifford. *The Interpretation of Culture*. London: Hutchinson, 1975. Print.

Giddens, Anthony. *Modernity and Self-identity: Self and Society in the Late Modern Age*. Stanford, CA: Stanford University Press, 1991. Print.

Giroux, Henry A. *Breaking into the Movies: Film and the Culture of Politics*. Oxford: Blackwell, 2002. Print.

Hall, Stuart. "Cultural Identity and Diaspora." *Identity: Community, Culture, Difference*. Ed. Jonathan Rutherford. London: Lawrence & Wishart, 1990: 222-37. Print.

Hall, Stuart. "Encoding/Decoding." *Culture, Media, Language*. Eds. Stuart Hall, Dorothy Hobson, Andrew Lowe and Paul Willis. London: Hutchinson, 1980. 128-38. Print.

Hetter, Katia. "Bedtime Story: Go the Bleep to Sleep." CNN 13 May 2011. Web. 26 May 2014.

Inglis, Fred. "Culture and Sentiment: Principles and Practice in Development." Atlantic Coast Opportunities Agency, Government of Canada Conference. Halifax, Nova Scotia: November 2005. Web. 12 April 2014.

Inglis, Fred. *A Short History of Celebrity*. Princeton, NJ: Princeton

University Press, 2010. Print.

"Inside Kate's Life as a Princess Mom!" *People* 21 April 2014: Cover. Print.

"It's a Boy!" *Hello!: Royal Baby Commemorative Edition* 3 (2013). Print.

"It's a Girl! Why the Nation is Cheering that the Royal Baby is a Princess." *The Telegraph* 6 May 2015. Web. 6 May 2015

"Kate Middleton Causes Diane Von Furstenberg Wrap Dress to Sell Out In Minutes." *The Huffington Post Canada* 17 April 2014. Web. 12 May 2014.

"Kate's Baby Days." *Hello!: Royal Baby Commemorative Edition* 2013: 60-7. Print.

"Kate's Pregnancy Parade." *Hello! Royal Baby Commemorative Edition* 2013: 68-73. Print.

KT. "12 Responses to '7 Children: A Body to Remember.'" *The Shape of a Mother*. BlogHer: Life Well Said, 10 March 2014. Web. 25 April 2014.

Mansbach, Adam. *Go the Fuck to Sleep*. New York: Akashic Books. 2011. Print.

McDowell, Edwin. "Publishing: Top Sellers among Books of 1984." *New York Times*. 18 January 1985. Web. 24 April 2014.

McRobbie, Angela. "Yummy Mummies Leave A Bad Taste for Young Women." *The Guardian*. 2 March 2006. Web. 11 May 2015.

Neill, Graeme. "Spoof Kids' Book to Canongate." *The Bookseller*. 13 May 2011. Web. 26 April 2014.

Podnieks, Elizabeth. "'The Bump is Back': Celebrity Moms, Entertainment Journalism, and the 'Media Mother Police." *Mediating Moms: Mothers in Popular Culture*. Montreal: McGill-Queen's University Press, 2012. 87-107. Print.

"Royal 'Mummy Tummy' Becomes a Role Model." *Insights on Therapy & Wellness* 25 July 2014. Web. 29 April 2014.

"The Royal Nursery." *Hello!: Royal Baby Commemorative Edition* 2013: 44-57. Print.

Senior, Jennifer. *All Joy and No Fun: The Paradox of Modern Parenting*. New York: Harper-Collins, 2014. Print.

Shields, Carmen. "Using Narrative Inquiry to Inform and Guide our (RE)Interpretations of Lived Experience." *McGill Journal of Education* 40.1 (2005): 179-188. Print.

Stacy. "7 Children: A Body to Remember." *The Shape of a Mother.* BlogHer: Life Well Said, 10 February 2014. Web. 25 April 2014.

Wade, Judy. "Raising a Royal Heir." *Hello!: Royal Baby Commemorative Edition* 2013: 78-85. Print.

Wade, Judy and Belinda Robey. "The Baby Brigade." *Hello!: Royal Baby Commemorative Edition* 2013: 92-99. Print.

White, Nancy. "It's So Chic to be Pregnant at Christmas." *Momnipotent.* Mouton Records, 1991. CD.

White, Nancy. "Momnipotent." *Momnipotent.* Mouton Records, 1991. CD.

About the Contributors

Elizabeth Allemang has been a practicing midwife in Toronto, Ontario since 1986 and is an Associate Professor at Ryerson University's Midwifery Education Program. Her research interests include the history of midwifery, childbirth in popular culture, and the learning and teaching process in midwifery clinical education.

Charley Baker is a Lecturer in Mental Health in the School of Health Sciences at the University of Nottingham. She is Associate Editor, Journal of Psychiatric and Mental Health Nursing. Recent books include the co-authored *Health Hunanities* (2015) and a co-edited volume *Our Encounters with Self Harm* (2013).

Cheryllee Bourgeois is a Cree / Métis Registered Midwife working with Seventh Generation Midwives Toronto since 2007. She is an instructor in Ryerson's Midwifery Education Program, sits on the core leadership of National Aboriginal Council of Midwives and helped establish the Midwife-Led and Indigenous governed Toronto Birth Centre. Cheryllee has three children.

Nadya Burton is a sociologist and Associate Professor in the Midwifery Education Program at Ryerson University in Toronto. As a social scientist within a clinical education program, her work focuses on issues of equity, social justice and diversity in midwifery, supporting future clinicians to work skilfully across differences of identity and social location. Her research addresses questions concerning midwifery as a practice of social justice, the provision of midwifery care to vulnerable and marginalized communities, and the intersection of informed choice, prenatal testing and disability rights.

Shelagh Cornish is a Senior Lecturer in Art Therapy at the University of Derby and an Art Therapist in Private Practice and clinical supervisor. She has extensive clinical experience as an art therapist, including work in children's services as a Lead Art Psychotherapist (CAMHS). http://www.heartening.co.uk/

Rachel Epp Buller is a feminist-art historian-printmaker-mama of three whose art and scholarship speak to the intersections of these roles. She lectures widely and curates exhibitions on themes of mothering. Her recent books include *Reconciling Art and Mothering* (2012) and *Mothering Mennonite* (2013). She is Associate Professor of Art at Bethel College (Kansas).

Lauren Cruikshank is an Assistant Professor in the Media Arts and Cultures program at the University of New Brunswick in Fredericton, Canada. She studies intersections of media, technology and embodiment, with specific interests in avatars, games and digital culture. More information about her work can be found at www.articulata.ca.

Deborah Dempsey is Senior Lecturer in Sociology at Swinburne University of Technology, Melbourne, Australia. Deb's research interests are in the sociology of families, relationships, personal life and ageing. She has a particular interest in relatedness in the era of assisted reproductive technologies (ART) and the socio-legal aspects of same-sex relationships. Recent publications include Dempsey, D. and Lindsay J. *Families, Relationships and Intimate Life*, 2nd edition, published in 2014.

Angela Dwyer is a senior lecturer in the School of Justice at the Queensland University of Technology. Her research focuses on queer communities' experience of criminal justice.

Alys Einion is a senior lecturer in midwifery. Her Ph.D. is in Creative Writing, in which she was able to explore representation of women through auto/biographical texts and women's life writing. Her academic focus is on the representation of women's lives, including pregnancy, birth and motherhood, lesbian parenting and on midwifery education.

Rebecca English is a lecturer in Education. Her research focuses on mothers' work, discourses of motherhood and the 'good mother', especially in relation to education.

Lynn Farrales is a bereaved mother, family physician and researcher. Her research interests are in the area of refugee health, health literacy, stillbirth bereavement and community-based participatory research. She actively volunteers with the community of bereaved families in Vancouver, British Columbia.

Claire Dion Fletcher is a Potawatomi-Lenape Registered Midwife practicing in Toronto. She recently graduated from the Midwifery Education Program at Ryerson University, and is currently practicing at Seventh Generation Midwives Toronto. Claire is committed to the growth of Aboriginal midwifery in Ontario and the expansion of Aboriginal content in the midwifery program.

Anna Hennessey is a Visiting Research Scholar in Philosophy at the University of California, Berkeley. Her current research takes an in-depth look at various religious, artistic, and philosophical dimensions of birth, with a focus on the way that women perform an ontological transition of art objects when they use them in birth as a rite of passage. Anna has an academic background in Religious Studies (Ph.D.), Art History (MA), and Philosophy (BA). She is Chair of the Religions of Asia section for the American Academy of Religion, Western Region. She is also the founder of visualizingbirth.org.

Susan Hogan is Professor of Cultural Studies and Art Therapy at the University of Derby and a Professorial Fellow at the Institute of Mental Health, University of Nottingham. She has written extensively on the relationship between the arts and insanity, and the role of the arts in rehabilitation, particularly in relation to the position of women. Her books include *Conception Diary: Thinking About Pregnancy & Childbirth*, and she is currently co-editing a volume entitled *Maternal Ambivalence*.

Raechel Johns is an Associate Professor in Marketing at the University of Canberra and the Head of the School of Management. Her research interest is on the ways that online communities influence families' consumption behaviour.

Natalie Jolly is a mother of four and an Assistant Professor of Sociology and Gender Studies at the University of Washington Tacoma. She is interested in pregnancy, childbirth, and motherhood and her research focuses on how women's experiences of these events are shaped by various social forces.

Marnie Kotak is a Brooklyn-based artist who makes multimedia works in which she presents everyday life being lived. Her "Found Performances," or works based on daily activities, experiences, or accomplishments, include *The Birth of Baby X* (2011), *Raising Baby X* (ongoing) and *Mad Meds* (2014) among others. She received her BA from Bard College and her MFA from Brooklyn College. Kotak is represented by Microscope Gallery in Brooklyn, New York.

Jennifer Long is an artist, curator and educator holding a BAA from Ryerson University and a MFA from York University. Long's artwork has been exhibited and published nationally and internationally and she has been the recipient of grants from the Toronto Arts Council, Ontario Arts Council, and The Canada Council for The Arts. She currently works at OCAD University as an Assistant Professor and the Associate Chair of Cross-Disciplinary Art Practices.

Jeanne Lyons, RM MA, has practiced midwifery for over 25 years and is one of the pioneer midwives who worked to legalize midwifery in British Columbia. Currently she is an Instructor (part-time) in the UBC Midwifery Program. She attended Rhode Island School of Design and is a practicing artist. She shows her work regularly and her work appears in numerous private collections throughout North America.

Paula McCloskey is a post-doctoral researcher, writer and artist. She has published on contemporary and feminist art and the maternal. Paula is co-founder of *A Place of Their Own* (www. aplaceoftheirown.org) and a member of *MeWe discussed above* (see http://meweart.org/projects/the-egg-the-womb-the-head-and-the-moon/).

Betty Ann Martin is a doctoral candidate in Educational Sustainability at Nipissing University, North Bay, Ontario. She is a teacher, mother, doula, and postpartum depression support co-ordinator with PSI (Postpartum Support International). Her research interests include the cultural mediation of maternal experience and identity, as well as the educational and therapeutic aspects of shared personal narrative.

Kory McGrath is a funeral director, student midwife and research assistant. Her work so far is based on experiences caring for babies born still and their bereaved families as a funeral director; volunteering with hospice and perinatal bereavement organizations in BC and Ontario; and facilitating perinatal bereavement education with doulas, midwives, and students.

Brescia Nember-Reid is a queer artist/zinester/performer, studying to be a midwife at Ryerson University. Brescia graduated from the Assaulted Women and Children's Counsellor/Advocate program of George Brown College. Brescia is a founder of Drawing With Knives Shadow Puppetry Co. Her work has been featured in the Rhubarb Festival, the Allied Media Conference and the Canadian Journal of Midwifery, among other venues.

Beth Osnes (Ph.D., University of Colorado Boulder) is an Assistant Professor of theatre at the University of Colorado Boulder. As cofounder of the former Mothers Acting Up (2002–2011), she toured a program, in partnership with Philanthropiece Foundation, entitled the MOTHER tour, to locations around the world to create a global community of mothers moving from concern to action on behalf of their most passionate concerns. In conjunction with that program, she is developing a methodology that is specific to gender equity in clean energy development, using theatre to include voices of women living in poverty in the planning and implementation of development projects in Panama, Guatemala, India, Nicaragua, and the Navajo Nation. She has presented that work at the 2010 World Renewable Energy Congress in Abu Dhabi, the 2012 World Renewable Energy Forum in Denver, and the 2012 United Nations Earth Summit in Rio. She also has conducted field research as a Fulbright Scholar in Malaysia; published books (including Theatre for Women's Participation in Sustainable Development) and many articles on women's vocal empowerment, gender equity in sustainable development, mothering, activism, and the performing arts; and she is featured in the award-winning documentary *Mother: Caring for 7 Billion* (www.motherthefilm.com).

Ara Parker is a Registered Art Therapist, Faculty Lecturer, and Chair of the Department of Psychotherapy and Spirituality at St. Stephen's College in Edmonton. She is also working on her Doctor of Ministry in spiritually-integrated art therapy. Ara is the grateful and proud solo parent (from the beginning) of her daughter Eliana.

Damien Riggs is an Australian Research Council Future Fellow (2013-2019) and an Associate Professor in social work at Flinders University. He teaches and researches in the areas of family studies, mental health, and gender/sexuality studies, and is the author of over 100 publications in these areas, including (with Victoria Clarke, Sonja Ellis and Elizabeth Peel) *Lesbian, Gay, Bisexual, Trans and Queer Psychology* (2010), which won the British Psychological Society book prize for 2013. Damien also works in private practice as a psychotherapist, where he specializes in working with young transgender people.

Rosie Rosenzweig author of *A Jewish Mother in Shangri-la*, about her journeys to meet her Buddhist son's Asian gurus, and *A Jewish Guide to Boston and New England*, is a Resident Scholar in Women's Studies at Brandeis University. Her latest publication is a chapter on Serach bat Asher in *Praise her Works: Conversations with Biblical Women* (Jewish Publication Society). She has contributed to a number of books and journals, including; *So that Your Values Live On: Ethical Wills; A Heart of Wisdom: Making the Jewish Journey from Mid-life through the Elder Years; Reading Between the Lines: New Stories from the Bible; All the Women Followed Her;* and *A Collection of Writings on Miriam the Prophet and the Women of Exodus*. She is an ordained meditation teacher, and is currently writing a book based on interviews with women artists through the lens of Buddhist psychology.

Mary Sharpe has been a practicing midwife in Ontario since 1979 and is Associate Professor, Midwifery Education Program at Ryerson University. Her research interests include: changes in midwifery practices following regulation; the confluence of text and practice; woman-midwife relationships; midwives as paid familial caregivers; the role and status of midwives internationally; intrapartum antibiotic prophylaxis for GBS; prenatal education for parenting; and home birth practice.

K. J. Surkan is birthparent and transdad to two amazing children, and has been teaching in the Program in Women's and Gender Studies at MIT for the past ten years. His research interests include new media activism and online social movements, feminist media studies, technology studies, queer/trans politics and representation, reproductive technologies, and most recently wearable technologies and epatient communities and health activism.

Michelle Walks, Ph.D., is a feminist medical anthropologist. In 2015 she completed a postdoctoral fellowship with the University of Ottawa researching "Transmasculine Individuals' Experiences with Pregnancy, Birthing, and Feeding Their Newborns: A Qualitative Study," funded through CIHR's Institute of Gender and Health. She is now an Adjunct Professor at the University of British Columbia, Okanagan campus, where she teaches Anthropology, Sociology and Gender & Women's Studies. Michelle resides in Kelowna, BC, with her spouse and their "queerling" son.

Lisa Watts is an artist with an eclectic practice that pivots around performance, sculpture and lens-based media. In the past, Channel 4 broadcast a documentary about her art, *Muscles* (1998) made in collaboration with artist Clare Charnley. Her film *Bun* (1997) made with artist Susan Gent has been a great success and been shown globally including: Canada, India, and Mexico, and broadcast in Europe such as Spain, Italy, and France. Watts toured performance and video art *More Funny Feelings* (2001) to Prema Arts Centre, Colchester Arts Centre, City Art Gallery, Leeds, and Tramway Arts Centre, Glasgow. She performed, *I Never Made it as a Sex Kitten* (1994) at Serpentine Gallery, London. She was commissioned by ACE, BBC, Saatchi and Saatchi's for *Escape Mechanism* (2001) made with artist Brian McClave. Recently she published her book *32 Significant Moments: An Artist's Practice as Research* and is currently writing a follow-up book, *Close-up Processes: An Artist's Practice as Research* (2017). Her next touring exhibition, *I Am Not a Decorator, But An Inventor,* will visit four galleries completing at John Hansard Gallery, Southampton, UK.